Diagnosis and Management of Eye Diseases

Diagnosis and Management of Eye Diseases

Edited by Anastasia Maddox

hayle
medical

New York

Hayle Medical,
750 Third Avenue, 9th Floor,
New York, NY 10017, USA

Visit us on the World Wide Web at:
www.haylemedical.com

ISBN: 978-1-63241-896-8

Cataloging-in-Publication Data

Diagnosis and management of eye diseases / edited by Anastasia Maddox.
p. cm.
Includes bibliographical references and index.
ISBN 978-1-63241-896-8
1. Eye--Diseases--Diagnosis. 2. Eye--Diseases--Treatment. 3. Eye--Abnormalities.
4. Eye--Care and hygiene. I. Maddox, Anastasia.
RE46 .D53 2020
617.7--dc23

Table of Contents

Preface

The world is advancing at a fast pace like never before. Therefore, the need is to keep up with the latest developments. This book was an idea that came to fruition when the specialists in the area realized the need to coordinate together and document essential themes in the subject. That's when I was requested to be the editor. Editing this book has been an honour as it brings together diverse authors researching on different streams of the field. The book collates essential materials contributed by veterans in the area which can be utilized by students and researchers alike.

The human eye provides a three-dimensional moving image that is normally colored during the daytime. There are many changes in the eye and its surrounding areas due to various disorders and diseases, and aging. Eye tumor, excessive tearing, dry eyes, macular degeneration, cataract, glaucoma, etc. are some of the common eye diseases caused by various internal and external factors. The aging process is one of the prominent reasons for certain changes in the eye. The most functionally important changes in the non-diseased eye are the loss of accommodation or focusing capability and a reduction in pupil size. From theories to research to practical applications, case studies related to all contemporary topics of relevance to ophthalmology have been included in this book. It presents the complex aspects of diagnosis and management of eye diseases in the most comprehensible and easy to understand language. The readers would gain knowledge that would broaden their perspective in this field of study.

Each chapter is a sole-standing publication that reflects each author´s interpretation. Thus, the book displays a multi-facetted picture of our current understanding of application, resources and aspects of the field. I would like to thank the contributors of this book and my family for their endless support.

Editor

1

Age Differences in Axial Length, Corneal Curvature, and Corneal Astigmatism in Marfan Syndrome with Ectopia Lentis

Jiahui Chen,[1,2] Qinghe Jing,[1,2] Yating Tang,[1,2] Dongjin Qian,[1,2] Yi Lu,[1,2] and Yongxiang Jiang[1,2]

[1] *Department of Ophthalmology and Vision Science, Eye & ENT Hospital of Fudan University, Shanghai, China*
[2] *Key Laboratory of Myopia of State Health Ministry and Key Laboratory of Visual Impairment and Restoration of Shanghai, Shanghai, China*

Correspondence should be addressed to Yongxiang Jiang; yongxiang_jiang@163.com

Academic Editor: Anna Nowinska

Purpose. To investigate the differences in axial length, corneal curvature, and corneal astigmatism with age in patients with Marfan syndrome (MFS) and ectopia lentis. *Methods.* A retrospective case series study was conducted. MFS patients with ectopia lentis were divided into groups according to age. Axial length, corneal curvature, and corneal astigmatism were measured. *Results.* This study included 114 MFS patients (215 eyes) with a mean age of 19.0 ± 13.9 years. Axial length differed significantly across age groups in MFS patients ($P < 0.001$), whereas corneal curvature did not ($P = 0.767$). Corneal astigmatism was statistically significant throughout the MFS cohort ($P = 0.009$), but no significant difference was found in young MFS patients ($P = 0.838$). With increasing age, the orientation of the corneal astigmatism changed from with-the-rule astigmatism to against-the-rule or oblique astigmatism ($P < 0.001$). A linear correlation analysis showed weak correlations between age and axial length for both eyes and with corneal astigmatism for the left eye, but there was no correlation between age and corneal curvature. *Conclusions.* In MFS, axial length varies with age, corneal curvature remains stable, and corneal astigmatism is higher in young patients and tends to shift toward against-the-rule or oblique astigmatism. Therefore, it is important to consider age when diagnosing MFS with ocular biometric data.

1. Introduction

Marfan syndrome (MFS) is an autosomal dominant inherited disease associated with systemic connective tissue disorders, particularly involving the ocular, cardiovascular, and skeletal systems. It is caused by the mutation of fibrillin-1 (FBN1) gene encoding fibrillin-1, which plays important roles in systemic connective tissues and has an integral role in maintaining ocular health [1, 2]. The estimated morbidity rate of MFS was reported to be 4.60–6.81 per 100,000 people [3–5].

Ectopia lentis (EL) affects 30.2%–87.0% of MFS patients [6–14]. Although the incidence of EL varies widely in prior studies, it is the major diagnostic criterion of the 2010 Revised Ghent Nosology [15]. Aside from EL, myopia of >3.0 diopters (D) is a minor ocular criterion for the diagnosis of MFS. Myopia, which is the most prevalent ocular disorder that develops rapidly in early childhood [16, 17], is strongly associated with increased axial length (AL) and decreased corneal curvature, which are common features in MFS patients. A long AL results in myopia; however, a flatter cornea may compensate for increased AL leading to a refractive error of <3.0 D.

Although the phenotype of MFS is becoming well documented in adults, it is incomplete in children, in whom the presence of ectopia lentis and aortic root dilatation are the best and most stable diagnostic features [18]. In young MFS patients, the incomplete phenotype limits the accurate detection of MFS and the timely interventions required to prevent severe complications. Many studies have demonstrated that some ocular biometric characteristics, such as increased AL, reduced corneal curvature, and high corneal astigmatism, have potential diagnostic values in MFS patients [8–10, 19–22]. Increased AL (>23.5 mm), reduced corneal curvature (<41.5 D), and high corneal astigmatism (>1.0 D) are common in MFS, but the differences across age groups have not been determined. Therefore, we investigated the differences in these parameters with age in MFS patients.

Our objective was to evaluate AL, corneal curvature, and the magnitude and orientation of corneal astigmatism in MFS patients with EL in different age subgroups and to determine the clinical diagnostic significance of these parameters for suspected MFS.

2. Methods

2.1. Ethics. The retrospective case series study was conducted at the Eye & ENT Hospital of Fudan University, Shanghai, China, by searching the medical records of patients treated between March 2012 and November 2017. The study was approved by the Human Research Ethics Committee of the Eye & ENT Hospital of Fudan University, and the research adhered to the tenets of the Declaration of Helsinki. Written informed consent was obtained from all patients.

2.2. Subjects. We included patients diagnosed with MFS based on the Ghent-2 criteria [15]. The study group comprised 114 MFS patients (215 eyes) with EL, who came from 15 provinces of China.70.2% of the patients came from the peripheral regions of Shanghai, where our hospital was located. Patients with a history of ocular surgery, corneal disease, uveitis, use of contact lenses within 2 weeks before examinations, or suspected (unconfirmed) MFS were excluded from this study. Both eyes of each subject were included.

2.3. Eye Examinations. All patients underwent thorough ophthalmic examinations of both eyes by experienced ophthalmologists. The patients' family and medical history were evaluated before the ocular examinations. We then used slit-lamp examination to determine the position of the lens in different gaze directions under complete pupillary dilation.

AL, corneal curvature, and corneal astigmatism were measured using an IOL Master (Carl Zeiss Meditec, Jena, Germany) or an auto refract keratometer (Nidek ARK-700A). The mean keratometry (Km; in D) was calculated as the mean value of Kmax and Kmin and was taken as the corneal curvature. The corneal astigmatism (AST) was calculated as Kmax–Kmin. The axis orientations of the corneal astigmatism were classified as "with the rule" (WTR) (the steepest corneal meridian was within $90^\circ \pm 30^\circ$) or "against the rule" (ATR) (the steepest corneal meridian was within 0°–30° or 150°–180°). If the astigmatism was outside these parameters, it was classified as oblique.

2.4. Data Analysis. To analyze the differences in these ocular biometric characteristics with age, we divided the MFS patients into five groups by age: G1 (≤10 years old), G2 (11–20 years old), G3 (21–30 years old), G4 (31–40 years old), and G5 (>40 years old). The MFS patients younger than 20 years old were further divided into four subgroups: Y1 (3–5 years old); Y2 (6–10 years old); Y3 (11–15 years old); and Y4 (16–20 years old).

Table 1: Demographic characteristics of the Marfan syndrome patients with ectopia lentis.

Subjects (eyes)	114 (215)
Mean age (range) (years)	19.0 ± 13.9 (3–54)
Gender (female : male)	56 : 58
Right : left	108 : 107
AL (range) (mm)	26.18 ± 3.11 (20.85–34.46)
Kmin (range) (D)	39.96 ± 1.70 (34.87–45.42)
Kmax (range) (D)	41.52 ± 1.86 (35.38–46.75)
Km (range) (D)	40.74 ± 1.72 (35.13–45.70)
AST (range) (D)	1.55 ± 0.93 (0.10–4.61)

AL: axial length; Kmin: minimum keratometry; Kmax: maximum keratometry; Km: mean keratometry; D: diopters; AST: corneal astigmatism.

Quantitative data passed the normal distribution test and were presented as the mean ± standard deviation (SD). We used the one-way analysis of variance, Kruskal–Wallis test, and chi-square test, as appropriate, to compare ocular biometric values between different age groups of MFS patients. To determine pairwise differences, a Bonferroni post hoc analysis was conducted when the groups were of equal sizes. Correlations between age and continuous variables were assessed by calculating Pearson's correlation coefficient (r). Values of $P < 0.05$ were considered statistically significant. All statistical analyses were performed using SPSS version 22.0 (IBM Corp., Armonk, NY, USA).

3. Results

The study included 215 eyes of 114 MFS patients with EL. The mean age of the subjects was 19.0 ± 13.9 years (range, 3–54 years), and 50.9% of them were male. The demographic characteristics of the MFS patients are listed in Table 1, and the distributions of elevated parameters are shown in Figure 1. In terms of the minor criteria, we determined the proportions of patients in the different age groups with increased AL, flat cornea, and high corneal astigmatism, which were defined as AL > 23.5 mm, Km < 41.5 D, and AST > 1.0 D, respectively (Figure 2).

3.1. Axial Length. The mean AL of the patients was 26.18 ± 3.11 mm (range, 20.85–34.46 mm) and included 174 eyes (80.9%) with a long AL (>23.5 mm). There were significant differences in AL among the age groups of MFS patients ($P < 0.001$; Table 2). The mean AL was significantly shorter in the G1 group (≤10 years old, 24.79 ± 2.46 mm) than those in the G2, G3, G4, and G5 groups ($P < 0.05$). Table 3 shows the ocular biometric data for the MFS patients younger than 20 years old. There were significant differences in the mean AL of the Y1 subgroup (3–5 years old) and those of the other subgroups ($P < 0.05$, Table 3). In the young MFS patients, the mean AL and the proportion of AL values > 23.5 mm increased significantly with increasing age (both $P < 0.001$, Table 3, and Figure 2(d)). An abnormally high AL (>23.5 mm) was observed in 60 eyes (65.9%) in the G1 group, in 41 eyes (93.2%) in the G2 group, in 32 eyes (91.4%) in

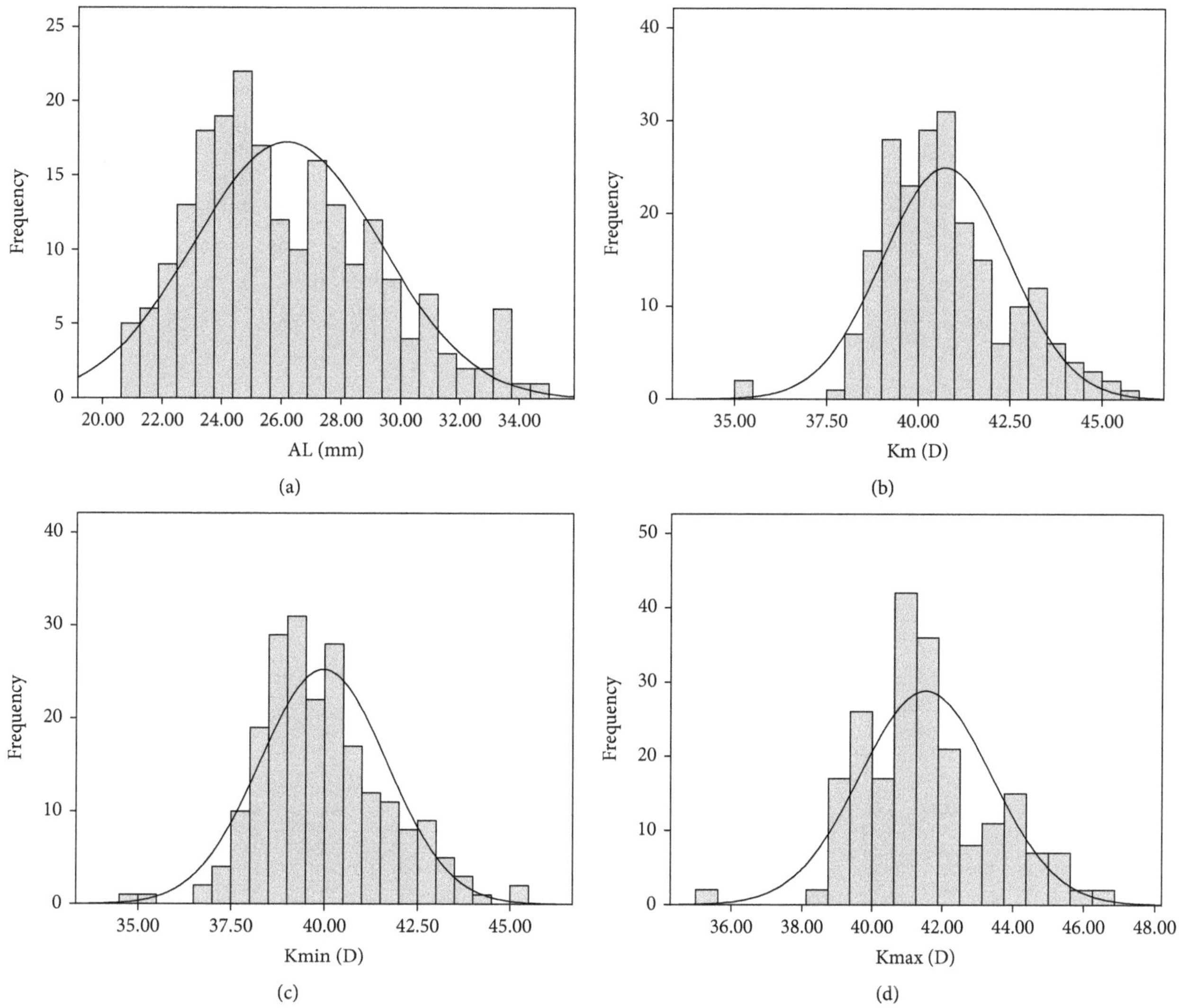

FIGURE 1: Distributions of axial length (a), Km (b), Kmin (c), and Kmax (d) for Marfan syndrome patients. AL: axial length; Km: mean keratometry; Kmin: minimum keratometry; Kmax: maximum keratometry; D: diopters.

the G3 group, in 22 eyes (88.0%) in the G4 group, and in 19 eyes (95.0%) in the G5 group ($P < 0.001$, Figure 2(a)). A linear correlation analysis showed a weak correlation between age and AL in MFS patients for the right eye ($r = 0.408$, $P < 0.001$; Figure 3(a)) and the left eye ($r = 0.360$, $P < 0.001$; Figure 3(a)).

3.2. Corneal Curvature. The mean corneal curvature (Km value) was 40.74 ± 1.72 D (range, 35.13–45.70 D) in the MFS patients with EL. Of the 215 eyes tested, 156 eyes (72.6%) had a flattened cornea, with Km < 41.5 D. The proportions of Km values < 41.5 D in the different age groups are shown in Figure 2(b) ($P = 0.144$). The proportion of Km values < 41.5 D decreased in young MFS patients with age, and the differences were statistically significant ($P = 0.026$; Figure 2(e)). The Km value did not change with age in MFS patients ($P = 0.767$, Table 2; $P = 0.269$, Table 3). No linear correlation was detected between age and corneal curvature ($P = 0.620$ for the right eye, $P = 0.918$ for the left eye, for the total group, Figure 3(b); $P = 0.686$ for the right eye, $P = 0.620$ for the left eye, for the young patients, Figure 3(e)).

3.3. Corneal Astigmatism. The mean corneal astigmatism in the MFS patients with EL was 1.55 ± 0.93 D (range, 0.10–4.61 D), and it was higher in the MFS patients < 20 years old (1.70 ± 0.97 D) than in the other patients. Corneal astigmatism differed significantly among the age groups ($P = 0.009$, Table 2), increasing in both the G1 group (age ≤ 10 years) and G2 group (11–20 years) and decreasing with age thereafter in the MFS patients. However, no significant differences were found in the corneal astigmatism of the young MFS patients ($P = 0.838$; Table 3). Figure 3(c) shows the weak correlation between age and corneal astigmatism in the total MFS patients in the left eye ($r = -0.274$, $P = 0.004$, Figure 3(c)), whereas no linear correlation was detected between age and corneal astigmatism in the young MFS patients (Figure 3(f)).

Among the 215 eyes of MFS patients examined, the type of corneal astigmatism was classified as WTR, ATR,

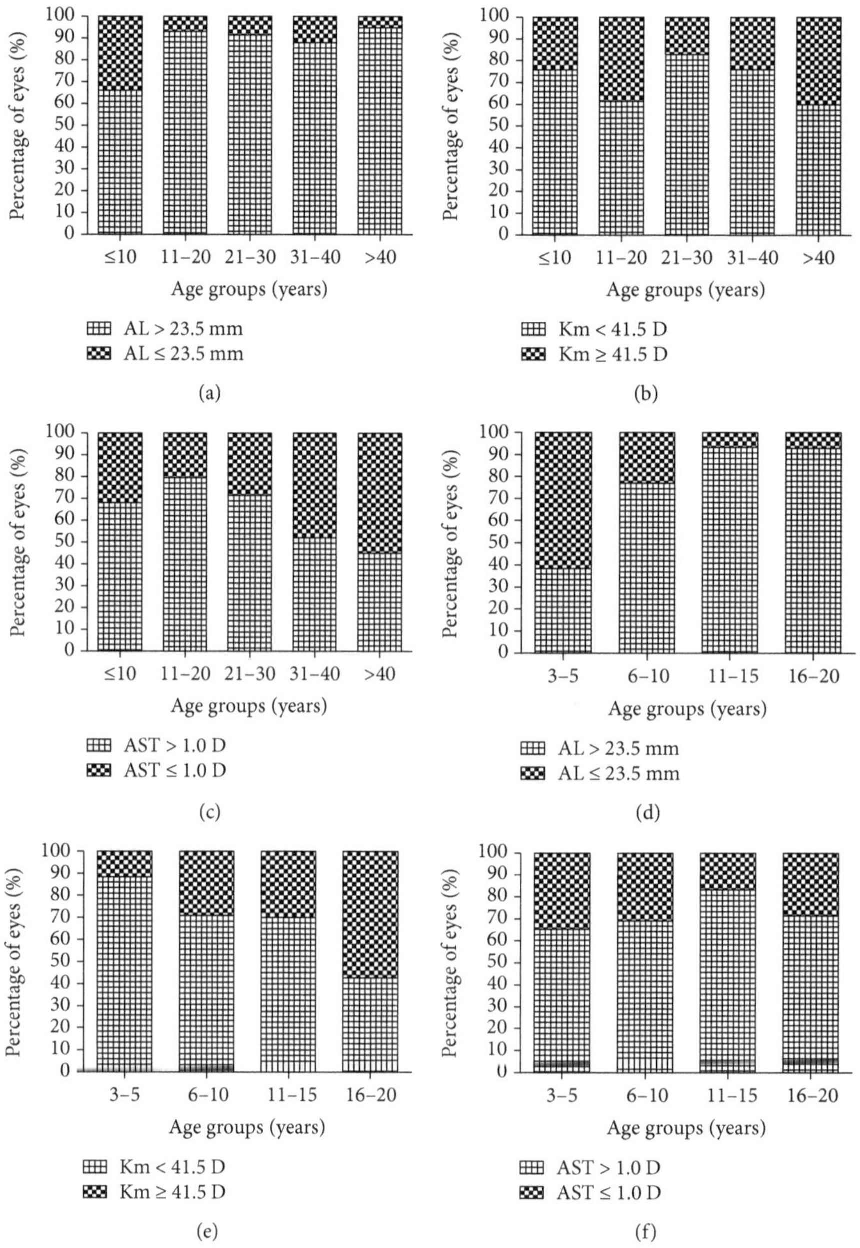

Figure 2: Proportions of increased axial length (a and d), reduced corneal curvature (b and e), and high corneal astigmatism (c and f) in different age groups of Marfan syndrome. AL: axial length; Km: mean keratometry; D: diopters; AST: corneal astigmatism.

Table 2: Demographic characteristics of the Marfan syndrome patients with ectopia lentis among different age groups.

Age group (years)	G1 (≤10)	G2 (11–20)	G3 (21–30)	G4 (31–40)	G5 (>40)	*P* value*
Eyes (*N*)	91	44	35	25	20	
Male/female	21/26	12/10	10/9	9/5	6/6	0.759
Right/left	45/46	22/22	19/16	12/13	10/10	0.990
AL (mm)	24.79 ± 2.46	26.32 ± 2.63	27.58 ± 3.34	27.75 ± 3.69	27.82 ± 2.85	<0.001
Km (D)	40.73 ± 1.84	40.90 ± 1.65	40.46 ± 1.45	40.69 ± 1.77	41.01 ± 1.75	0.767
AST (D)	1.68 ± 1.00	1.74 ± 0.90	1.44 ± 0.67	1.36 ± 1.08	1.00 ± 0.55	0.009

AL: axial length; Km: mean keratometry; D: diopters; AST: corneal astigmatism; *P values represent general differences among groups.

Table 3: Demographic characteristics of the young Marfan syndrome patients with ectopia lentis among different age subgroups.

Age groups (years)	Y1 (3–5)	Y2 (6–10)	Y3 (11–15)	Y4 (16–20)	*P* value*
Eyes (*N*)	26	65	30	14	
Male/female	6/7	15/19	8/7	4/3	0.890
Right/left	13/13	32/33	15/15	7/7	1.000
AL (mm)	23.55 ± 2.11	25.28 ± 2.43	26.31 ± 2.67	26.36 ± 2.66	<0.001
Km (D)	40.59 ± 1.43	40.78 ± 1.99	40.56 ± 1.49	41.63 ± 1.78	0.269
AST (D)	1.55 ± 0.93	1.73 ± 1.03	1.78 ± 0.88	1.68 ± 0.96	0.838

AL: axial length; Km: mean keratometry; D: diopters; AST: corneal astigmatism; **P* values represent general differences among subgroups.

or oblique in 74.9%, 11.2%, or 13.9% of eyes, respectively. The corresponding values were 82.9%, 6.7%, or 10.4% for the eyes of the young MFS patients. Figure 4 shows the distributions of the orientations of corneal astigmatism in each age group and subgroup. With increasing age, the orientation of corneal astigmatism shifted from WTR astigmatism to ATR or oblique astigmatism ($P < 0.001$, Figure 4(a)), whereas the distribution of corneal astigmatism in the young patient subgroups was primarily WTR astigmatism and did not differ significantly between the subgroups ($P = 0.395$, Figure 4(b)).

4. Discussion

In 1981, Maumenee [14] first reported distinctive ocular manifestations of MFS, including globe enlargement, corneal flattening, and lens dislocation. Since then, several studies have demonstrated these ocular biometric characteristics in MFS patients with or without EL [6, 8, 9, 19, 20]. Recently, Kinori et al. [20] reported that the corneas of children with established MFS were flattened to at least the same degree as in adults. It seems that the ocular phenotype of MFS patients displays age-related differences. In this study, we recruited MFS patients with EL to investigate these age differences in AL, corneal curvature, and corneal astigmatism, to provide a better overview of some ocular biometric characteristics of MFS patients of all ages.

In previous studies, AL was reported to be longer in MFS patients with or without EL [6, 20, 21], and we found that 80.9% of MFS eyes with EL had AL > 23.5 mm. The average AL of the patients recruited was 26.18 ± 3.11 mm, which is relatively longer than that of healthy patients in population studies [23, 24] and is consistent with previous reports. Although a longer AL is no longer considered a criterion for the diagnosis of MFS, MFS should be suspected in patients with longer AL. Among the different age groups, the mean AL was significantly longer in older MFS patients, and AL was shorter in the Y1 group (3–5 years old) than in the other MFS patients less than 20 years old. Moreover, a weak correlation between age and AL indicated that AL varies with age in MFS patients with EL. Both the values of AL and the proportions of eyes with AL > 23.5 mm changed with increasing age. Therefore, we propose that AL is less important in the diagnosis of MFS in young patients than in older patients.

Ocular parameters generally have complex and mutual effects on ocular refraction [23, 25]. The length of the globe increases significantly with increasing age, but the anterior segment of the eyeball changes negligibly. The corneal curvature did not differ between the different age groups of MFS patients, whereas the average corneal curvature value (40.74 ± 1.72 D) was low and 156 eyes (72.6%) of our patients had a flat cornea (Km < 41.5 D). Corneal curvature differed significantly in neither the young nor the old MFS patients, which is contrary to a previous study that showed flatter corneas in children with MFS [20]. The Km value did not change with increasing age, and no linear correlation was detected between age and corneal curvature, so corneal curvature remained relatively stable in most MFS patients (mean value < 41.5 D). Therefore, corneal curvature might be useful in the diagnosis of MFS or could represent a warning sign when evaluating patients with suspected MFS.

Several recent studies have highlighted the importance of high corneal astigmatism in the diagnosis of MFS [9, 20]. It has been suggested that any deviation arising from advanced EL and zonule defects, which are very frequent in MFS patients, might increase corneal astigmatism [9, 20, 26]. It has also been proposed that defects in the *FBN1* gene might affect the zonule and corneal connective tissues, resulting in greater corneal astigmatism [9]. When the MFS patients were divided into five groups by age, corneal astigmatism was greater in the young MFS patients and differed significantly between the age groups of MFS patients. Therefore, it is important to take the patient's age into account when assessing corneal astigmatism in MFS patients. Although previous studies have reported that corneal astigmatism is higher in MFS patients with EL than in those without EL [9, 20], MFS patients generally display more corneal astigmatism than healthy people. Therefore, our results imply that higher corneal astigmatism can be considered a positive symptom in the diagnosis of MFS in young patients.

Corneal astigmatism was classified as WTR in most eyes in each subgroup of MFS patients younger than 20 years old. The astigmatic orientation of the cornea in the total cohort of MFS patients tended to shift from WTR to ATR or oblique astigmatism with advancing age, consistent with previous studies of healthy eyes [27, 28]. However, the number of patients in our study was relatively small, which limited our capacity to detect age-related differences in corneal astigmatism. The age-related shift in astigmatism orientation is believed

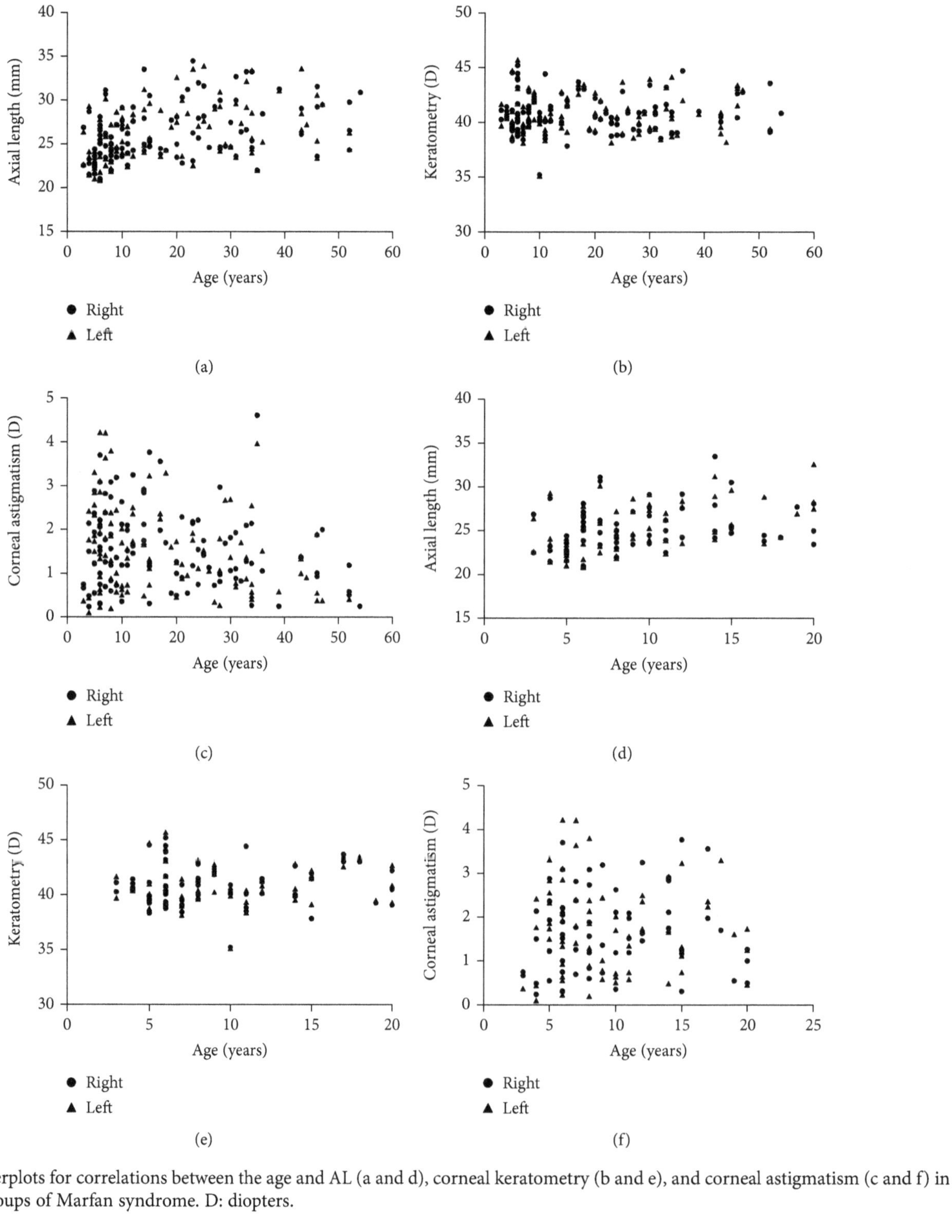

FIGURE 3: Scatterplots for correlations between the age and AL (a and d), corneal keratometry (b and e), and corneal astigmatism (c and f) in different age groups of Marfan syndrome. D: diopters.

to involve reduced lid tension, increased intraocular pressure, age-related changes in extraocular muscle tension, and changes to the corneal structure [29]. Toric intraocular lenses (IOLs) are perhaps not beneficial for patients with high corneal astigmatism when we consider the shift from WTR to ATR with increasing age, because toric IOLs will not correct corneal astigmatism unless they are correctly aligned along the steep meridian [30]. Therefore, toric IOLs may be unsuitable in MFS patients with high corneal astigmatism, especially young children with EL.

In the revised Ghent criteria, myopia > 3.0 D is a minor ocular criterion for the diagnosis of MFS [15]. However, myopia is the most prevalent ocular disorder in the world, developing rapidly in early childhood and affecting many healthy people. We know that AL is strongly associated with the development of myopia [17]. However, a refractive

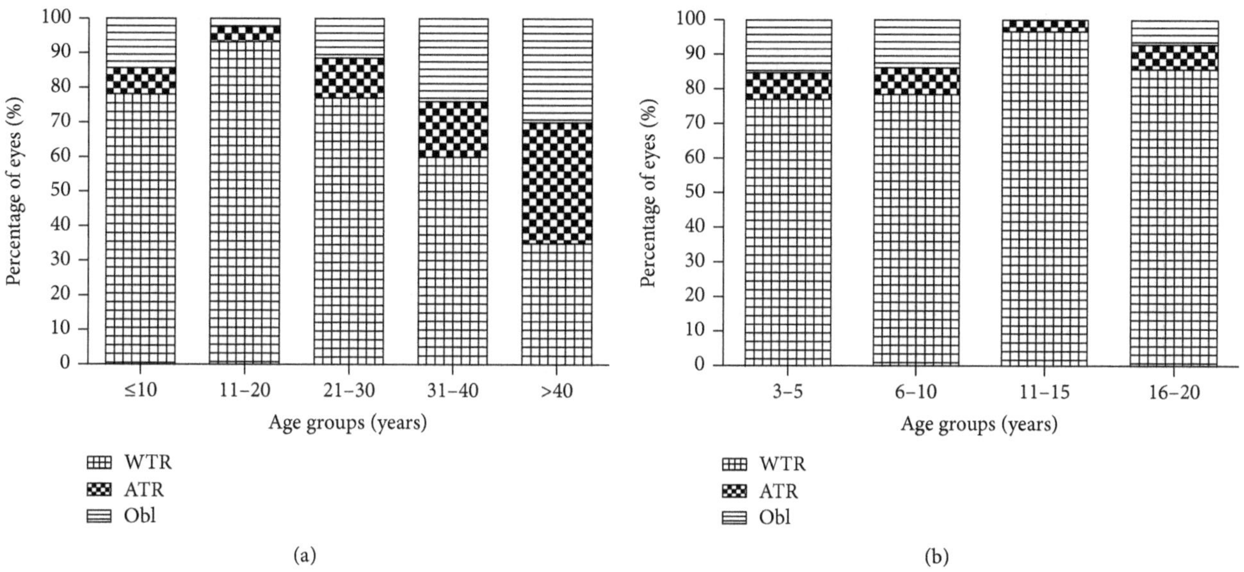

FIGURE 4: Distributions of the orientations of corneal astigmatism in each age group (a) and subgroup (b) of Marfan syndrome. WTR: with the rule; ATR: against the rule; Obl: oblique.

error of <3.0 D in patients with MFS may be accompanied by corneal flattening. Therefore, myopia > 3.0 D may not be diagnostically useful in children with MFS, despite increased AL. Corneal flattening and increased AL are probably more relevant to the diagnosis of MFS than myopia. Furthermore, advanced EL and zonule defects, which are very frequent in MFS patients, will result in higher myopia and astigmatism [9, 20]. Therefore, a suspicion of MFS should be considered seriously in children with high corneal astigmatism.

There are two limitations to our study. First, our cohort of MFS patients all had EL, which prevented us from detecting differences in patients without EL for early diagnosis. Second, we must acknowledge that not all the patients diagnosed with MFS underwent genetic testing for confirmation. However, it is necessary to assess the ocular characteristics in MFS patients in order to better understand the age differences of this disease.

In conclusion, AL varies with age and MFS should be suspected in older patients with long AL; high corneal astigmatism appears to have utility in the diagnosis of MFS in young patients, and reduced corneal curvature may also be a useful marker in the diagnosis of MFS. With advancing age, the orientation of corneal astigmatism in MFS patients tends to shift from WTR astigmatism to ATR astigmatism or oblique astigmatism. Therefore, age should be considered in the diagnosis of patients with suspected MFS. We propose that AL, corneal curvature, and corneal astigmatism should be measured in the clinical context for patients in whom MFS is suspected based on ocular biometric data.

Conflicts of Interest

The authors declare that there is no conflict of interest regarding the publication of this paper.

Acknowledgments

This study was funded by the National Natural Science United Foundation of China (Grant U1503124) and the National Natural Science Foundation of China (Grant 81770908).

References

[1] B. Loeys, J. De Backer, P. Van Acker et al., "Comprehensive molecular screening of the FBN1 gene favors locus homogeneity of classical Marfan syndrome," *Human Mutation*, vol. 24, no. 2, pp. 140–146, 2004.

[2] H. C. Dietz, C. R. Cutting, R. E. Pyeritz et al., "Marfan syndrome caused by a recurrent de novo missense mutation in the fibrillin gene," *Nature*, vol. 352, no. 6333, pp. 337–339, 1991.

[3] J. Fuchs, "Marfan syndrome and other systemic disorders with congenital ectopia lentis. A Danish national survey," *Acta Paediatrica*, vol. 86, no. 9, pp. 947–952, 1997.

[4] J. R. Gray, A. B. Bridges, M. J. Faed et al., "Ascertainment and severity of Marfan syndrome in a Scottish population," *Journal of Medical Genetics*, vol. 31, no. 1, pp. 51–54, 1994.

[5] K. A. Groth, H. Hove, K. Kyhl et al., "Prevalence, incidence, and age at diagnosis in Marfan Syndrome," *Orphanet Journal of Rare Diseases*, vol. 10, no. 1, p. 153, 2015.

[6] L. Drolsum, S. Rand-Hendriksen, B. Paus, O. R. Geiran, and S. O. Semb, "Ocular findings in 87 adults with Ghent-1 verified Marfan syndrome," *Acta Ophthalmologica*, vol. 93, no. 1, pp. 46–53, 2015.

[7] A. Chandra, V. Ekwalla, A. Child, and D. Charteris, "Prevalence of ectopia lentis and retinal detachment in Marfan syndrome," *Acta Ophthalmologica*, vol. 92, no. 1, pp. e82–e83, 2014.

[8] T. R. Konradsen and C. Zetterström, "A descriptive study of ocular characteristics in Marfan syndrome," *Acta Ophthalmologica*, vol. 91, no. 8, pp. 751–755, 2013.

[9] T. R. Konradsen, A. Koivula, M. Kugelberg, and C. Zetterström, "Corneal curvature, pachymetry, and endothelial cell density in Marfan syndrome," *Acta Ophthalmologica*, vol. 90, no. 4, pp. 375–379, 2012.

[10] M. Heur, B. Costin, S. Crowe et al., "The value of keratometry and central corneal thickness measurements in the clinical diagnosis of Marfan syndrome," *American Journal of Ophthalmology*, vol. 145, no. 6, pp. 997–1001.e1, 2008.

[11] E. Arbustini, M. Grasso, S. Ansaldi et al., "Identification of sixty-two novel and twelve known FBN1 mutations in eighty-one unrelated probands with Marfan syndrome and other fibrillinopathies," *Human Mutation*, vol. 26, no. 5, p. 494, 2005.

[12] G. Sultan, C. Baudouin, O. Auzerie et al., "Cornea in Marfan disease: Orbscan and in vivo confocal microscopy analysis," *Investigative Ophthalmology & Visual Science*, vol. 43, no. 6, pp. 1757–1764, 2002.

[13] L. Faivre, G. Collod-Beroud, A. Child et al., "Contribution of molecular analyses in diagnosing Marfan syndrome and type I fibrillinopathies: an international study of 1009 probands," *Journal of Medical Genetics*, vol. 45, no. 6, pp. 384–390, 2008.

[14] I. H. Maumenee, "The eye in the Marfan syndrome," *Transactions of the American Ophthalmological Society*, vol. 79, pp. 684–733, 1981.

[15] B. L. Loeys, H. C. Dietz, A. C. Braverman et al., "The revised Ghent nosology for the Marfan syndrome," *Journal of Medical Genetics*, vol. 47, no. 7, pp. 476–485, 2010.

[16] B. T. Tinkle, H. M. Saal, and the COMMITTEE ON GENETICS, "Health supervision for children with Marfan syndrome," *Pediatrics*, vol. 132, no. 4, pp. e1059–e1072, 2013.

[17] E. A. H. Mallen, Y. Gammoh, M. Al-Bdour, and F. N. Sayegh, "Refractive error and ocular biometry in Jordanian adults," *Ophthalmic and Physiological Optics*, vol. 25, no. 4, pp. 302–309, 2005.

[18] C. Stheneur, F. Tubach, M. Jouneaux et al., "Study of phenotype evolution during childhood in Marfan syndrome to improve clinical recognition," *Genetics in Medicine*, vol. 16, no. 3, pp. 246–250, 2014.

[19] L. C. Beene, E. I. Traboulsi, I. Seven et al., "Corneal deformation response and ocular geometry: a noninvasive diagnostic strategy in Marfan syndrome," *American Journal of Ophthalmology*, vol. 161, pp. 56–64.e1, 2016.

[20] M. Kinori, S. Wehrli, I. S. Kassem, N. F. Azar, I. H. Maumenee, and M. B. Mets, "Biometry characteristics in adults and children with Marfan syndrome: from the Marfan eye consortium of Chicago," *American Journal of Ophthalmology*, vol. 177, pp. 144–149, 2017.

[21] P. Gehle, B. Goergen, D. Pilger, P. Ruokonen, P. N. Robinson, and D. J. Salchow, "Biometric and structural ocular manifestations of Marfan syndrome," *PLoS One*, vol. 12, no. 9, article e0183370, 2017.

[22] J. Luebke, D. Boehringer, P. Eberwein, and T. Reinhard, "Corneal K-values as a diagnostic screening tool for Marfan syndrome," *Cornea*, vol. 36, no. 6, pp. 700–703, 2017.

[23] T. Olsen, A. Arnarsson, H. Sasaki, K. Sasaki, and F. Jonasson, "On the ocular refractive components: the Reykjavik Eye Study," *Acta Ophthalmologica Scandinavica*, vol. 85, no. 4, pp. 361–366, 2007.

[24] C. Shufelt, S. Fraser-Bell, M. Ying-Lai, M. Torres, and R. Varma, "Refractive error, ocular biometry, and lens opalescence in an adult population: the Los Angeles Latino Eye Study," *Investigative Ophthalmology & Visual Science*, vol. 46, no. 12, p. 4450, 2005.

[25] D. O. Mutti, G. L. Mitchell, L. A. Jones et al., "Axial growth and changes in lenticular and corneal power during emmetropization in infants," *Investigative Opthalmology & Visual Science*, vol. 46, no. 9, pp. 3074–3080, 2005.

[26] H. Radhakrishnan and W. N. Charman, "Refractive changes associated with oblique viewing and reading in myopes and emmetropes," *Journal of Vision*, vol. 7, no. 8, p. 5, 2007.

[27] T. Miyake, K. Shimizu, and K. Kamiya, "Distribution of posterior corneal astigmatism according to axis orientation of anterior corneal astigmatism," *PLoS One*, vol. 10, no. 1, article e0117194, 2015.

[28] D. D. Koch, S. F. Ali, M. P. Weikert, M. Shirayama, R. Jenkins, and L. Wang, "Contribution of posterior corneal astigmatism to total corneal astigmatism," *Journal of Cataract & Refractive Surgery*, vol. 38, no. 12, pp. 2080–2087, 2012.

[29] J.-D. Ho, S.-W. Liou, R. J.-F. Tsai, and C.-Y. Tsai, "Effects of aging on anterior and posterior corneal astigmatism," *Cornea*, vol. 29, no. 6, pp. 632–637, 2010.

[30] R. S. Hoffman, M. E. Snyder, U. Devgan et al., "Management of the subluxated crystalline lens," *Journal of Cataract and Refractive Surgery*, vol. 39, no. 12, pp. 1904–1915, 2013.

2

Efficacy and Safety of Intravitreal Conbercept, Ranibizumab, and Triamcinolone on 23-Gauge Vitrectomy for Patients with Proliferative Diabetic Retinopathy

Jinglin Cui,[1,2] Hong Chen,[1] Hang Lu,[1] Fangtian Dong,[3] Dongmei Wei,[1] Yan Jiao,[2] Steve Charles,[4,5] Weikuan Gu,[2,6] and Lin Wang[1]

[1]*Center of Integrative Research, The First Hospital of Qiqihar City, Qiqihar, Heilongjiang 161005, China*
[2]*Department of Orthopedic Surgery and BME-Campbell Clinic, University of Tennessee Health Science Center, Memphis, TN 38163, USA*
[3]*Department of Ophthalmology, Peking Union Medical College Hospital, Beijing 100730, China*
[4]*Department of Ophthalmology, University of Tennessee Health Science Center, Memphis, TN 38163, USA*
[5]*Charles Retina Institute, Germantown, TN 38138, USA*
[6]*Research Service, Veterans Affairs Medical Center, 1030 Jefferson Avenue, Memphis, TN 38104, USA*

Correspondence should be addressed to Weikuan Gu; wgu@uthsc.edu and Lin Wang; Wanglinqsdyyy@126.com

Academic Editor: Yoshihiro Takamura

Introduction. To compare the effect and safety of intravitreal conbercept (IVC), intravitreal ranibizumab (IVR), or intravitreal triamcinolone acetonide (IVTA) injection on 23-gauge (23-G) pars plana vitrectomy (PPV) for proliferative diabetic retinopathy (PDR). *Methods.* Fifty patients (60 eyes) of varying degrees of PDR were randomly grouped into 3 groups (1 : 1 : 1) ($n = 20$ in each group). The 23-G PPV was performed with intravitreal conbercept or ranibizumab injection 3–7 days before surgery or intravitreal TA injection during surgery. The experiment was randomized controlled, with a noninferiority limit of five letters. Main outcome measures included BCVA, operation time, incidence of iatrogenic retinal breaks, endodiathermy rate, and silicone oil tamponade. *Results.* At 6 months after surgery, there were no significant differences of BCVA improvements, operation time, incidence of iatrogenic retinal breaks, endodiathermy rate, silicone oil tamponade, vitreous clear-up time, and the incidence of intraoperative bleeding between the IVC and IVR groups (all P values ≥ 0.05), but they were significantly different from the IVTA group (all P values < 0.05). IOP increases did not show significant differences between the IVC and IVR groups, but both were significantly different with the IVTA group. More patients had higher postoperative IOP in the IVTA group. *Conclusions.* The intravitreal injection of conbercept, ranibizumab, or TA for PDR had a significant different effect on outcomes of 23-G PPV surgery. Conbercept and ranibizumab can reduce difficulty of the operation, improve the success rate of PPV surgery, and decrease the incidence of postoperative complications.

1. Introduction

Proliferative diabetic retinopathy (PDR) is the leading cause of blindness among DR in diabetic patients [1–6]. PDR can lead to vitreous hemorrhage, traction detachment from fibrous proliferation, or neovascular glaucoma [7]. The current standard treatment for PDR is panretinal photocoagulation (PRP), combined with PPV whenever necessary. However, PRP is naturally destructive and has several potential adverse effects on visual function, including constriction of the peripheral visual field and reductions in night vision, contrast sensitivity, and color perception. Furthermore, it has been known that in the absence of intravitreal administration of ranibizumab or triamcinolone acetonide (TA), PRP can negatively affect vision and macular thickness in patients with diabetic macular edema (DME) [8]. In the surgery of advanced PDR, the occurrence of intraoperative hemorrhage when dissecting epiretinal neovascular membrane will seriously affect visualization of the surgical field. In addition, repeated bleeding can prolong the operation time, increase the frequency of instrument exchange, and greatly increase the occurring rate of complications [9].

In order to reduce the chance of complications, a variety of drugs have been utilized in PPV for PDR. TA (Kenalog, Bristol-Myers Squibb Company, Princeton, NJ) (Kenakolt-A, Bristol Pharmaceuticals KK, Tokyo, Japan) is a water-insoluble steroid that inhibits various inflammatory reactions. It has been confirmed that it can aid visualization of transparent vitreous, reduce the degree of postoperative inflammation, and decrease the incidence of reoperation owing to epiretinal membrane formation in TA-assisted PPV for PDR [10–12]. In recent years, the important role of excessive release of vascular endothelial growth factor (VEGF) in many retinal vascular diseases has been unanimously recognized worldwide, including in PDR surgery [13–15]. Ranibizumab (Lucentis; Genentech Inc., South San Francisco, CA) and bevacizumab (Avastin; Genentech Inc., South San Francisco, CA) are monoclonal antibodies, militating by block VEGF-A. Studies showed that both of them can result superior visual acuity and central retinal thickness, reduce the duration of surgery, achieve fewer retinal breaks, and lessen intraoperative bleeding and also lead fewer endodiathermy applications [16]. However, bevacizumab has not been approved for use in intraocular injections in China. Conbercept (Langmu; Kanghong Inc., Sichuan, China) is a VEGF receptor (VEGFR) fusion protein. In late 2013, it received the new drug certificate, drug registration approval, and GMP certification from State Food and Drug Administration in China and has been widely used, accompanied by neovascularization vitreoretinopathy, such as neovascular age-related macular degeneration (AMD). It functions by competitively inhibiting the binding of VEGF with its receptor by blocking multiple targets, VEGF-A, VEGF-B, and placental insulin-like growth factor (PlGF) [17]. Most recently, conbercept has been reported to be an effective adjunct for the intravitreal conbercept (IVC) injection before vitrectomy for proliferative diabetic retinopathy (PDR) [18]. Thus, TA has traditionally been used PPV for PDR. Conbercept has been recently tested for its benefit when it was used PPV for PDR, mostly in Europe. Conbercept has been mostly tested in China. These three of them have never been directly compared. This study aims to compare the efficacy and safety of PPV when assisted by conbercept, ranibizumab, and TA intravitreal injection for PDR.

2. Methods

2.1. Study Population. This study adheres to the guidelines of the Declaration of Helsinki. The study was approved by the Institutional Review Board of the First Hospital of Qiqihar City. The protocol number is 2006-04. Patients' consents were given to all participants, and all patients signed the consents before participating the study. Between Jan 2015 and Dec 2015, 60 eyes from 53 patients were collected of varying degrees of PDR in the First Hospital of Qiqihar. There were 33 (55%) male and 27 (45%) female. The age was between 29 and 78 years old, with the average age of 58.83 (±3.62). Mean duration of DM was 26.57 ± 5.82 years. All patients had a history of DM, with 14 (23.3%) cases of type 1 DM and 46 (76.7%) cases of type 2 DM. Visual acuity was tested using Early Treatment Diabetic Retinopathy Study (ETDRS) charts at 4 m [18]. The BCVA was from HM to 20/80 as determined by protocol trial lens refraction. Other examinations included slit lamp directly, indirect ophthalmoscopy, IOP measurement, B-scan ultrasonography, fundus fluorescein angiography (FFA), and optical coherence tomography (OCT). Patients were selected for the PPV treatments (Table 1) based on the existence of extent of vitreous hemorrhage, retinal proliferation or traction retinal detachment, and other serious PDR. Exclusion criteria included those who received prior intravitreal injection, underwent vitreous or retinal surgeries, and glaucoma. Patients with abnormal blood coagulation indexes and other diseases of surgical contraindication were also excluded [19]. Before treatment, patients were provided with informed consent, the risks of surgery, and intraocular injection, and surgical complications related to the treatments were discussed. All patients understood the content and signed the informed consent. The study was approved by the First Hospital of Qiqihar Committees for Medical and Health Research.

2.2. Study Procedures. Patients were randomly divided into IVC, IVR, and IVTA groups (1 : 1 : 1) ($n = 20$ eyes in each group). Mean BCVA was 27.83 ± 6.78, 25.31 ± 4.23, and 28.46 ± 7.55 (ETDRS letters) in the IVC, IVR, and IVTA groups, respectively. The IVC group were 20 eyes in 17 patients, including 11 eyes (9 cases, 55%) of male and 9 eyes (8 cases, 45%) of female. Patients received 0.5 mg (0.05 ml, 10 mg/ml) intravitreal injections of conbercept [20] while the IVR group were 20 eyes of 20 patients, including 14 eyes (14 cases, 70%) of male and 6 eyes (6 cases, 30%) of female. Patients received 0.5 mg (0.05 ml, 10 mg/ml) intravitreal injections of ranibizumab [21]. PPV in both IVC and IVR groups was completed within 3–7 days after injection, and TA was not used during the surgery in both groups. The IVTA group were 20 eyes in 16 patients, including 12 eyes (11 cases, 60%) of male and 8 eyes (5 cases, 40%) of female. Patients received 4 mg (0.5 ml, 8 mg/ml) intravitreal injections of TA during the PPV [22]. The TA in the group of IVTA was removed during the surgery, with no remaining in the vitreum at the end of surgery. Three drugs were acquired commercially, and batch numbers for all vials used in the study were registered. Sterile techniques were used for every injection. Ophthalmic antibiotics and prophylactic peri-intravitreal injection were not used. Topical anesthetics were used (0.4% oxybuprocaine hydrochloride eye drops, Santen Pharmaceutical Co. Ltd.). The periocular skin, eyelids, and eyelashes were disinfected with 10% povidone-iodine swabs, and 5% povidone-iodine ophthalmic solution was applied to the ocular surface. All the patients received 23-G (Gauge) PPV (Alcon). The surgeries were performed by two experienced vitreoretinal specialist (Fangtian Dong and Hang Lu), who were masked from the patient information. The choice of tamponade was made between C3F8 gas or silicone oil depending on the difficulty and complexity of

Table 1: Baseline characteristics of participants with or without conbercept pretreatment.

	IVC ($n = 20$)	IVR ($n = 19$)	IVTA ($n = 19$)	P value
Sex				0.759
Male (eyes, %)	9 (11, 55%)	13 (13, 68.4%)	10 (11, 57.9%)	
Female (eyes, %)	8 (9, 45%)	6 (6, 31.6%)	5 (8, 42.1%)	
Age (yrs)				
Mean (SD)	60.74 ± 2.63	55.28 ± 5.16	57.49 ± 4.22	0.246
Type of diabetes (case, %)				0.527
1	3 (15.0)	4 (21.1)	2 (10.5)	
2	12 (6.0)	10 (52.6)	14 (73.7)	
Uncertain		5 (25.0)	5 (26.3)	3 (15.8)
Ocular profile (case, %)				
Study eye (left/right)	13/7 (65.0/35.0)	8/11 (42.1/57.9)	6/13 (31.6/68.4)	0.138
Previous history of laser	4 (20.0)	2 (10.5)	2 (10.5)	0.495
Lens status	3 (15.0)	4 (21.1)	2 (10.5)	0.663
Pathogeny (case, %)				
Nonclearing vitreous hemorrhage	9 (45.0)	9 (47.4)	8 (42.1)	0.914
Diffuse fibrovascular proliferation	4 (20.0)	3 (15.8)	5 (26.3)	0.125
Traction retinal detachment	7 (35.0)	7 (36.8)	6 (31.6)	0.573
Extent of vitreoretinal adhesion grade (case, %)				0.416
0	0 (0.0)	0 (0.0)	0 (0.0)	
1	2 (10.0)	4 (21.1)	5 (26.3)	
2	12 (60.0)	9 (47.4)	10 (52.6)	
3	6 (30.0)	6 (31.6)	4 (21.1)	
Duration of diabetes (y)				
Mean (SD)	24.25 ± 6.33	28.76 ± 5.27	25.98 ± 4.6	0.227
Mean BCVA (ETDRS letters)			0.531	
Mean (SD)	27.83 ± 6.78	25.31 ± 4.23	28.46 ± 7.55	
Snellen equivalent (range)	20/100–HM	20/100–20/2000	20/80–HM	
IOP (mmHg)				
Mean (SD)	15.24 ± 4.67	$.64 \pm 6.21$	16.35 ± 2.89	0.395
Cardiovascular condition (case, %)	12 (60.0)	10 (52.6)	13 (68.4)	1.103
Hypertension (case, %)	15 (75.0)	11 (57.9)	14 (73.7)	0.587
Cerebral vascular disease (case, %)	5 (25.0)	7 (36.8)	4 (21.1)	0.862

the surgery, such as the severity of traction, size and number of retinal breaks or detachment, presence of iatrogenic breaks, retinectomy, severe bleeding, and other intraoperative complications [21]. Intraoperative panretinal endolaser photocoagulation was used, whenever necessary, at the end of the PPV surgery [23]. Ophthalmic antibiotics (5% levofloxacin eye drops, Santen, Japan) were used from the first day after surgery for 3 days, 4 times/d. Follow-up time was 6 months.

2.3. Data and Statistical Analysis. The primary outcomes were mean BCVA (ETDRS chart) monthly, operation time, incidence of iatrogenic retinal breaks, endodiathermy rate, and silicone oil tamponade. Secondary outcomes included average vitreous clearing time and the frequency of intraoperative and postoperative bleeding, PRP completion rate, reoperation probability, and intraocular pressure (IOP) in each group. Vitreous clearing time was defined as the interval between the end of surgery and the time at which the vitreous cleared up completely. Increased IOP was defined as an intraocular pressure > 21, which occurred within 24 hours after injections. To prevent effect of silicone oil on postoperative visual acuity, the final results of BCVA were determined after silicone oil removal. For patients with cataract after surgery, BCVA was measured after cataract extraction combined with intraocular lens implantation. Complications of cataract surgery were not included in this study.

The margin of clinical noninferiority was defined as five letters on the ETDRS visual acuity chart. Statistical analysis of the primary outcome variable, the mean change in BCVA from baseline to 6 m follow-up, was performed on data from the per protocol population (patients attending the 6 m visits). The mean scores of the primary outcome variables in three treatment groups were compared to each other using the independent samples t-test. The same statistical procedure was applied when analyzing the data according to the

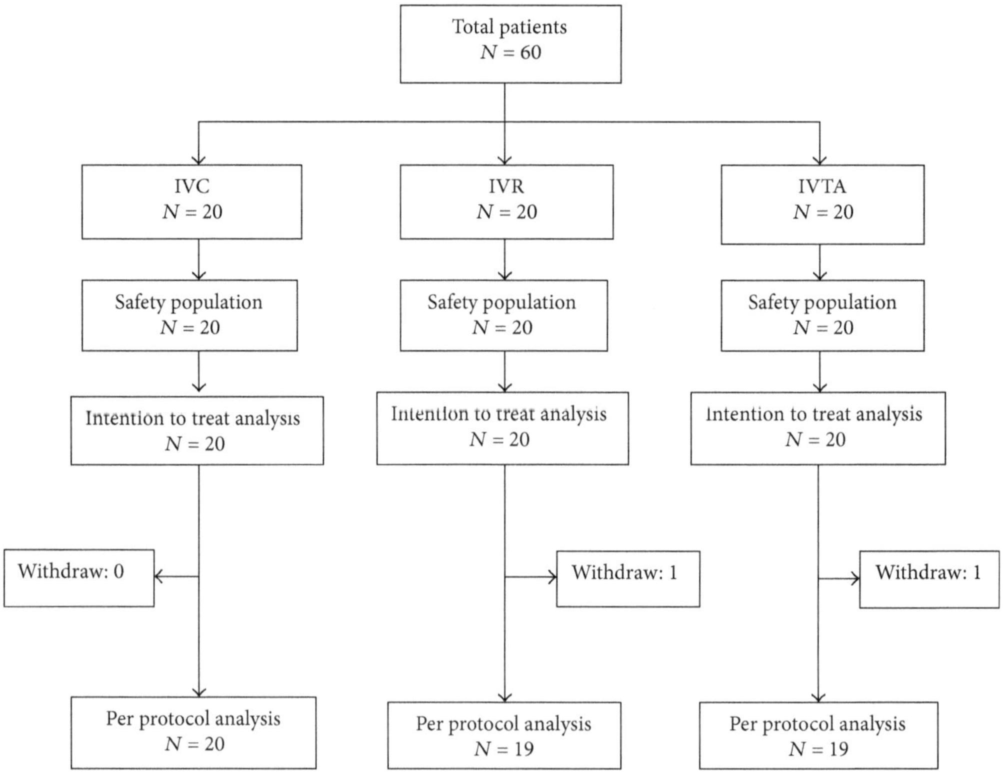

Figure 1: Study flow chart.

intent-to-treat principle, using multiple imputing to replace missing observations at 6 m follow-up.

Statistical analysis of secondary outcomes was performed only on data from the per protocol population, the operation time by independent samples t-test; if $p < 0.05$, the difference was considered statistically significant.

3. Results

3.1. Patients and Treatments. 60 patients were included in the treatment and safety analysis. The 6-month visits were completed by 58 (96.7%) patients (Supplementary Table 1). Two (3.3%) patients were lost to follow-up (one was in the IVR group and the other in the IVTA group). The primary analysis followed the intent-to-treat principle and included all randomized eyes (Figure 1). There were no substantial differences among the groups regarding age, sex, IOP, BCVA, and DR degree of severity in baseline characteristics (Table 1). To obtain 3 homogeneous groups of surgical complexity, we assigned scores from 0 to 3 for the following preoperative parameters: (1) vitreous hemorrhage (VH), (2) previous retinal laser photocoagulation, and (3) morphological types of retinal detachment, such as hammock, central diffuse, and table-top [24]. There was no significant difference in these scores. All patients did not receive PPV or intravitreal injection treatment, but some of them have received PRP treatment (cases were 4, 2, and 2 in 3 groups, resp.) (Table 2). The means and standard deviation of three groups showed that there was no difference among them.

3.2. Primary Outcomes. At the end of 6 m follow-up, the mean improvements in the IVC, IVR, and IVTA groups, respectively, were as follows (Figure 2): BCVA (ETDRS charts) was 25.10 ± 3.73, 26.32 ± 4.06, and 17.16 ± 2.87; the mean operation time was 56.65 ± 6.52, 54.89 ± 6.46, and 77.32 ± 6.36; the incidence of iatrogenic retinal breaks was 2 (10.0%), 2 (10.5%), and 8 (42.1%) cases; the endodiathermy rate was 5 (25.0%), 6 (31.6%), and 12 (63.2%) cases; and silicone oil tamponade was 9 (45.0%), 9 (47.4%), and 15 (78.9%) cases. There were no significant differences in BCVA improvements, operation time, incidence of iatrogenic retinal breaks, endodiathermy rate, and silicone oil tamponade between the IVC and IVR groups (all P values ≥ 0.05). However, each of these two groups showed significant difference with the IVTA group (all P values < 0.05) (Table 3).

3.3. Secondary Outcomes. The average vitreous clear-up time was 6.10 ± 1.52, 6.32 ± 1.57, and 11.11 ± 2.38 in the IVC, IVR, and IVTA groups, respectively (Figure 3); the incidence of intraoperative bleeding was 2 (10.0%), 3 (15.8%), and 9 (47.4%) cases in the three groups, respectively; postoperative bleeding was 1 (5.0%), 1 (5.3%), and 3 (15.8%) cases in the three groups, which occurred at 5 d, 1 w, and 1.5 m, respectively. Three patients required reoperation. Two cases were treated with Chinese drugs (He Xue Ming Mu Pian and Hong Hua Huang Se Su). BCVA was measured at 3 months after treatments. PRP completion rate was 11 (55.0%), 10 (52.6%), and 6 (31.6%) cases in the IVC, IVR, and IVTA groups, respectively. Four patients needed reoperation with the distribution of 1 (5.0%), 1 (5.3%), and 2 (10.5%) in the

Table 2: Baseline complexity surgery score of DR patients.

Surgery		IVC		IVR		IVTA
	Cases ($n = 20$)	Complexity surgery Score	Cases ($n = 19$)	Complexity surgery Score	Cases ($n = 19$)	Complexity Score
VH						
Absent (0)	11	0	10	0	11	0
Mild (+1)	2	2	3	3	2	2
Moderate (+2)	5	10	4	8	5	10
Severe (+3)	2	6	2	6	1	3
Amount of previous						
Retinal photocoagulation						
Complete PRP (0)	1	0	0	0	0	0
Incomplete PRP (+1)	2	2	1	1	2	2
Focal (+2)	1	2	1	2	0	0
None (+3)	16	48	17			1
Configuration of retinal detachment						
Absent (0)	13	0	12	0	13	0
Hammock (+1)	4	4	3	3	2	2
Central diffuse (+2)	3	6	4	8	4	8
Table-top (+3)	0	0	0	0	0	0
Total complexity surgery score	20	80	19	82	19	78
Means (SD)		4.00 ± 13.38		4.32 ± 14.23		4.11 ± 14.39
P		0.67 (IVC versus IVTA)		0.39 (IVR versus IVTA)		

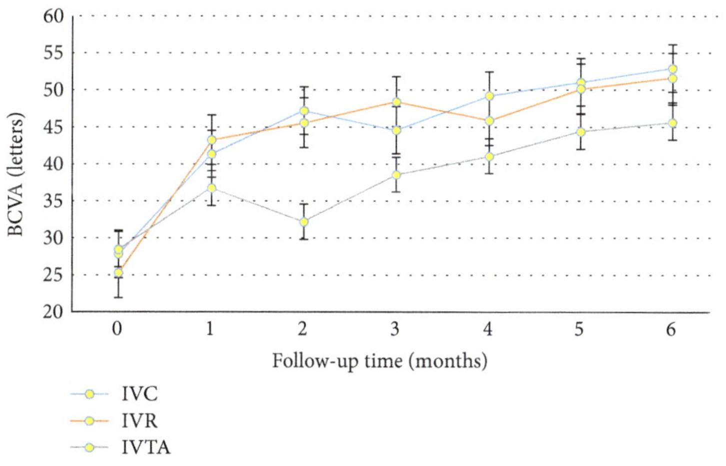

Figure 2: The mean changes in BCVA from baseline in IVC, IVR, and IVTA groups over 6 m were as indicated by the ETDRS chart letters. BCVA gradually increased after treatments in all three groups. The increases of BCVA were the most at the end of the first month. At the end of 6 m, the mean BCVA was improved by 25.10 ± 3.73, 26.32 ± 4.06, and 17.16 ± 2.87 letters in IVC, IVR, and IVTA groups, respectively (all P values < 0.05).

three groups, respectively. Three of them were caused by postoperative bleeding, and 1 was caused by silicone oil emulsified into the anterior chamber. There were no significant differences in vitreous clear-up time and the incidence of intraoperative bleeding between the IVC and IVR groups, while both of these groups were significantly different from the IVTA group. However, there were no significant differences in the incidence of postoperative bleeding, PRP completion rate, and reoperation probability among the 3 groups (Table 4).

3.4. Adverse Events. IOP increase is defined as an intraocular pressure > 25 mmHg, which appeared within 24 hours after injections. If IOP increased, subjects were monitored until intraocular pressure at 25 mmHg or less. The cases with increased IOP were 3 (15.0%), 2 (10.5%), and 9 (47.4%) in the IVC, IVR, and IVTA groups, respectively (Figure 4). There were no significant differences of IOP rate between the IVC and IVR groups, but both groups were significantly less than that in the IVTA group. Thus, more patients are at high IOP level in the IVTA group than

Table 3: Primary outcomes (Mean ± SD).

	IVC	IVR	IVTA	*P* value*
Mean BCVA improvement (ETDRS letters)				
(Mean ± SD)	25.10 ± 3.73	26.32 ± 4.06	17.16 ± 2.87	0.337, <0.01, <0.01
Operation time (minutes)				
(Mean ± SD)	56.65 ± 6.52	54.89 ± 6.46	77.32 ± 6.36	0.404, <0.01, <0.01
Incidence of iatrogenic retinal breaks (cases, %)	2 (10.0)	2 (10.5)	8 (42.1)	0.958, 0.024, 0.027
Endodiathermy rate (cases, %)	5 (25.0)	6 (31.6)	12 (63.2)	0.659, 0.014, 0.049
Silicone oil tamponade (cases, %)	9 (45.0)	9 (47.4)	15 (78.9)	0.885, 0.029, 0.045

**P* value of IVC versus IVR, IVC versus IVTA, and IVR versus IVTA.

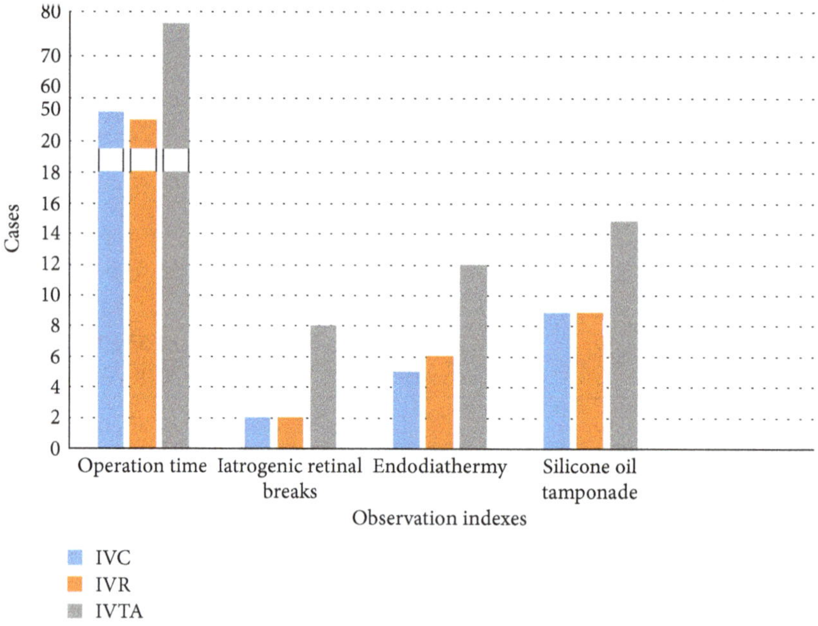

Figure 3: Comparison of outcomes of IVC, IVR, and IVTA groups at 6 m. There were no significant differences in operation time, incidence of iatrogenic retinal breaks, endodiathermy rate, and silicone oil tamponade between IVC and IVR groups. However, each of these two groups showed significant difference with the IVTA group.

Table 4: Secondary outcomes and IOP.

	IVC	IVR	IVTA	*P* value*
Vitreous clear-up time (days)				
(Mean ± SD)	6.10 ± 1.52	6.32 ± 1.57	11.11 ± 2.38	0.66, <0.01, <0.01
Intraoperative bleeding (cases, %)	2 (10.0)	3 (15.8)	9 (47.4)	0.602, 0.010, 0.04
Postoperative bleeding (cases, %)	1 (5.0)	1 (5.3)	3 (15.8)	0.971, 0.287, 0.305
PRP completion rate (cases, %)	11 (55.0)	10 (52.6)	6 (31.6)	0.886, 0.147, 0.199
Reoperation probability (cases, %)	1 (5.0)	1 (5.3)	2 (10.5)	0.971, 0.534, 0.560
IOP increase (case, %)	3 (15.0)	2 (10.5)	9 (47.4)	0.684, 0.031, 0.011

**P* value of IVC versus IVR, IVC versus IVTA, and IVR versus IVTA.

the other two groups after surgeries. Among IOP patients, 5 were given anterior chamber tap, while others were treated with IOP-lowering drugs. The IOP of all of these patients decreased to normal ranges within 2 weeks. There were no significant differences in hypertension, cardiovascular, and cerebral vascular diseases among the 3 groups, compared with baselines (Table 5). No endophthalmitis, iris neovascularization, or TRD progression were observed during the follow-up period.

4. Discussion

PDR usually is extremely complicated with intraocular hemorrhage and TRD. Because of the existence of hemorrhage,

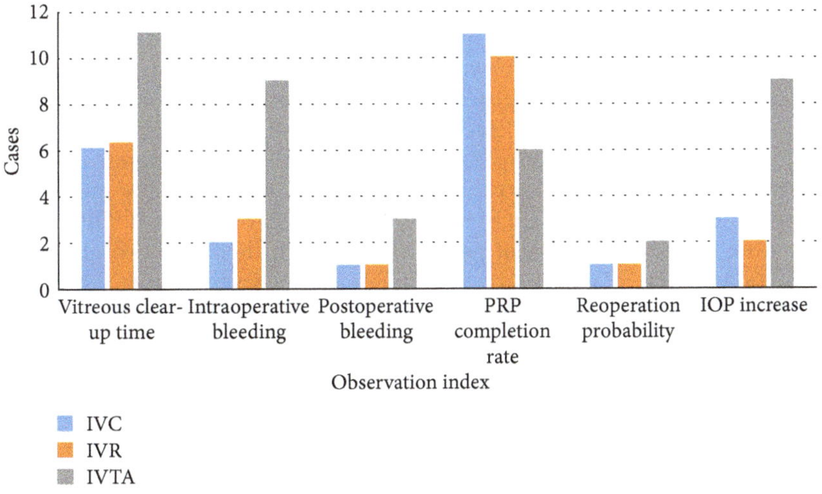

Figure 4: Secondary outcomes and adverse events of the IVC, IVR, and IVTA groups at 6 m. There were no significant differences in vitreous clear-up time and the incidence of intraoperative bleeding between IVC and IVR groups, while both of these groups were significantly different from IVTA group. More patients were at high IOP level in the IVTA group than the other two groups after surgeries. However, there were no statistically significant differences in the incidence of postoperative bleeding, PRP completion rate, and reoperation probability among 3 groups.

Table 5: System adverse events compared with baseline.

IVC	IVR	IVTA	P value*	
Cardiovascular disease (case, %)	14 (70.0)	13 (68.4)	14 (73.7)	0.519, 0.333, 0.729
Hypertension (case, %)	15 (75.0)	12 (63.2)	16 (84.2)	1.000, 0.748, 0.439
Cerebral vascular disease (case, %)	6 (30.0)	7 (36.8)	5 (26.3)	0.731, 1.000, 0.712

*P value of IVC, IVR, and IVTA.

exudation, and proliferation membrane during surgery in severe PDR, structures of retina are not easily identified and surgical difficulty and complexity are increased. Several studies have confirmed that VEGF plays a very important role in complex PDR [25, 26]. Due to long-term hypoxia in the occurrence and development of PDR, secretion of VEGF by retinal cells is increased, which causes new vessel hyperplasia, vitreous hemorrhage, and fibrovascular membranes and eventually leading to the TRD and severe damage to vision or even blindness [27, 28]. Clinical trials concluded that preoperative intravitreal injection of anti-VEGF drugs can reduce the intravitreal VEGF level, inhibit the activity of VEGF partially, and decrease retinal vascular leakage and neovascularization [29, 30]. Anti-VEGF drugs can also reduce the incidence of bleeding and iatrogenic holes during epiretinal membrane dissection [31, 32]. The VEGF family consists of VEGF-A, VEGF-B, VEGFC, VEGF-D, and placental growth factor (PIGF), which are related to receptors VEGFR-1, VEGFR-2, and VEGFR-3. VEGF-A can activate both VEGFR-1 and VEGFR-2. Meanwhile, VEGF-B and PIGF only bind to VEGFR-1. Also, VEGF-C and VEGF-D only bind to VEGFR-3 [33]. However, the monoclonal antibodies such as ranibizumab and bevacizumab had been found to bind VEGF-A only and lasted for only a short time [34]. Conbercept is a humanized soluble VEGFR protein which comprises extracellular domain 2 of VEGFR-1 and extracellular domains 3 and 4 of VEGFR-2, all of which are combined with the Fc region of human immunoglobulin G1 simultaneously. Based on its structure, it is predicted that it inhibits the binding of multiple VEGF receptors. Previous studies have demonstrated that extracellular domain 4 of VEGFR-2 can enhance the three-dimensional structure and efficiently advance dimerization [35]. Therefore, it is relatively stable and long lasting, in comparison with that of monoclonal antibodies. Also, preclinical studies have presented higher affinity of conbercept for VEGF than bevacizumab [36].

In addition, postoperative inflammation is also one of the major causes of postoperative complications, such as proliferative vitreoretinopathy (PVR). The postoperative inflammatory cells can secrete varieties of chemical mediators and cytokines, which stimulate the invasion of secondary inflammatory cells into the vitreoretinal tissue and activate the retinal glial cells and retinal pigment epithelium cells. These activated cells cause the proliferation of themselves, produce extracellular matrix, and contract the epiretinal membrane, thus leading to a secondary retinal detachment [37, 38]. Therefore, a reduction of postoperative inflammation is a logical strategy to prevent postoperative complications.

IVC, IVR, and IVTA are three commonly used procedures to improve the PDR operation in China. Only a single injection of TA was used early. Currently, anti-VEGF drugs in this study have been used in conjunction with PPV for PDR in China. Early studies showed that intravitreal injection of TA successfully inhibited experimental PVR in the rabbit and optic disk neovascularization in the pig [39, 40]. In the study by Enaida et al., 62 Patients with PVR, diabetic macular edema (DME), PDR, rhegmatogenous retinal detachment (RRD), and macular hole retinal detachment (MHRD) were treated with TA-assisted PPV surgeries. Results showed that 49% of patients had improved vision and a lower incidence of reoperation caused by preretinal fibrous membrane formation [41]. Also, a study showed that performing intravitreal TA injection during PPV can increase the intraoperative visualization of vitreous; therefore, it may facilitate both removal of epiretinal membrane and separation of vitreous, especially in patients with undetached vitreous [42]. TA also was confirmed sufficient to reduce postoperative inflammation, as TA particles were left on the retinal surface for a few days [43]. Ranibizumab is a humanized monoclonal antibody fragment, which lacks an Fc domain, that functions by blocking all VEGF-A isoforms [44]. Conbercept is a different VEGFR fusion protein with multiple binding targets [45]. Large randomized controlled trials (RCTs) have authenticated principally the role of anti-VEGF agents in age-related macular degeneration, retinal vascular occlusion, and diabetic macular edema [46–49]. Studies in recent years have explored the role of anti-VEGF agents in PDR either as stand-alone therapy or as an adjunct to laser or PPV. Meta-analysis suggests that the addition of IVR to PRP results in improved structural and functional outcomes at 3 months/16 weeks and supports the assertion that application of intravitreal anti-VEGF therapy before PPV has the effect of reducing operating times, increasing the ease of surgery [50]. These facts support the use of anti-VEGF agents as adjunctive therapy in patients requiring PRP or vitrectomy for complicated PDR.

In our study, 60 eyes of PDR which combined with vitreous hemorrhage in different degrees and TRD were selected. Patients were randomly divided into three groups, ignoring the severity of the disease. The results showed that the preoperative application of intravitreal injections of conbercept and ranibizumab had equal effect in improvement of visual acuity, operation time, incidence of iatrogenic retinal breaks, endodiathermy rate, frequency of silicone oil tamponade, vitreous clearing time, and the incidence of intraoperative bleeding. Compared with the IVTA group, the IVC and IVR groups had more visual acuity gains after surgeries and increased operation safeties. In PPV surgery of the IVC and IVR groups, the fibrous proliferative membranes were easily separated from the retina with a few individual of bleeding. The advantages of the IVC and IVR groups are time saving for operations and reduced risks of surgical complications.

However, the posterior hyaloid can be clearly seen after the injection of TA suspension that enhanced visualization of vitreous in the IVTA group. Nevertheless, considering the potential increased risk of glaucoma and cataract associated with the use of intravitreal corticosteroids, the use of intravitreal corticosteroid preparations to reduce the likelihood of retinopathy worsening does not seem warranted [7].

Our data indicated that there were no significant differences among the three groups in the incidence of postoperative bleeding, PRP completion rate, and reoperation probability. Thus, although IVC, IVR, and IVTA may function in variable degrees, they all improved postoperative conditions and reduced complication occurrence of PPV. Conbercept, ranibizumab, and TA also improved the completion rate of postoperative PRP, prevented the development of DR, and greatly improved the patient's prognosis. The number of eyes with IOP increase was more in the IVTA group than the other two groups, suggesting that although TA was believed able to be removed from vitreous after PPV [40], its effect on IOP continually exists to a certain extent. There were no significant differences in other adverse events, such as hypertension, cardiovascular, and cerebral vascular diseases among the 3 groups compared with baselines, suggesting that there is very little or no influence on the system events from intravitreal injections of these three drugs. The early postoperative bleeding usually was relevant to the dissection of fibrovascular membranes in surgery which occurred typically within 1 week of surgery [51]. Pretreatment with conbercept surely facilitated the reducing of postoperative bleeding early after surgery due to the regression of neovascularization, cessation of hemorrhage from all potential bleeding sources, and reintegration of retinal vascular tissue. However, due to the short-time effect of anti-VEGF drugs injected before surgery, it did not affect late VH incidence [20]. Thus, due to the short duration of time of the anti-VEGF drug pretreatment in the eye, there were no significant differences in the incidence of postoperative bleeding among the three groups.

It has been controversial on the optimal timing of preoperative injection of anti-VEGF drugs before vitrectomy. In our study, PPV was completed during 3–7 days after intravitreal injection. Data indicated that drugs were effective and patient postoperative conditions were significantly improved. Furthermore, no significant development of proliferative lesions was observed in 6 m. Since the blood glucose level is one of the important factors that affect the development of PDR [52], in our study, all patients were asked to actively control blood glucose before and after surgeries, preventing hyperglycemia leading to surgical failure. Several studies reported that drugs caused the retinal pigment epithelium (RPE) tears [53, 54]. However, in our study, no RPE tears were found after intravitreal injection during follow-up. Since there are many factors in the formation of cataract, for example, silicone oil intraocular filling can also lead to cataract, our study did not include cataract as one of the surgical complication [7].

In conclusion, this study suggested that in a developing country such as China, PDR patients living in rural areas usually could not receive early and effective treatment due to inconvenient transportation and inadequate community health care services; therefore, it is essential to reduce the cost of surgical complications, reoperation, and long-term treatment. 23-G PPV surgery assisted by intravitreal injection of conbercept, ranibizumab, or TA for PDR had a significant impact on patient health condition and economic burden. The application of these drugs can reduce difficulty of the operation, improve the success rate of PPV surgery, and decrease the incidence of postoperative complications, therefore reducing the patient's economic burden in China. Conbercept and ranibizumab have equal effectiveness and achieved better results than TA. The safety and efficacy of the anti-VEGF drugs were confirmed in the treatment of complex PDR. However, our research is limited, as the observation time is short, the long-term effects and complications of drugs had not been well reflected. Function mechanism of these drugs is also not completely understood. In addition, the number of cases in this study is inadequate for a definitive conclusion. Therefore, these results also need to be proved by clinical trials of large sample sizes and extended follow-up period.

Disclosure

The funding organization had no role in the design or conduct of this research.

Conflicts of Interest

The authors declare that they have no competing interests.

Authors' Contributions

Jinglin Cui, Weikuan Gu, and Hong Chen had full access to all the data in the study and take responsibility for the integrity of the data and the accuracy of the data analysis. Jinglin Cui, Lin Wang, Weikuan Gu, and Hong Chen were responsible for the study concept and design. Jinglin Cui, Hang Lu, and Fangtian Dong performed the clinical treatment and data collection. All authors performed the acquisition, analysis, or interpretation of data. Jinglin Cui, Weikuan Gu, and Steve Charles were responsible for the drafting of the manuscript. All authors helped in the critical revision of the manuscript for important intellectual content. Jinglin Cui, Yan Jiao, and Weikuan Gu performed the statistical analysis. Jinglin Cui, Lin Wang, Dongmei Wei, and Weikuan Gu performed the literature search. Yan Jiao, LinWang, Weikuan Gu, Steve Charles, and Hong Chen obtained funding. Lin Wang, Dongmei Wei, Hang Lu, and HongChen were responsible for administrative, technical, or material support. Hong Chen, Lin Wang, and Dongmei Wei supervised the study.

Acknowledgments

This work was partially supported by the funding from the First Hospital of Qiqihar City, Heilongjiang, China, the National Natural Science Foundation of China (Project 81372996 to Yan Jiao), the U.S. Department of Veterans Affairs (1IPIBX001607-01), and the Veterans Administration Medical Center at Memphis, TN.

References

[1] F. Boscia, "Current approaches to the management of diabetic retinopathy and diabetic macular oedema," *Drugs*, vol. 70, no. 16, pp. 2171–2200, 2010.

[2] W. Yang, J. Lu, J. Weng et al., "Prevalence of diabetes among men and women in China," *The New England Journal of Medicine*, vol. 362, no. 12, pp. 1090–1101, 2010.

[3] L. Liu, X. Wu, L. Liu et al., "Prevalence of diabetic retinopathy in mainland China: a meta-analysis," *PLoS One*, vol. 7, no. 9, article e45264, 2012.

[4] D. S. Fong, L. Aiello, T. W. Gardner et al., "Retinopathy in diabetes," *Diabetes Care*, vol. 27, Supplement 1, pp. S84–S87, 2004.

[5] V. L. Tseng, P. B. Greenberg, I. U. Scott, and K. L. Anderson, "Compliance with the American Academy of Ophthalmology Preferred Practice Pattern for Diabetic Retinopathy in a resident ophthalmology clinic," *Retina*, vol. 30, no. 5, pp. 787–794, 2010.

[6] F. M. Li, "Chinese ophthalmology," in *Systemic disease and retinopathy; Part1, diabetic retinopathy*, vol. 2, pp. 2165–2171, People's Medical Publishing House, Beijing, 2005.

[7] S. B. Bressler, H. Qin, M. Melia et al., "Exploratory analysis of the effect of intravitreal ranibizumab or triamcinolone on worsening of diabetic retinopathy in a randomized clinical trial," *JAMA Ophthalmology*, vol. 131, no. 8, pp. 1033–1040, 2013.

[8] J. Googe, A. J. Brucker, N. M. Bressler et al., "Randomized trial evaluating short-term effects of intravitreal ranibizumab or triamcinolone acetonide on macular edema after focal/grid laser for diabetic macular edema in eyes also receiving panretinal photocoagulation," *Retina*, vol. 31, no. 6, pp. 1009–1027, 2011.

[9] T. Liu, A. M. Xie, X. Y. Tian, M. Chen, and J. Wei, "Drug assisted vitrectomy for the treatment of proliferative diabetic retinopathy," *International Journal of Ophthalmology*, vol. 8, pp. 1681–1684, 2008.

[10] G. A. Peyman, R. Cheema, M. D. Conway, and T. Fang, "Triamcinolone acetonide as an aid to visualization of the vitreous and the posterior hyaloid during pars plana vitrectomy," *Retina*, vol. 20, no. 5, pp. 554-555, 2000.

[11] T. Sakamoto, M. Miyazaki, T. Hisatomi et al., "Triamcinolone-assisted pars plana vitrectomy improves the surgical procedures and decreases the postoperative blood-ocular barrier breakdown," *Graefe's Archive for Clinical and Experimental Ophthalmology*, vol. 240, no. 6, pp. 423–429, 2002.

[12] H. Enaida, Y. Hata, A. Ueno et al., "Possible benefits of triamcinolone-assisted pars plana vitrectomy for retinal diseases," *Retina*, vol. 23, no. 6, pp. 764–770, 2003.

[13] J. Zhu, Y. S. Wang, and Y. N. Hui, "Growth and inhibition of choroidal neovascularization," *Recent Advances in Ophthalmology*, vol. 24, pp. 57–60, 2004.

[14] Q. D. Nguyen, S. Tatlipinar, S. M. Shah et al., "Vascular endothelial growth factor is a critical stimulus for diabetic macular edema," *American Journal of Ophthalmology*, vol. 142, no. 6, pp. 961–969.e4, 2006.

[15] P. Kroll, E. Büchele Rodrigues, and S. Hoerle, "Pathogenesis and classification of proliferative diabetic vitreoretinopathy," *Ophthalmologica*, vol. 221, no. 2, pp. 78–94, 2007.

[16] M. P. Simunovic and D. A. L. Maberley, "Anti-vascular endothelial growth factor therapy for proliferative diabetic retinop-

athy: a systematic review and meta-analysis," *Retina*, vol. 35, no. 10, pp. 1931–1942, 2015.

[17] H. Lu, J. Cui, H. Dong, B. Luo, W. Xiu, and H. Li, "Clinical observation of a new anti-VEGF drugs conbercept for wet age-related macular degeneration," *Chinese Journal of Ophthalmology*, vol. 51, no. 11, pp. 818–821, 2015.

[18] X. Yang, J. Xu, R. Wang et al., "A randomized controlled trial of conbercept pretreatment before vitrectomy in proliferative diabetic retinopathy," *Journal of Ophthalmology*, vol. 2016, Article ID 2473234, 8 pages, 2016.

[19] T. Li, Z. Zheng, B. Q. Zheng, S. Z. Zhao, W. Chen, and L. S. Ni, "Effect of bevacizumab combined 23G vitrectomy in the treatment of severe proliferative diabetic retinopathy," *Progress in Modern Biomedicine*, vol. 13, pp. 4488–4491, 2013.

[20] X. Zhang, C. Wu, L. J. Zhou, and R. P. Dai, "Observation of optic disc neovascularization using OCT angiography in proliferative diabetic retinopathy after intravitreal conbercept injections," *Scientific Reports*, vol. 8, article e3972, 2018.

[21] F. Dong, C. Yu, H. Ding, L. Shen, and D. Lou, "Evaluation of intravitreal ranibizumab on the surgical outcome for diabetic retinopathy with tractional retinal detachment," *Medicine*, vol. 95, no. 8, p. e2731, 2016.

[22] W. M. Munir, J. S. Pulido, M. C. Sharma, and B. M. Buerk, "Intravitreal triamcinolone for treatment of complicated proliferative diabetic retinopathy and proliferative vitreoretinopathy," *Canadian Journal of Ophthalmology*, vol. 40, no. 5, pp. 598–604, 2005.

[23] L. Su, X. Ren, H. Wei et al., "Intravitreal conbercept (kh902) for surgical treatment of severe proliferative diabetic retinopathy," *Retina*, vol. 36, no. 5, pp. 938–943, 2016.

[24] R. di Lauro, P. De Ruggiero, R. di Lauro, M. T. di Lauro, and M. R. Romano, "Intravitreal bevacizumab for surgical treatment of severe proliferative diabetic retinopathy," *Graefe's Archive for Clinical and Experimental Ophthalmology*, vol. 248, no. 6, pp. 785–791, 2010.

[25] R. Keshavamurthy, P. Venkatesh, and S. Garg, "Ultrasound biomicroscopy findings of 25 G transconjuctival sutureless (TSV) and conventional (20G) pars plana sclerotomy in the same patient," *BMC Ophthalmology*, vol. 6, no. 1, p. 7, 2006.

[26] J. T. Durham and I. M. Herman, "Microvascular modifications in diabetic retinopathy," *Current Diabetes Reports*, vol. 11, no. 4, pp. 253–264, 2011.

[27] R. J. Van Geest, S. Y. Lesnik-Oberstein, H. S. Tan et al., "A shift in the balance of vascular endothelial growth factor and connective tissue growth factor by bevacizumab causes the angiofibrotic switch in proliferative diabetic retinopathy," *British Journal of Ophthalmology*, vol. 96, no. 4, pp. 587–590, 2012.

[28] D. S. Fong, F. L. Ferris III, M. D. Davis, E. Y. Chew, and Early Treatment Diabetic Retinopathy Study Research Group, "Causes of severe visual loss in the early treatment diabetic retinopathy study: ETDRS report no. 24," *American Journal of Ophthalmology*, vol. 127, no. 2, pp. 137–141, 1999.

[29] J. A. S. Ribeiro, A. Messias, and R. Jorge, "Antiangiogenic drugs and advanced proliferative diabetic retinopathy," *Arquivos Brasileiros de Oftalmologia*, vol. 74, no. 2, pp. 143–146, 2011.

[30] R. L. Avery, J. Pearlman, D. J. Pieramici et al., "Intravitreal bevacizumab (Avastin) in the treatment of proliferative diabetic retinopathy," *Ophthalmology*, vol. 113, no. 10, pp. 1695–1705.e6, 2006.

[31] R.-I. Kohno, Y. Hata, Y. Mochizuki et al., "Histopathology of neovascular tissue from eyes with proliferative diabetic retinopathy after intravitreal bevacizumab injection," *American Journal of Ophthalmology*, vol. 150, no. 2, pp. 223–229.e1, 2010.

[32] E. Chen and C. H. Park, "Use of intravitreal bevacizumab as a preoperative adjunct for tractional retinal detachment repair in severe proliferative diabetic retinopathy," *Retina*, vol. 26, no. 6, pp. 699-700, 2006.

[33] S. Takahashi, "Vascular endothelial growth factor (VEGF), VEGF receptors and their inhibitors for antiangiogenic tumor therapy," *Biological and Pharmaceutical Bulletin*, vol. 34, no. 12, pp. 1785–1788, 2011.

[34] C. C. Wykoff and S. M. Hariprasad, "Comparing aflibercept, bevacizumab, and ranibizumab for DME: analysis of DRCR protocol T," *Ophthalmic Surgery, Lasers and Imaging Retina*, vol. 46, no. 3, pp. 302–305, 2015.

[35] K. Suto, Y. Yamazaki, T. Morita, and H. Mizuno, "Crystal structures of novel vascular endothelial growth factors (VEGF) from snake venoms: insight into selective VEGF binding to kinase insert domain-containing receptor but not to *fms*-like tyrosine kinase-1," *Journal of Biological Chemistry*, vol. 280, no. 3, pp. 2126–2131, 2005.

[36] M. Zhang, J. Zhang, M. Yan, H. Li, C. Yang, and D. Yu, "Recombinant anti-vascular endothelial growth factor fusion protein efficiently suppresses choridal neovascularization in monkeys," *Molecular Vision*, vol. 14, pp. 37–49, 2008.

[37] J. F. Arevalo, M. Maia, H. W. Flynn et al., "Tractional retinal detachment following intravitreal bevacizumab (Avastin) in patients with severe proliferative diabetic retinopathy," *British Journal of Ophthalmology*, vol. 92, no. 2, pp. 213–216, 2008.

[38] P. Wiedemann, "Growth factors in retinal diseases: proliferative vitreoretinopathy, proliferative diabetic retinopathy, and retinal degeneration," *Survey of Ophthalmology*, vol. 36, no. 5, pp. 373–384, 1992.

[39] B. M. Glaser, A. Cardin, and B. Biscoe, "Prolieferative vitreoretinopathy: the mechanism of development of vitreoretinal traction," *Ophthalmology*, vol. 94, no. 4, pp. 327–332, 1987.

[40] Y. Tano, D. B. Chandler, B. W. McCuen, and R. Machemer, "Glucocorticosteroid inhibition of intraocular proliferation after injury," *American Journal of Ophthalmology*, vol. 91, no. 2, pp. 184–189, 1981.

[41] Y. Tano, D. Chandler, and R. Machemer, "Treatment of intraocular proliferation with intravitreal injection of triamcinolone acetonide," *American Journal of Ophthalmology*, vol. 90, no. 6, pp. 810–816, 1980.

[42] C. N. Meyer, "Current treatment approaches in diabetic macular edema," *Ophthalmologica*, vol. 221, no. 2, pp. 118–131, 2007.

[43] A. Ueno, H. Enaida, Y. Hata et al., "Long-term clinical outcomes and therapeutic benefits of triamcinolone-assisted pars plana vitrectomy for proliferative vitreoretinopathy: a case study," *European Journal of Ophthalmology*, vol. 17, no. 3, pp. 392–398, 2007.

[44] A. Mańkowska, R. Rejdak, K. Nowomiejska, and Z. Zagórski, "Efficacy of intravitreal triamcinolone acetonide in the visualization of the vitreous during pars plana vitrectomy," *Klinika Oczna*, vol. 108, no. 1-3, pp. 24–27, 2006.

[45] D. M. Brown, P. K. Kaiser, M. Michels et al., "Ranibizumab versus verteporfin for neovascular age-related macular degen-

eration," *The New England Journal of Medicine*, vol. 355, no. 14, pp. 1432–1444, 2006.

[46] X. Sun and X. Lu, "Profile of conbercept in the treatment of neovascular age-related macular degeneration," *Drug Design, Development and Therapy*, vol. 9, pp. 2311–2320, 2015.

[47] CATT Research Group, D. F. Martin, M. G. Maguire et al., "Ranibizumab and bevacizumab for neovascular age-related macular degeneration," *The New England Journal of Medicine*, vol. 364, no. 20, pp. 1897–1908, 2011.

[48] P. A. Campochiaro, J. S. Heier, L. Feiner et al., "Ranibizumab for macular edema following branch retinal vein occlusion: six-month primary end point results of a phase III study," *Ophthalmology*, vol. 117, no. 6, pp. 1102–1112.e1, 2010.

[49] M. Michaelides, A. Kaines, R. D. Hamilton et al., "A prospective randomized trial of intravitreal *bevacizumab* or *laser therapy* in the management of diabetic macular edema (BOLT study): 12-month data: report 2," *Ophthalmology*, vol. 117, no. 6, pp. 1078–1086.e2, 2010.

[50] J. G. Gross and A. R. Glassman, "A Novel Treatment for Proliferative Diabetic Retinopathy: Anti-Vascular Endothelial Growth Factor Therapy," *JAMA Ophthalmology*, vol. 134, no. 1, pp. 13-14, 2016.

[51] G. A. Peyman, *Vitreoretinal Surgical Techniques*, MartinDunitz, London, UK, 2001.

[52] P. Tangjai, P. Chingchana, and R. Taweerutchana, "Glycated haemoglobin and diabetic retinopathy in type 2 diabetic patients in HRH Princess Maha Chakri Sirindhorn Medical Center," *Journal of the Medical Association of Thailand*, vol. 98, pp. 135–42m, 2015.

[53] C. A. Moreira Jr, L. A. Arana, and R. J. Zago, "Long-term results of repeated anti-vascular endothelial growth factor therapy in eyes with retinal pigment epithelial tears," *Retina*, vol. 33, no. 2, pp. 277–281, 2013.

[54] E. T. Cunningham Jr, L. Feiner, C. Chung, L. Tuomi, and J. S. Ehrlich, "Incidence of retinal pigment epithelial tears after intravitreal ranibizumab injection for neovascular age-related macular degeneration," *Ophthalmology*, vol. 118, no. 12, pp. 2447–2452, 2011.

3

Internal Limiting Membrane Flaps for Coexistent Macular Hole and Retinal Detachment in Eyes with Proliferative Diabetic Retinopathy

San-Ni Chen[1,2,3] and Chung-May Yang[4,5]

[1]*Department of Ophthalmology, Changhua Christian Hospital, Changhua, Taiwan*
[2]*Department of Optometry, Da-Yeh University, Changhua, Taiwan*
[3]*College of Medicine, Chung-Shan Medical University, Taichung, Taiwan*
[4]*Department of Ophthalmology, National Taiwan University Hospital, Taipei, Taiwan*
[5]*College of Medicine, National Taiwan University, Taipei, Taiwan*

Correspondence should be addressed to Chung-May Yang; chungmay@ntu.edu.tw

Academic Editor: Elad Moisseiev

Purpose. To evaluate logical surgical approaches to closing macular holes in eyes with proliferative diabetic retinopathy with retinal detachment. *Methods.* Retrospective, interventional case series. *Results.* 10 eyes in 10 patients were included in this study. The inverted internal limiting membrane (ILM) flap technique was used in 2 eyes, while inverted ILM insertion was used in 5 eyes, and free ILM flaps in 3 eyes. Closed macular holes and retinal reattachment were observed in all eyes. Best corrected visual acuity improved from 1.33 ± 0.39 preoperatively to 1.02 ± 0.36 postoperatively ($p = 0.03$). *Conclusion.* Various surgical approaches utilized in managing macular holes may effectively close macular holes and reattach retinas. This trial is registered with NCT 03618498.

1. Introduction

Macular holes (MH) associated with retinal detachment (RD) most commonly occur in eyes with high myopia. Conventional surgery with vitrectomy and complete internal limiting membrane (ILM) peeling results in an unsatisfactory macular closure rate [1]. Recently, several surgical techniques have been developed, including the use of epiretinal ILM flap covering the hole [2, 3]; ILM flap insertion into the hole, with or without the adjunct of blood clot and viscoelastic agents [4–6]; or even free ILM flaps [7]. High MH closure rates can be achieved. Other than high myopia, MH with RD may appear in several other conditions, such as severe vitreomacular traction, proliferative diabetic retinopathy (PDR) [8, 9], or complicated rhegmatogenous retinal detachment (RRD) from peripheral breaks [10–12].

In eyes of PDR, the combination of MH and RD usually signifies severe and complex vitreoretinal traction; thus, the closure rate of MH after conventional ILM peeling surgery may, as a consequence, also be less satisfactory [8, 9]. Thus, in this retrospective study, we aim to study whether using various techniques including epiretinal ILM flap, ILM insertion, or free ILM flap may effectively close MHs and reattach retinas where MH coexists with RD in PDR eyes.

2. Materials and Methods

From September 2014 to January 2018, clinical charts were reviewed of patients with PDR suffering from MH with RD who had been treated with vitrectomy combined with inverted epiretinal ILM flap, inverted ILM flap insertion technique, or free ILM flaps. Two experienced surgeons (SN Chen and CM Yang, from Changhua Christian Hospital and

National Taiwan University Hospital, respectively) performed the operations. The study was approved by the ethics committees and research boards of the two hospitals. The severity of RD was separated into 3 types: within the arcade; beyond the arcade but within the equator; and beyond the equator. Active fibrovascular proliferation (FVP) was defined as FVP containing visible neovascularization tissue or associated with any degree of VH; otherwise, it was regarded as "mainly fibrotic." The extent of FVP was separated into 4 grades based on the severity of vitreoretinal adhesion as previously described [13]: multiple-point adhesions with or without 1 site plaque-like broad adhesion (Grade 1); broad adhesions in more than 1 but fewer than 3 sites, located posterior to the equator (Grade 2); broad adhesions in more than 3 sites, located posterior to the equator or extending beyond the equator within 1 quadrant (Grade 3); and broad adhesions extending beyond the equator into more than 1 quadrant (Grade 4). Distribution of fibrous tissue was separated into 2 types: fibrous tissue along the arcade and fibrous tissue along the arcade and other areas.

Each patient underwent thorough ophthalmological examinations before and after surgery. The patients' demographic data, records of ophthalmological examinations, and surgical procedures were collected, including best corrected visual acuity (BCVA) before and after operation, fundus changes, presence or absence of proliferative vitreoretinopathy, and MH repairing techniques. The macular structure and presence of vertical vitreomacular traction were evaluated via optical coherence tomography, both pre- and postoperatively (Stratus OCT or Cirrus OCT; Carl Zeiss Meditec, Inc, Dublin, CA, or RTVue Premier; Optovue, Inc, Fremont, CA). All patients had a follow-up duration of more than 3 months following reattachment surgery.

2.1. Surgical Techniques. Standard 3-port 23- or 25-gauge pars plana vitrectomy was performed. After core vitrectomy, anterior-posterior-oriented traction and all fibrovascular tissues were removed as thoroughly as possible. Any epiretinal membrane causing fixed retinal folds was removed using forceps. The peripheral vitreous was detached as far anteriorly as could be safely done. A 25-gauge blunt-tipped needle connected with a syringe containing Viscoat® (Alcon laboratories, Fort Worth, TX) was placed within the macular hole, just below the level of the macular hole. A small amount of Viscoat® was injected into and around the hole. An ICG solution (25 mg ICG in 15 ml 5% glucose-water solution, final concentration = 1.7 mg/ml) was then carefully applied around the macular hole within the arcade. Excessive ICG was immediately removed via suction. ILM at the parafoveal area was peeled in a circular fashion. Care was taken not to peel the ILM flap across the hole edge. If possible, at least 1.5 to 2 times the disc area of partially detached ILM around the hole was left in place, with the central part remaining attached to the edge of the hole. Further anterior ILM peeling was performed up to the arcade along with the overlying epiretinal membrane (ERM). The pieces of ILM flap removed were saved in a balanced salt solution-soaked sponge for possible later use. The peripheral retina was then examined for possible breaks. Using microforceps, the ILM flap anchoring on the hole edge was inverted and used to cover the hole. If possible, a large semicircular flap (about 180 degrees and 2 disc diameters in size) was created superiorly as previously described [3]. Otherwise, temporal side ILM flap was used. However, if the risk of the ILM flipping back was judged to be high, ILM insertion instead of ILM hole coverage was adopted [5]. If the size of the ILM flaps was judged inadequate, the double ILM insertion technique was used [6], done by adding a piece of previously obtained free ILM flap on top of the inverted ILM tissue until it was securely in place. If, however, the ILM flaps around the hole edge were difficult to create, or ILM tissue adjacent to the hole had been torn away inadvertently or along with ERM, 2 to 3 pieces of free ILM flap were inserted sequentially into the hole instead after copious Viscoat® agent was injected in and around the MH [7]. Fluid-air exchange (FAX) up to the detached margin was performed for localized RD within the arcade. For RD extending to or beyond the equator, a drainage retinotomy was made with the vitreous cutter at the temporal upper detached retina for internal drainage and fluid-air exchange. No complete fluid-air exchange was intended, to avoid disturbance of the inserted ILM flaps. Laser photocoagulation was done around the iatrogenic break. Finally, the air was replaced with a 20% C_3F_8 infusion or silicon oil into the vitreous cavity. Patients were kept in a facedown position overnight and were allowed to take any position except supine for approximately one week.

2.2. Statistics. The decimal visual acuity was converted to logarithm of a minimal angle of resolution (logMar) for visual acuity (VA). The difference in logMar VA before and after operation was calculated via the Wilcoxon signed-rank test.

3. Results

There were 10 eyes (M : F = 5 : 5, age: 51.30 ± 10.58 years) included in this study. The demographic data are listed in Table 1. In the 10 eyes, 3 had active FVP and 7 were mainly fibrotic. Minor vitreous hemorrhage which only minimally obscured the posterior fundus view was present in 2 of the 3 eyes with active FVP (cases 4 and 5). All eyes had previous panretinal photocoagulation. Intravitreal injection of bevacizumab 1.25 mg three days before operation was performed in cases of active FVP (cases 3–5). The severity of FVP was grade 2 in the majority. FVP was noted along the arcade in all cases; 4 of the 10 eyes also had ERM across the macula noted. One post-SO removal case also had thickened ERM on the temporal upper and temporal lower arcade. Severity of fibrovascular traction and extent of retinal detachment are listed in Table 1. Only 1 eye had a bullous characteristic (Case 1). OCT showed cystic changes at the MH margin in 9 eyes. Vitreomacular traction on the macular hole was noted in 8 eyes (Figure 1). The average size of MH was 406.50 ± 223.28 microns. Iatrogenic retinal breaks encountered while dissecting FVP occurred in 2 of the 10 eyes, without affecting the final results. The inverted

Table 1: Demographic data of patients.

Case number	Age/sex/eye	MH size	Active/fibrotic	Severity	Distribution	RD extent	Initial	Final	F/U duration	MH closure	Procedure
1	56/M/L	500	F	1	1	3	ND/50 cm	0.03	5M	+	2
2	52/F/R	500	F	2	2	2	0.1	0.05	15M	+	2
3	49/M/R	480	A	1	1	1	0.05	0.05	12M	+	2
4	33/M/R	200	A	2	2	2	0.04	0.25	12M	+	2
5	52/F/L	200	A	3	2	2	0.05	0.05	16M	+	2
6	71/F/R	900	F	1	1	1	0.1	0.1	10M	+	3
7	49/F/L	200	F	2	1	1	0.1	0.2	6M	+	3
8	63/M/L	200	F	2	2	2	0.01	0.05	5M	+	3
9	42/F/L	510	F	2	2	2	0.05	0.2	18M	+	1
10	46/M/L	375	F	2	2	1	0.1	0.3	5M	+	1

BCVA: best corrected decimal visual acuity; F/U: follow-up; MH: macular hole; M: male; F: female; FVP: fibrovascular proliferation; ERM: epiretinal membrane; RD: retinal detachment; L: left; R: right; ND: number of digits. Procedure: (1) inverted internal limiting membrane (ILM) flaps covering macular hole; (2) inverted ILM flaps insertion; (3) free ILM flaps insertion. Severity scale of FVP: Grade 1: multiple-point adhesions with or without 1 site plaque-like broad adhesion; Grade 2: broad adhesions in more than 1 but fewer than 3 sites, located posterior to the equator; Grade 3: broad adhesions in more than 3 sites, located posterior to the equator or extending beyond the equator within 1 quadrant; Grade 4: broad adhesions extending beyond the equator for more than 1 quadrant. Distribution of fibrous tissue: (1) arcade; (2) arcade and other area. RD extent: extent of retinal detachment—(1) within the arcade; (2) beyond the arcade, within the equator; (3) beyond the equator.

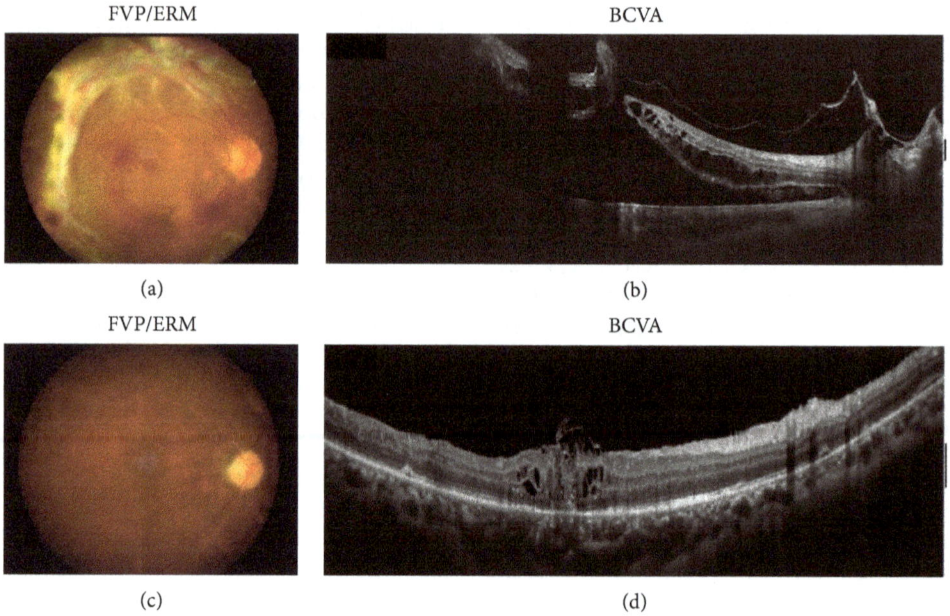

Figure 1: A 33-year-old man with proliferative diabetic retinopathy and active fibrovascular proliferation (case 4) had progressive loss of vision in the right eye. Preoperative fundus (a) and horizontal OCT scan images (b), showing retinal detachment and macular hole. After vitrectomy, internal limiting membrane insertion, air-fluid exchange, and gas tamponade, postoperative fundus (c) and horizontal OCT scan images (d).

epiretinal ILM flap technique was used in 2 cases; the inverted ILM flap insertion technique (including the double ILM flap technique; see Surgical Techniques) was used in 5 cases (Figure 1); and free ILM flap insertion was used in 3 cases. 20% C_3F_8 was infused in 9 eyes and silicon oil in 1 eye as a tamponade at the end of surgery. All eyes had retina reattachment and type 1 MH closure after 1 operation. None of the cases had recurrent vitreous hemorrhage noted during the follow-up period. Demographic data are shown in Figure 1. The best corrected logMar VA improved from 1.33 $\pm$ 0.39 preoperatively to 1.02 $\pm$ 0.36 postoperatively ($p = 0.03$, Wilcoxon signed-rank test).

4. Discussion

Multiple traction forces, such as posterior bulging, ERM and ILM tangential traction, or posterior hyaloid oblique traction, are involved in MH with RD in highly myopic eyes. Similarly, multidirectional forces and strong vitreomacular adhesion are required to produce MH with RD in cases of PDR. However, there are some differences in the pathogenesis of MH formation between MH associated with RD in HM and coexisting MH with RD in PDR. In HM, RD generally develops secondary to MH formation. Even after cortical vitreous stripping and ILM peeling, the retinal surface is often insufficient to meet the choroid surface area and allows the hole to close. In contrast, in coexisting MHs with RD in PDR, a long-term vitreomacular traction from VMT or a tangential traction from fibrovascular tissue predisposes MH formation [8, 9] and secondary retinal detachment. In our cases of PDR, the clinical findings suggest that, to induce MH and RD in PDR, the major factors may not be the severity of FVP but the distribution of FVP/fibrotic tissue. All our cases had fibrous tissue distributed at the arcade. The traction force around the arcade that exerts oblique traction on the posterior macula, in addition to the adherent epiretinal membrane usually found in such conditions, may be the primary force that induces RD when an MH forms. These changes create multidirectional traction and testify to the complexity of vitreoretinal relationships.

Although the pathogenesis of MH formation and RD development may be different in highly myopic and PDR patients, both severe traction and tissue degeneration of the fovea are present in both types of cases; thus, a lower rate of MH closure than with idiopathic MH cases is expected after surgical repair with the traditional techniques of membrane peeling and ILM peeling [1, 8]. Uemoto et al. have reported that after ILM peeling, MHs closed in 72.7% of highly myopic eyes with MH-related RD. Yeh et al. have reported that, after release of fibrovascular tissue with or without ILM peeling, MHs were closed in 82.6% of eyes with PDR-related MH [8]. Whether the MH in a specific case will successfully close after conventional surgery, however, has not been predictable. Traction and relative ischemic status predispose toward tissue degeneration of the macula. When severe, complex, long-standing traction and the resultant tissue degeneration are present, macular tissue around the hole might lose its ability to achieve hole closure even after traction force had been released. We postulate the above reasoning as one of the major causes for the unsatisfactory closure rate. In the current study, we offered ILM tissue within or above the macular holes as a bridging tissue in our cases of PDR, as what has recently been adopted in macular holes with high myopia. This technique has proven to be effective in improving the unpredictable MH closure results in coexistent macular hole and retinal detachment in eyes with PDR.

In this series, the initial choice to close the macular hole was always the inverted epiretinal ILM flap technique because this approach interferes least with the photoreceptor regeneration and best avoids possible dye toxicity on the retinal pigment epithelial cells after surgery. Inverted ILM flap insertion or free flaps were used when the size and the integrity of the ILM flap were judged insufficient for adequate MH coverage. When even the ILM insertion, including the addition of a free ILM flap, could not be done, multiple ILM flaps were used. The latter technique did not require a meticulous fovea-spared ILM peeling and was best suited to small MHs [7].

In our case series, only two had inverted epiretinal ILM flaps; others had either inverted ILM insertion (5 cases) or free ILM flaps (3 cases). Because complex traction condition existed in the PDR cases, with multilayered ERM adhered and exerting vertical and/or horizontal traction on the macula, adequately large ILM tissue to cover the MH could not be consistently obtained. Thus, the other techniques were chosen for more secure ILM positioning. Indeed, all 10 of our cases had MH closure with reattached retina.

In our series, only 3 eyes with active fibrovascular proliferation had preoperative intravitreal injection of antivascular endothelial growth factors (anti-VEGFs). Although pretreatment with anti-VEGF agents may reduce bleeding tendency during the operation, it may also aggravate the tractional force of the fibrovascular tissue, and thus it should be judiciously used in eyes with fibrous components.

In this study, we showed that all eyes had type 1 macular hole closure and retina reattachment. Statistically improved visual acuity was also noted. However, the final BCVA was still far less than that observed with idiopathic macular holes. The possible reasons for the limited visual improvement after hole closure may be predisposed disease status, including macular ischemia, cystoid changes secondary to microvascular anomalies in PDR, or schisis changes secondary to long-term traction from the FVP, which irreversibly damage the foveal structure. ICG toxicity to the photoreceptors and the retinal pigment epithelium may also be contributing factors. The limitations of this study are the small group of patients, and the lack of a control group. A larger case number with a proper control study is necessary to clarify whether the closure rate is higher with our present techniques, risk factors for MH closure, and whether closure of macular hole helps further improvement of VA in this difficult group of patients.

Conflicts of Interest

There are no conflicts of interest in connection with this work.

References

[1] R. Uemoto, S. Yamamoto, I. Tsukahara, and S. Takeuchi, “Efficacy of internal limiting membrane removal for retinal detachments resulting from a myopic macular hole,” *Retina*, vol. 24, no. 4, pp. 560–566, 2004.

[2] S. Kuriyama, H. Hayashi, Y. Jingami, N. Kuramoto, J. Akita, and M. Matsumoto, “Efficacy of inverted internal limiting membrane flap technique for the treatment of macular hole in high myopia,” *American Journal of Ophthalmology*, vol. 156, no. 1, pp. 125–131, 2013.

[3] S. N. Chen, “Large semicircular inverted internal limiting membrane flap in the treatment of macular hole in high myopia,” *Graefe’s Archive for Clinical and Experimental Ophthalmology*, vol. 255, no. 12, pp. 2337–2345, 2017.

[4] C. C. Lai, Y. P. Chen, N. K. Wang et al., “Vitrectomy with internal limiting membrane repositioning and autologous blood for macular hole retinal detachment in highly myopic eyes,” *Ophthalmology*, vol. 122, no. 9, pp. 1889–1898, 2015.

[5] S. N. Chen and C. M. Yang, "Inverted internal limiting membrane insertion for macular hole associated retinal detachment in high myopia," *American Journal of Ophthalmology*, vol. 162, pp. 99–106, 2016.

[6] S. N. Chen and C. M. Yang, "Double internal limiting membrane insertion for macular hole-associated retinal detachment," *Journal of Ophthalmology*, vol. 2015, Article ID 3236516, 5 pages, 2017.

[7] S. N. Chen, Y. T. Hsieh, and C. M. Yang, "Multiple free internal limiting membrane flaps insertion in the treatment of macular hole associated retinal detachment in high myopia," *Ophthalmologica*, vol. 240, no. 3, pp. 143–149, 2018.

[8] P. T. Yeh, C. K. Cheng, M. S. Chen, C. H. Yang, and C. M. Yang, "Macular hole in proliferative diabetic retinopathy with fibrovascular proliferation," *Retina*, vol. 29, no. 3, pp. 355–361, 2009.

[9] T. Amemiya and H. Yoshida, "Macular hole in diabetic maculopathy," *Ophthalmologica*, vol. 177, no. 4, pp. 188–191, 1987.

[10] D. Shukla, A. Rajendran, R. Maheshwari, and K. B. Naresh, "Early closure of macular hole secondary to rhegmatogenous retinal detachment with internal limiting membrane peeling," *Ophthalmic Surgery, Lasers, and Imaging*, vol. 39, no. 1, pp. 81–85, 2008.

[11] P. Riordan-Eva and A. H. Chignell, "Full thickness macular breaks in rhegmatogenous retinal detachment with peripheral retinal breaks," *British Journal of Ophthalmology*, vol. 76, no. 6, pp. 346–348, 1992.

[12] A. M. O'Driscoll, R. R. Goble, and G. R. Kirkby, "Vitrectomy for retinal detachments with both peripheral retinal breaks and macular holes. An assessment of outcome and the status of the macular hole," *Retina*, vol. 21, no. 3, pp. 221–225, 2001.

[13] C. M. Yang, P. T. Yeh, C. H. Yang, and M. S. Chen, "Bevacizumab pretreatment and long-acting gas infusion on vitreous clear-up after diabetic vitrectomy," *American Journal of Ophthalmology*, vol. 146, no. 2, pp. 211–217, 2008.

4

Patient and Surgeon Satisfaction Levels after using an Acrylic, Hydrophobic, Monofocal IOL and the Malyugin Ring in Pseudoexfoliation Syndrome Patients

Andreas F. Borkenstein and Eva-Maria Borkenstein

Private Practice, Privatklinik der Kreuzschwestern Graz, Kreuzgasse 35, 8010-Graz, Austria

Correspondence should be addressed to Andreas F. Borkenstein; crustalith@gmx.at

Academic Editor: Van C. Lansingh

Purpose. The purpose of this prospective analysis was to evaluate the patient and surgeon satisfaction levels after using a fully preloaded acrylic, hydrophobic, monofocal "premium" IOL in pseudoexfoliation syndrome. *Materials and Methods.* 42 eyes of twenty-eight patients with progressed cataract formation and pseudoexfoliation syndrome (PXF) or pseudoexfoliation glaucoma and best corrected distance visual acuity (BCDVA) between 0.30–1.00 logMAR were enrolled. After a detailed preexamination, they underwent phacoemulsification and implantation of the acrylic, hydrophobic, heparin-coated, single-piece, monofocal intraocular lens (CT LUCIA 601P, Zeiss, Germany) with 360° square edge and ultraclear purity aspheric ZO optic. We evaluated the visual performance of the IOL and the patient satisfaction. We also evaluated the intraoperative handling of the injector and the behavior of the IOL in these complicated cases (PXF). *Results.* The BCDVA increased from mean 0.48 logMAR (range 0.30–1.00 logMAR) preoperatively to -0.05 ± 0.13 logMAR postoperatively. The mean IOL power was 23.5 D (range 16.5–27.5 D). The target refraction using the Haigis formula within ±0.5 D was reached by 92.9% ($n = 39$) and by 100% ($n = 42$) within 1.0 D of all cases, respectively. Patient satisfaction was very high, and no halos or glare were reported in any case. The fully preloaded injector system enabled an easy IOL preparation and safe implantation. *Conclusion.* Our results show that the implantation of the fully preloaded CT LUCIA 601P (Zeiss, Germany) is safe and enhances OR workflow in complicated cases as pseudoexfoliation. In these cases, an adapted approach (special preoperative, intraoperative, and postoperative regime) with considering possible complications is necessary to achieve best outcomes.

1. Introduction

The pseudoexfoliation syndrome (PXF) was first described in 1917 by the Finnish ophthalmology resident Lindberg. Lindberg modified a Zeiss microscope and constructed a slit lamp on his own because slit lamps were not commercially available at that time. He conducted a study of more than 200 patients and recorded his findings with skilful hand drawings (Figures 1 and 2), and his conclusions still stand valid today [1]. Unfortunately, Lindberg was not cited in subsequent research projects by his colleagues as he was a modest gentleman who did not complain [2].

The prevalence of PXF increases with age; it is seldom seen before the age of 50. Pseudoexfoliation syndrome has been reported from all over the world, although prevalence varies between countries and even between local geographical areas. Prevalence rates may depend on the diagnostic criteria used and the age group of the population studied [3]. PXF syndrome and PXF glaucoma, which must be promptly detected to avoid surgical complications, are frequent in patients scheduled for cataract surgery. Regarding a study of consecutive cases, in 25.2% of patients, exfoliation was detected in the preoperative examination [4].

Cataract surgery in eyes with pseudoexfoliation syndrome is associated with higher rates of complications. Therefore, accurate preoperative precautions and exact intraoperative care are required to ensure a successful and safe surgery with the best postoperative outcomes [5, 6].

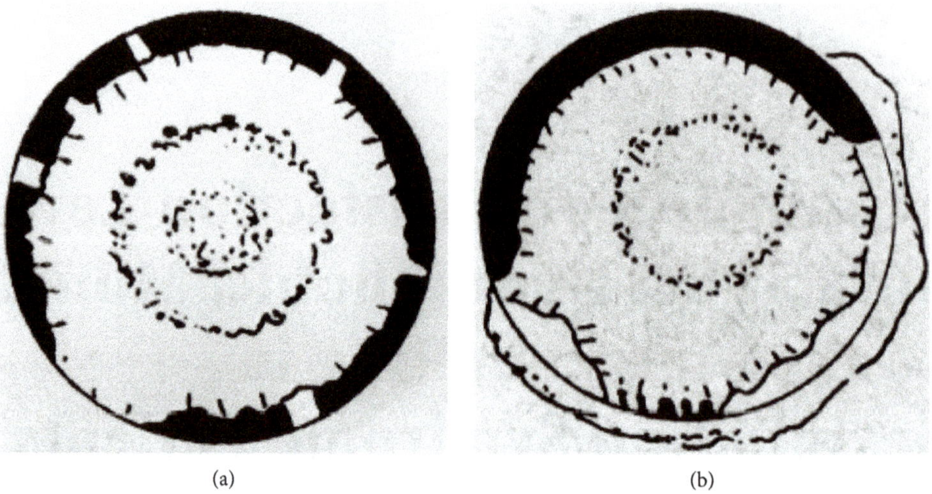

FIGURE 1: Hand drawings of Lindberg: The central disc and peripheral band are illustrated as well as the degeneration of the pupillary border.

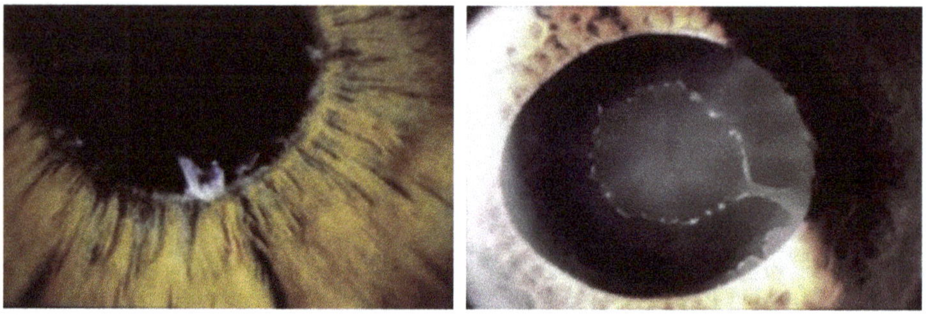

FIGURE 2: Pseudoexfoliation syndrome with grey-whitish flakes and PXF disc.

2. Materials and Methods

In this prospective analysis, 42 eyes with progressed cataract formation (senile cataract) and a best corrected distance visual acuity (BCDVA) between 0.30 and 1.00 logMAR were enrolled. The main inclusion criteria was an existing and detectable pseudoexfoliation syndrome with its characteristic findings in the anterior segment which includes the typical PXF disc with its fluffy deposits on the anterior lens capsule, the transillumination defect on the pupillary borders, and the poor pupillary dilation (maximum pupil diameter 3.5 mm in spite of medical-induced mydriasis). The intraoperative application of the 6.25 mm Malyugin ring to enlarge the pupil was mandatory, which is another inclusion criterion. 27 eyes were diagnosed with pseudoexfoliation glaucoma, high intraocular pressure (IOP) regulated with topical glaucoma medication, and pathognomonic glaucoma-associated defects in optic nerve disc with visual field loss. The cloudy lenses were graded with the "LOCS III" (Lens Opacities Classification System) in nuclear, cortical, and subcapsular opacities. Exclusion criteria included other severe eye pathologies such as corneal dystrophy, posttraumatic corneal wound scar, diabetic proliferative retinopathy, age-related macular degeneration, or retinal dystrophy. In all cases, phacoemulsification and removing of the cloudy lens were performed with the same phacomachine (Abbott Signature Whitestar) by the same surgeon in the same facility. Repeated measurements were performed preoperatively to avoid or minimize complications of cataract extraction and get the best outcomes in these PXF eyes. An increased awareness was required because of the problem this disorder may induce. Biometry was performed with the IOLMaster 500 (Zeiss, Germany) twice to increase accuracy even in hard nuclear or dense subcapsular cataracts. In 4 cases, ultrasound measurement of the axial length (Axis) was necessary. In all cases, Scheimpflug measurement with the Pentacam AXL (Oculus, Germany) for exact evaluation of the corneal topography, keratometry, and pachymetry was performed. Objective measurements of the refractive error including autorefraction and IOP measurements with Goldmann tonometry were performed at least 3 times (1–12 weeks) before surgery. Perimetry results (visual field) were meaningful and utilizable in just 8 cases, and in all the other cases, the dense cataract had already blocked too much light and the visual acuity was worse. A special preoperative procedure of eye drops was applied: 3 days prior to surgery, patients received bromfenac (NSAID) eye drops (2 times daily) and cyclopentolate eye drops 3 hours prior to surgery. Tetracaine eye drops (4x) as topical anesthesia were instilled 30 minutes before surgery, and disinfecting eye drops were used several times. In all cases, the fully preloaded, acrylic, hydrophobic, heparin-coated, single-piece, monofocal, "premium IOL"-CT LUCIA 601P (Zeiss, Germany) was implanted without any complications (Figure 3). The lens had an overall diameter of 13 mm (C-loop with 5° angulation) and a 360° square edge design with clear, aspheric ZO optic. Additionally, in all cases, the 6.25 mm "Malyugin ring" was inserted through the main incision and placed to provide a large and round pupil. Control examinations including visual tests for BCDVA, slit lamp exam, IOP measurement, and Scheimpflug measurement for effective lens position were performed after 1, 4, 7, 28, and 84 days. In addition, imaging (photograph documentation) of the IOL and optical coherence tomography (OCT) of the macula were done one week and three months after surgery. In all cases, the postoperative medication included acetazolamide 250 mg tablets 1 × 1 for the first 2 days, bromfenac eye drops (2 weeks), and betamethasone sodium phosphate eye drops for 4 weeks.

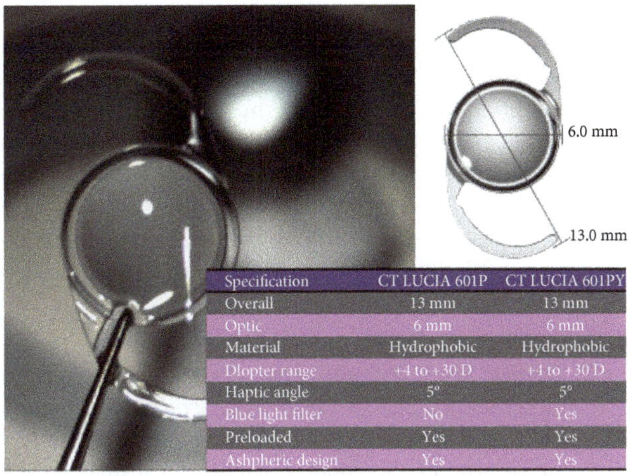

FIGURE 3: Specifications of the acrylic, hydrophobic CT LUCIA 601(P) (Zeiss, Germany).

3. Results

42 eyes of twenty-eight patients (19 female, 9 male) with dense cataracts and pseudoexfoliation syndrome were included. The mean age of the participants was 77.9 years ± 7.5 years. The cloudy lenses (cataracta senilis) were graded with the "LOCS III" (Lens Opacities Classification System) in 16 nuclear (8x NC5 and 8x NC6), 14 cortical (3x C3, 5x C4, and 6x C5), and 12 subcapsular posterior (5x P4 and 7x P5) lens opacities. The best corrected distance visual acuity (BCDVA) increased from mean 0.48 logMAR (range 0.30–1.00 logMAR) preoperatively to −0.05 ± 0.13 logMAR postoperatively. The mean IOL power was 23.5 D (range 16.5–27.5 D). The target refraction with Haigis formula was reached within ± 0.5 D by 92.9% (n = 39) and within 1.0 D by 100% (n = 42) of all cases, respectively. Patient satisfaction was very high, and no halos or glare were reported in any of the cases. The fully preloaded injector system (Zeiss, Germany) enabled an easy and safe IOL preparation and good OR workflow (Figure 4). The implantation of the CT LUCIA 601P was performed "wound-assisted" (just the tip of the nozzle goes in the corneal tunnel) through a 2.4 mm clear cornea incision. The insertion of the acrylic, hydrophobic, single-piece IOL was achieved, despite the small pupil and Malyugin ring without touching the iris or the ring directly into the capsular bag without further manipulation. The IOL-unfolding process was slow, controlled, analogue, and independent of the IOL power. The unfolding of the trailing haptic did not interfere with the Malyugin ring, and no "handshake phenomenon" (sticking of the haptics to the optic) was recognized. The desired lens orientation and positioning was achieved fast with very minimal capsular and zonular stress. No complications (n = 0) in terms of posterior capsule defects or (sub)luxation of the lens were experienced. Intraocular pressure (IOP) was independent from medications in pseudoexfoliation syndrome patients, and pseudoexfoliation glaucoma patients showed lower values after lens extraction with a mean decrease of 4 mmHg 3 months postoperatively. These findings showed a significant correlation to the anterior chamber depth measured with the Pentacam (mean 2.95 mm preoperative versus 4.08 mm postoperative values). The lens position image analysis of retroillumination photos of 40 eyes showed well-centered IOLs, and the effective lens position (ELP) did not change significantly over the postoperative course of 3 months. In two cases, an intense capsular phimosis (8 weeks after surgery) with "myopic shift effect" led to a slight displacement of the IOL in the direction of the anterior chamber with resulting myopia (−1.0 D). The slit lamp exam and retroillumination photo showed a clear acrylic optic with high purity without any glistenings.

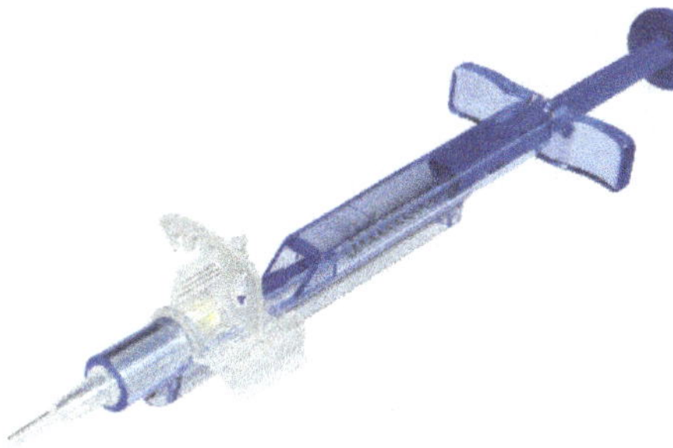

FIGURE 4: Fully preloaded injector.

4. Discussion

Pseudoexfoliation syndrome is a systemic, age-related disease and occurs worldwide, but the prevalence varies between different regions. PXF is a risk factor for both glaucoma (≈30%) and cataract formation. Moreover, several studies have verified that PXF is correlated with an increased risk of intraoperative and/or postoperative complications [7]. The deposition of extracellular fibers results in alterations of tissues in the anterior segment of the eye which makes cataract surgery potentially challenging [8]. Surgeons must be aware of numerous preoperative, intraoperative, and postoperative issues in managing the PXF eyes. For extensive surgical considerations in matters of the pathophysiology of PXF, the changes and their impact should include the following:

(1) A smaller pupil with posterior synechiae causes reduced visualization and complicates the procedure. NSAIDs can be given preoperatively to discourage intraoperative miosis. The application of

the Malyugin ring through the main incision (2.2 mm) is a very elegant and time-saving method to achieve a round, large pupil without damaging the iris sphincter and without the need of making extra paracentesis. Especially in the PXF eyes, the surgical procedure should be as gentle as possible. To enlarge the pupil and to separate the synechiae, cohesive viscoelastic devices (OVDs) can be used. The use of trypan blue for staining the anterior capsule can be very wise in cases of poor red-reflex in dense subcapsular cataracts.

(2) Zonular weakness and phacodonesis can make the capsulorhexis, phacoemulsification,irrigation/aspiration, and implantation of the IOL challenging. Depending on the severity of the zonular dialysis, a capsular tension ring (CTR) should be used in the intraoperative course as soon as possible to facilitate the situation.

(3) Less anterior capsule tension makes the capsulorhexis in the PXF eyes more difficult. The filling of the anterior chamber with OVD should be repeated, and the rhexis should be done with a sharp needle or forceps very slowly and carefully to generate as less pressure to the zonules as possible. The size and design of the rhexis is most important for good IOL centration because of potential postoperative shrinkage and phimosis in the PXF eyes.

(4) Phacoemulsification has to be performed with special respect for the weak zonules and the thinner posterior lens capsule. A chopping technique with low ultrasound energy and low irrigation/aspiration adjustments is recommended. The cortical removal is a crucial step in the PXF eyes. The "Hurricane I/A technique" allows a tangential vector resultant voltage on the zonules smaller than the conventional radial suction. In some cases, the "dry" removal of cortex with a cannula (stripping technique) is the best way to preserve zonular fibers.

(5) Several studies have confirmed that the acrylic, hydrophobic IOLs are the best choice in pseudoexfoliation syndrome. Considerations should include the diameter of the lens, the haptic design and IOL stability, the edges regarding the PCO rate, and the surface of the lens. There are studies with controversial results regarding the effect of a heparin coat, and its benefit has not been confirmed till now [9]. Further investigations have to be done. However, we are certain that the clarity and purity of the optic is most important. Any inclusions in the lens material such as glistenings can also lead to light scatter effects, halos, and glare. In the PXF eyes, the possibility of IOL exchange is limited because of the higher risk of surgical trauma to the tissues [10]. When we are afraid of the higher likelihood of postoperative decentration and tilt of the IOL (caused by phimosis or pseudophacodonesis), we should not select negative aspheric aberrated IOLs because if the optic position is not well aligned, other higher order aberrations (HOAs), such as coma, could occur and reduce contrast sensitivity and effect quality of vision.

(6) The implantation of the IOL should be as harmless as possible with a minimum of stress to the zonules, less manipulation in the anterior chamber, and fast orientation/centration of the IOL in the capsular bag [11]. Therefore, the right injector is also important. The ideal insertion of the IOL should be as harmless as possible regarding the weak zonules and altered capsular bag. Sometimes, it is advantageous to form a kind of "viscoshield" (combination of cohesive and dispersive OVD) in the capsular bag just before implantation. Hence, the posterior capsule is protected from the unfolding process of the leading haptic which is slower and more controllable for the surgeon. Any additional manipulation with instruments (spatula, Sinsky hooks, and so on) should be avoided. Moreover, especially in complicated cases, a good OR workflow can improve the atmosphere in the operating room and the mood of the surgeon and the scrub nurse subsequently. Best results can be achieved with careful and slow approach.

(7) It is well known that, in pseudoexfoliation, the intraocular pressure may rise up rapidly 2 hours after surgery. Persistent intraocular pressure elevations and persistent inflammation in the first postoperative period are very common [12]. Therefore, a special adapted postoperative regime is recommended. Rebound tonometry without topical anesthesia, which is fast, simple, safe, and reliable can be done either in the sitting or lying position. Intraocular pressure should be measured before discharge and the first morning after surgery.

(8) With the rising life expectancy, the zonules are finally lost from the epithelium and the bag with the IOL may loose into the vitreous. It was found that 6-7 years following cataract surgery, posterior chamber intraocular lenses were positioned lower in pseudoexfoliation syndrome than in control eyes [13]. Due to possible (sub)luxation of the lens, photodocumented slit lamp examinations should be performed carefully and more frequently. In this way, a prompt intervention can be initiated.

5. Conclusion

Pseudoexfoliation syndrome is a common disorder, and every cataract surgeon has to face the special challenges associated with it. Careful preoperative considerations and special intraoperative care to ensure safe surgery are necessary to get the best postoperative outcomes.

Our prospective analysis in cataract patients with pseudoexfoliation syndrome and dense cataracts showed that the implantation of the fully preloaded CT LUCIA 601P (Zeiss, Germany) is safe and enhances OR workflow in complicated cases. Postoperatively, no halos or glare were reported by the patients. We have not observed a single case of glistenings till now, and therefore, we fully recommend the CT LUCIA 601P in complicated cases, and we believe that the label of "premium" is appropriate.

Conflicts of Interest

The authors declare that they have no conflicts of interest.

References

[1] J. G. Lindberg, "Clinical investigations on depigmentation of the pupillary border and translucency of the iris in cases of senile cataract and normal eyes in elderly persons," *Acta Ophthalmologica*, vol. 190, pp. 1-96, 1998.

[2] A. Vogt, "Ein neues Spaltlampenbild des Pupillargebietes: Heilblauer Pupillarsaumfilz mit Häutchenbildung auf der Linsenvorderkapsel," *Klein Monatsbl Augenhk*, vol. 75, pp. 1–12, 1925.

[3] L. Drolsum, A. Ringvold, and B. Nicolaissen, "Cataract and glaucoma surgery in pseudoexfoliation syndrome: a review," *Acta Ophthalmologica Scandinavica*, vol. 85, no. 8, pp. 810–821, 2007.

[4] J. Hietanen, T. Kivelä, E. Vesti, and A. Tarkkanen, "Exfoliation syndrome in patients scheduled for cataract surgery," *Acta Ophthalmologica*, vol. 70, no. 4, pp. 440–446, 1992.

[5] G. O. Naumann, U. Schlötzer-Schrehardt, and M. Küchle, "Pseudoexfoliation syndrome for the comprehensive ophthalmologist: intraocular and systemic manifestations," *Ophthalmology*, vol. 105, no. 6, pp. 951–968, 1998.

[6] S. Kastelan, M. Tomic, R. Kordic, M. Kalauz, and J. Salopek-Rabatic, "Cataract surgery in eyes with pseudoexfoliation (PEX) syndrome," *Journal of Clinical & Experimental Ophthalmology*, vol. 2013, no. S1, p. 009, 2013.

[7] G. O. Naumann, "Exfoliation syndrome as a risk factor for vitreous loss in extra-capsular cataract surgery. Erlanger-Augenblätter Group," *Acta Ophthalmologica. Supplement*, vol. 184, pp. 129–131, 1988.

[8] C. Zetterström, G. Olivestedt, and A. Lundvall, "Exfoliation syndrome and extracapsular cataract extraction with implantation of posterior chamber lens," *Acta Ophthalmologica*, vol. 70, pp. 85–90, 1992.

[9] S. Maedel, N. Hirnschall, Y. A. Chen, and O. Findl, "Effect of heparin coating of a foldable intraocular lens on inflammation and capsular bag performance after cataract surgery," *Journal of Cataract & Refractive Surgery*, vol. 39, no. 12, pp. 1810–1817, 2013.

[10] G. U. Auffarth, K. Tsao, T. A. Wesendahl, A. Sugita, and D. J. Apple, "Centration and fixation of posterior chamber intraocular lenses in eyes with pseudoexfoliation syndrome: an analysis of explanted autopsy eyes," *Acta Ophthalmologica Scandinavica*, vol. 74, no. 5, pp. 463–467, 1996.

[11] D. J. Apple, M. Escobar-Gomez, B. Zaugg, G. Kleinmann, and A. F. Borkenstein, "Modern cataract surgery: unfinished business and unanswered questions," *Survey of Ophthalmology*, vol. 56, no. 6, pp. S3–S53, 2011.

[12] A. Turalba, T. Cakiner-Egilmez, A. R. Payal et al., "Outcomes after cataract surgery in eyes with pseudexfoliation: results from the Veterans Affairs Ophthalmic Surgery Outcomes Data Project," *Canadian Journal of Ophthalmology*, vol. 52, no. 1, pp. 61–68, 2017.

[13] A. Ostern, G. Sandvik, and L. Drolsum, "Positioning of the posterior intraocular lens in the long term following cataract surgery in eyes with and without pseudoexfoliation syndrome," *Acta Ophthalmologica*, vol. 92, no. 3, pp. 253–258, 2014.

5

Clinical and Genetic Features of Tubulointerstitial Nephritis and Uveitis Syndrome with Long-Term Follow-Up

Hiroaki Kanno,[1] Kyoko Ishida,[2] Wataru Yamada,[1] Ikumi Shiraki,[1] Hiroki Murase,[3] Yuka Yamagishi,[4] and Kiyofumi Mochizuki[1]

[1]Department of Ophthalmology, Gifu University Graduate School of Medicine, 1-1 Yanagido, Gifu-shi, Gifu 500-1194, Japan
[2]Department of Ophthalmology, Toho University Ohashi Medical Center, 2-17-6, Ohashi, Meguro-ku, Tokyo 153-8515, Japan
[3]Murase Eye Clinic, 17-1 Hanaike, Hagiwaracho, Gero-shi, Gifu 509-2515, Japan
[4]Department of Infection Control and Prevention, Aichi Medical University, 1-1 Karimata, Iwasaku, Nagakute-shi, Aichi 480-1195, Japan

Correspondence should be addressed to Kyoko Ishida; kyoko.ish@gmail.com

Academic Editor: Anna Nowinska

Purpose. To investigate the clinical manifestations, prognosis, and HLA-type of tubulointerstitial nephritis and uveitis syndrome (TINU) with long-term follow-up. *Methods.* Clinical data of five patients with TINU were retrospectively reviewed. *Results.* The mean age was 15.8 years. The mean follow-up periods were 54.0 months. The initial subjective symptoms were bulbar injection (100%), ocular pain (80%), and blurred vision (60%). The medical department that the patients visited first was ophthalmology in 4 (80%) cases. Urinalysis showed the characteristic increase of the $\beta 2$ microglobulin in all (100%) patients. Uveitis and nephritis were diagnosed within 1 week from each other. Although two showed recurrences, the topical and systemic steroid treatment with mean duration of 14.1 months brought the resolution of nephritis and uveitis in all patients. Recurrence-free periods ranged from 12 to 71 months. The final visual outcome was 20/20 or better in all cases. HLA-DR4 or the allele of DRB1 *04 was present in all (100%) patients. *Conclusions.* TINU should be considered in the differential diagnosis in young patients with uveitis of unknown origin and renal dysfunction. Urinary $\beta 2$ microglobulin level and HLA typing may help in the diagnosis of TINU. The prognosis for patients with TINU is generally good with steroid treatment.

1. Introduction

The tubulointerstitial nephritis and uveitis syndrome (TINU) is a specific form of intraocular inflammation (uveitis) combined with kidney disease that was first described in 1975 by Dobrin et al. [1] in two patients. It affects approximately 1-2% of the patients who visit uveitis clinics and, however, may represent up to a third of bilateral acute anterior uveitis in patients younger than 20 years old [2–6]. In a prospective multicenter epidemiological study of uveitis in Japan in 2009, TINU accounted only for 0.4% of the 2556 patients with uveitis [7]. Since TINU is considered relatively to be a rare disease, it is still unfamiliar to most ophthalmologists, pediatricians, or nephrologists [2, 4].

Generally, renal dysfunction in TINU is mild, and uveitis tends to recur [8, 9]. Patients younger than 20 years of age are more prone to chronic uveitis than the adult population [8]. Although the uveitis can relapse during and after therapy, long-term follow-up reports are few and lacking (The mean follow-up of 17.8 [10], 19.6 [11], 25.4 [5], and 54.8 months [12]).

The pathogenesis of TINU is still unknown. TINU has been reported to have an association with human leukocyte antigen (HLA), and HLA alleles have been implicated as susceptibility risk factors [8, 13–16]. However, the distribution of the HLA haplotypes varies considerably in Japan [3, 17].

We had 5 cases of TINU with a mean age of 15.8 years old and a mean follow-up of 54.0 months. TINU is a rare disease

[4]; however, it may be far more common than currently appreciated, especially in young patients whom mild renal disease does not become symptomatic and/or if diagnostic tests regarding renal involvement are not performed at the time of presentation. Moreover, no guidelines or recommendations for screening have been made to date in patients with interstitial nephritis [2]. In this report, we described clinical findings, long-term treatment outcomes, and the HLA haplotype in TINU cases.

2. Materials and Methods

This was a retrospective study of 5 patients with TINU who were examined in the Department of Ophthalmology of Gifu University Graduate School of Medicine or branch hospital, the Chuno Kosei Hospital between January 2001 and December 2015. The study followed the tenets of the Declaration of Helsinki and was approved by the affiliated hospitals' institutional review boards.

The diagnostic criteria for TINU were based on the reports of Mandeville et al. [8] and Mackensen and Billing [4]. Two patients with definite TINU and 3 with probable TINU were included in the study. Patients with sarcoidosis, Behçet's disease, Vogt-Koyanagi-Harada disease, Wegener's granulomatosis, and juvenile idiopathic arthritis-associated uveitis were excluded [2]. The following information was collected from their medical records with special attention given to the gender, age, initial manifestations, ocular findings, laboratory findings, treatment, visual prognosis, follow-up and treatment periods, and HLA typing.

3. Results

3.1. Basic Demographics (Table 1). There were 2 males (40%) and 3 females (60%). Patient age at the first visit to the hospital ranged from 13 years to 24 years (mean 15.8 years, median 14 years). The ages of four patients (80%) were between 13 and 15 years. One of the patients had diabetes, and the others did not have any systemic diseases.

3.2. Initial Signs and Symptoms (Table 1). The clinical department that the patients first visited for detailed examinations was ophthalmology in 4 (80%) and pediatrics in 1 (20%) patient. The median interval between the onset of subjective symptoms and the day that patients first visited the hospital was 7 days (range 7–90 days). All patients reported sudden onset of disease and initially had subjective ocular symptoms. The initial signs and symptoms were eye redness in 5 (100%), eye pain in 4 (80%), and a decrease in vision in 3 patients (60%). Both eyes were affected in all patients (100%). None had general symptoms, for example, fatigue, weight loss, fever, anorexia, abdominal or flank pain, and arthralgias at the onset of this disease [4]. However, two patients (cases 1 and 3) had been incidentally found to have proteinuria without any general symptoms by annual medical examinations at school or work, before the appearance of subjective eye symptoms.

3.3. Ocular Findings (Table 1). The initial visual acuity was better than 20/20 in 7 eyes (70%) and deteriorated to 12/20 in one eye (10%) of the patients. The initial intraocular pressure (IOP) was lower than 15 mmHg in all eyes. Anterior segment findings included conjunctival injection, iridocyclitis, and fine keratic precipitates in all patients (100%), but severe inflammation with more than 3+ cells (by the grading of inflammation described by the SUN working groups) [18] was not seen. Posterior synechiae were seen in one patient (20%, case 3). Posterior segment findings included cells in the anterior vitreous (40%, cases 3 and 4), peripheral vasculitis (20%, case 4), retinal exudates (40%, cases 3 and 4), and optic disk swelling (40%, cases 3 and 4).

3.4. Laboratory Findings (Table 1). Blood tests and urinalysis were administered to investigate the cause of uveitis. The blood counts and liver function were normal. The blood urea nitrogen (BUN) level was normal in all patients, and the serum creatinine level was slightly increased at 1.0 mg/dl (normal range 0.3 to 0.9 mg/dl) in 2 (40%) patients. Antinuclear antibody and rheumatoid factor were negative in all patients. The level of angiotensin-converting enzyme was normal, and hepatitis B and C antibodies were not detected. The estimated glomerular filtration rate (eGFR) was outside normal limits in 2 (40%) patients (normal range $60 \leq \text{eGFR} < 90\,\text{mL/mim/1.73m}^2$).

Urinalysis was positive for proteinuria in 3 patients (60%) and positive for glycosuria in 4 patients (80%). The urinal $\beta 2$ microglobulin was increased in all patients (100%), with values at least 10 times higher than upper normal limits (<230 μg/L). N-Acetylglucosaminidase (normal range <7.0 U/L) was increased in 3 patients (75%, not measured in one patient). Chest X-rays and computed tomography scans were normal in all cases.

3.5. Renal Biopsy, Classification, and Cause (Tables 1 and 2). All patients have consulted pediatricians or nephrologists after abnormal urinary test. Two patients (cases 1 and 3) had a renal biopsy, and the histopathological findings showed focal tubulointerstitial inflammatory infiltrations containing lymphocytes and nonspecific histiocytes. From these results, these 2 patients (cases 1 and 3) were confirmed to have definite TINU. The 3 other patients (cases 2, 4, and 5) were diagnosed with probable TINU. They did not receive a renal biopsy because pediatricians did not justify this invasive procedure for renal dysfunction level in each patient. The uveitis and nephritis were diagnosed within 1 week from each other in all patients.

TINU may be triggered by infectious disease and numerous medications, but the causes were unknown in all cases.

3.6. Treatment and Outcomes (Table 2). Depending on the severity of the disease conditions, topical corticosteroids were used to treat the anterior uveitis and systemic steroids were used for renal indications and/or the posterior uveitis. Two (40%, cases 2 and 5) of 5 patients without posterior uveitis were treated with topical or subconjunctival steroids alone, and the remaining 3 (60%, cases 1, 3, and 4) patients had the topical steroids combined with systemic corticosteroids prescribed by internists or pediatricians mainly for the tubulointerstitial nephritis. Initial

Table 1: Patient data 1.

Case	Type	Age	Gender	Side	Family history	Days between the first sign of uveitis and consultation (day)	Presenting symptoms	First sign uveitis or TIN	Uveitis			Visual acuity		IOP	Urinalysis		Blood test		Renal biopsy
									Anterior	Posterior		Initial	Last	Initial (mmHg)	Initial $\beta 2$-MG ($\mu g/L$)	Initial NAG (U/L)	Initial Cr (mg/dl)	Initial eGFR (l/min/ 1.73m^2)	
1	Definite	24	Female	Both	Grandmother: renal failure Brother: diabetes mellitus	9	Eye pain Eye redness	TIN (proteinuria)	+	–	R L	30/20 30/20	30/20 30/20	10 10	32700	20.6	1.00	57.6	+
2	Probable	14	Female	Both	Mother: glaucoma	7	Eye pain eye Redness decreased in vision	Uveitis	+	–	R L	14/20 30/20	30/20 30/20	9 9	2340	13.8	0.65	105.6	–
3	Definite	13	Female	Both	–	90	Eye redness Decreased in vision	TIN (proteinuria)	+ Posterior synechiae	Cells in the anterior vitreous, retinal exudates, and optic disk swelling	R L	18/20 12/20	30/20 24/20	11 11	2630	5.2	0.80	87.7	+
4	Probable	15	Male	Both	–	7	Eye pain Eye redness decreased in vision	Uveitis	+	Cells in the anterior vitreous, vasculitis, and optic disk swelling	R L	20/20 20/20	30/20 24/20	10 11	9600	19.5	1.00	89.2	–
5	Probable	13	Male	Both	–	2	Eye pain Eye redness	Uveitis	+	–	R L	30/20 30/20	30/20 30/20	13 11	3460	n.d.	0.80	n.d.	–

TIN: tubulointerstitial nephritis; IOP: intraocular pressure; R: right eye; L: left eye; n.d.: not done; $\beta 2$-MG: $\beta 2$ microglobulin; NAG: N-acetylglucosaminidase; Cr: creatinine; eGFR: estimated glomerular filtration rate.

dose of corticosteroid determined by internists or pediatrician ranged from 15 to 60 mg (15 mg for case 1, 30 mg for case 3, and 60 mg for case 4).

After a reduction of the steroid dosage, two patients (40%, cases 3 and 4) who had developed complicated posterior segment findings had a recurrence or exacerbation of the nephritis. Numbers of recurrence or exacerbation were none in 3 patients (cases 1, 2, and 5), twice in case 3, and once in case 4, respectively. Dose of systemic steroids was increased whenever a recurrence or exacerbation was observed. One patient (case 4) developed ocular hypertension during the topical steroid therapy. Average follow-up periods were 54.0 months (range 23–86 months). The mean number of attack per year was 1.6 in the 1st year and 0 thereafter. After the mean steroid treatment duration of 14.1 months (range 11–18 months), no recurrences were observed. The nephritis and uveitis were resolved in all patients, and the last recorded visual acuity was at least 20/20 in both eyes in all patients. Recurrence-free periods ranged from 12 to 71 months.

3.7. HLA Types (Table 2). The A locus had A24, 26, and 31 in 2 (40%) patients, and the DR locus had DR4 in 1 (20%) patient. The DRBI allele was DRB1*01 in 2 (40%) patients and DRB1*04 in 4 (80%) patients. The DQ was not tested in 3 patients and was DQ A1*01/B1*05 in 1 patient.

4. Discussion

Mandeville et al. [8] were the first to provide structured diagnostic criteria for TINU. Definite TINU syndrome is diagnosed when acute tubulointerstitial nephritis (TIN) is firmly established and the patient has bilateral anterior uveitis of sudden onset. Acute TIN is diagnosed either by histologic examination of renal biopsy specimens or by all three criteria as follows: (1) abnormal renal function (increased serum creatinine or decreased creatinine clearance); (2) abnormal urinalysis: increased $\beta 2$ microglobrin, low-grade proteinuria, presence of urinary eosinophils, pyuria or hematuria without infection, urinary white cell casts, or normoglycemic glucosuria; and (3) asystemic illness lasting ≥ 2 weeks, characterized by a combination of the following symptoms and laboratory findings: (a) signs and symptoms: fever, weight loss, anorexia, malaise, fatigue, rash, abdominal or flank pain, arthralgias, or myalgias; and (b) laboratory findings such as the evidence of anemia, abnormal liver function, eosinophilia, or a Westegren erythrocyte sedimentation rate > 40 mm/h. When two of the 3 criteria are fulfilled and typical uveitis is present, a diagnosis is probable for TINU. When one of the clinical findings meets the criteria and typical uveitis coexists, a diagnosis is possible for TINU [4]. We diagnosed TINU in our five patients using their criteria [4, 8]. Since the renal function does not change significantly between patients with and without treatment with prednisolone, a renal biopsy as an invasive diagnostic method remains controversial [12, 19]. According to Goda et al.'s data [3], all (100%) of the 12 patients with biopsy-proven TINU met criterion 2 for abnormal urinalysis (all patients had increased urinary $\beta 2$ microglobulin), but only 3 (25%) met criterion 1 (increased serum creatinine). Similar to them, all (100%) patients had increased urinary $\beta 2$ microglobulin, but 2 (40%) patients had increased serum creatinine in our cases. Mackensen et al. [20] reported that creatinine levels were more likely to be elevated in patients older than 40. Average age of patients in Goda et al.'s [3] and our study were 21.2 and 15.8, respectively. The sensitivity and specificity of elevated $\beta 2$ microglobulin were 87.5% and 70%, respectively, with positive predictive values and negative predictive values of urinary $\beta 2$ microglobulin greater than 1000 μg/L being 88 and 97%, respectively [21]. Takemura et al. [22] reported that the histologic grade of TIN was correlated with urinary $\beta 2$ microglobulin levels. Urinary $\beta 2$ microglobulin is a very sensitive marker for tubular damage, and its analysis is helpful in the diagnosis of TINU syndrome [4, 20, 21], especially when a renal biopsy is not indicated.

We had only 5 cases in 15 years at our medical institutions that provide medical support to a population of approximately 500,000. The median age of the onset of TINU is 15 years and is dominant in young girls in the Mandeville et al.'s review [8]. In our cohort, the median age was 14 years, and 3 (60%) of the 5 were girls. Ocular effects seen with uveitis are limited to the anterior chamber in 80% of cases; both eyes are affected in 77% of cases in Aguilar et al.'s review [6]. In our cases, anterior uveitis and bilateral uveitis were observed in 60% and 100%, respectively.Uveitis in TINU syndrome may cause severe complications in approximately 20% of patients, the most common being posterior synechia in about 70% of patients, optic disc swelling in 25%, cataract in 20%, and secondary glaucoma in 20% [8]. Complications including posterior synechiae, optic disk swelling, and secondary glaucoma were observed in two (40%) of five patients in our cohorts.

Uveitis may occur before the presentation of acute interstitial nephritis in approximately 20% of cases, but in most cases (65%), nephritis precedes uveitis, and in 15%, the two conditions occur simultaneously [8]. In our cohort, two (40%) patients were incidentally pointed to have proteinuria by annual medical examinations at school or work. However, eye redness was the most common subjective symptom before abnormal results of urea were seen upon precise testing at the hospital. Asystemic illness lasting ≥ 2 weeks was only observed in 33% in Goda et al.'s biopsy-proven Japanese TINU cases [3], and none in our cohorts. On the other hand, nineteen Finnish children with a biopsy-proven TIN had no ocular symptom in 50%, fatigue in 95%, and loss of appetite in 84% of patients [5]. Thus, most of the Japanese patients might initially present with ophthalmic findings or mild symptoms of TIN of which they are unaware. In fact, 4 of 5 patients visited an ophthalmologist first in our cohort. Thus, ophthalmologists play an important role in the initial diagnosis of patients with the TINU syndrome. TINU should be considered in the differential diagnosis especially in young patients with anterior uveitis of unknown origin.

In general, TINU responds to steroids. Topical corticosteroids were used to treat the anterior uveitis, and systemic steroids were used for renal indications and/or the posterior uveitis [2]. TIN can be resolved spontaneously and dialysis therapy is not usually required [23]. Steroid therapy (1 mg/

Table 2: Patient data 2.

Case	Type	Steroid			Secondary glaucoma	Recurrence	Last follow-up data			HLA				
		Topical	Subconjunctival	Systemic (initial dose) [dose after recurrence]			Blood test Cr (mg/dl)	Urinalysis $\beta 2$-MG (μg/L)	Follow-up (months)	HLA-A	HLA-B	HLA-C	HLA-DQ	HLA-DR
1	Definite	+	–	+ (15 mg)	–	–	0.69	n.d.	23	A24:02 A26:01 : 01	B40:02 : 01 B48:01 : 01	C03:04 : 01 C08:03 : 01	DQA1*03 : 01 : 01 DQA1*03 : 03 DQB1*03 : 02 : 01 DQB1*04 : 01 : 01	DRB1*04 : 05 DRB1*08 : 02 DPB1*02 : 02 DPB1*05 : 01
2	Probable	+	+	–	–	–	0.49	54	47	A31	B60/B55	–	–	DRB1*04 DRB1*14
3	Definite	+	–	+ (30 mg) [80 mg] [80 mg]	–	3 and 6 months	0.50	125	86	A2/A31	B7/B40	–	DQA1*01 DQA1*03 DQB1*05 DQB1*04	DRB1*01 DRB1*04
4	Probable	+	+	+ (60 mg) [20 mg]	+	3 months	0.70	94	69	A11	B54(22)/ B35	Cw1/Cw3	–	DR4
5	Probable	+	–	–	–	–	0.70	102	46	A24/A26	B7/B56	C0401 C0702	–	DRB1*01 DRB1*04

n.d.: not done; $\beta 2$-MG: $\beta 2$ microglobulin.

kg per day for 2-3 weeks with subsequent taper) is often administered when renal function impairment is severed or prolonged [22]. Few cases characterized by prolonged or recurrence of interstitial nephritis are treated with high-dose corticosteroids or steroid-sparing immunosuppressives [24]. Legendre et al. [10] reported that the median number of attack per patient per year was 1.0 (range 0.1–4.6) for eye symptoms and 0.8 (range 0.2–2.0) for renal symptoms in cases with French adult TINU. According to the review of 133 cases with TINU, 54% of patients developed recurrences, 17% were treated with topical steroids alone, 80% required systemic steroids, and 9% needed immunosuppressive treatment [8]. In our cases, recurrences or exacerbation were found in two (40%) cases; however, all cases were resolved with systemic steroids by the end of the observation periods. Since the inflammation in TINU syndrome can relapse during and after therapy, a long-term follow-up is required. The prolonged use of adequate treatment with the mean treatment duration of 29.5 months (range 13–40 months) improved the recurrence-free periods [12]. On the other hand, patients were needed on a low-dose topical treatment regime for months but this was hardly ever necessary for more than a year [4]. After the mean treatment duration of 14.1 months (range 11–18 months) in our cases, TINU had not relapsed for more than 12 months (range 12 to 71 months). Further investigations with longer follow-up periods are needed to clarify the optimum treatment regime.

The pathogenesis of TINU is not clear; however, it is thought to be the result of an autoimmune process that might involve cellular and humoral autoimmunity [13, 25]. Autoimmune diseases such as rheumatoid arthritis, thyroidism, and Sjögren syndrome, infectious and iatrogenic factors have been reported to accompany TINU cases [2, 8, 20, 21]. We did not find such association in our case.

Several studies have reported that renal tubulointerstitial infiltrations are composed of activated lymphocytes, predominantly helper/inducer T-cell subset [26, 27]. Immunohistochemical kidney analysis in TINU patients demonstrated that the interstitium is infiltrated mainly by T-cells, together with monocytes/macrophages [22, 28]. Otherwise, ciliary body and renal tubular epithelium share some similar functions including those pertaining to electrolyte transporters sensitive to carbonic anhydrase inhibitors [8]. Thus, they might share cross-active autoantigens. In fact, the high prevalence of serum anti-modified CRP (mCRP) autoantibodies were detected in TINU syndrome in active phase of nephritis [25]. Tan et al. [25] also found that the staining of mCRP and human IgG was colocalized in renal and ocular tissues. Although, these findings are impressive, we have no data of mCRP in our patients.

Genetic markers for TINU also have been reported to be related to the risk of development of the syndrome. Loss of T-cell tolerance is suggested by several reports identifying a strong link between TINU and human leukocyte antigen (HLA) [15, 16]. In the report of Goda et al. [3], 7 (87.5%) of 8 patients in Hokkaido, Japan, were HLA-A2, 3 (37.5%) of 8 patients were HLA-A24, 2 (25%) of 8 patients were HLA-A31, and 2 (25%) of 8 patients were HLA-DR4. Mandeville et al. [8] reported that HLA-A2 and HLA-A24 were important antigens associated with TINU in Japanese individuals. On the other hand, Matsumoto et al. [17] compared 22 Japanese adult cases of previous reported TINU to 50 healthy Japanese adults and concluded that there were no significant differences in HLA-A2 and HLA-A24 between those with and without the disease. In our cases, the A locus was A24, 26, and 31 in 2 (40%) patients, and A2 in 1 (20%).

Levinson et al. [15] found that HLA-DQA1*01, HLA-DQB1*05, and HLA-DQB1*01 were associated with TINU and concluded that HLA-DQA1*01/HDQB1*05 may be related to the risk of development of the disease in their population. We found DQ A1*01/B1*05 in one patient with the definite type.

The HLA-DR4 serotype, and its corresponding allele HLA-DRB1*04, has been reported to be a risk factor for Vogt-Koyanagi-Harada (VKH) disease [29]. In our cohorts, HLA-DR4 or the allele of DRB1*04 was present in all (100%) patients. It was also reported that VKH patients are sensitized to melanocyte epitopes [30]. HLA-DR is an MHC class II cell surface receptor which displays peptide antigens produced from the HLA-DRB1 gene to the immune system. If the immune system recognizes a peptide induced by a virus, bacteria, or environmental substances, it triggers a response to attack these invading factors [24]. A common antibody may be produced against ocular and renal proteins, subsequently a crossed autoimmune reaction could induce the renal and ocular alterations in TINU. HLA-DR4 or the allele of DRB1*04 may be involved in these reactions. HLA typing may be helpful in diagnosing TINU; however, further research on this association is required.

Our study has several limitations. First, its retrospective nature may have introduced a degree of bias. Second, as mentioned earlier, it might have been underdiagnosed if mild renal disease does not become symptomatic and/or if diagnostic tests regarding renal involvement are not performed at the time of presentation. Prospective long-term follow-up of more subjects is needed as a creation of the guideline for screening and treatment strategy in patients with TINU.

In conclusion, we reported clinical findings, treatment outcomes, and the HLA haplotype in 5 cases of TINU syndrome with a mean follow-up of 54.0 months. Although recurrences or exacerbation is observed, the prognosis for patients with TINU is good with steroid treatment. Since some Japanese patients might initially present with ophthalmic findings or mild symptoms of TIN of which they are unaware, TINU should be considered in the differential diagnosis especially in young patients with anterior uveitis of unknown origin and renal dysfunction. Examination for urinary $\beta 2$ microglobulin and HLA typing may be helpful in diagnosing TINU.

Conflicts of Interest

All the authors have declared no competing interest.

References

[1] R. S. Dobrin, R. L. Vernier, and A. J. Fish, "Acute eosinophilic interstitial nephritis and renal failure with bone marrow-

lymph node granulomas and anterior uveitis," *The American Journal of Medicine*, vol. 59, no. 3, pp. 325–333, 1975.

[2] K. Pakzad-Vaezi and K. L. Pepple, "Tubulointerstitial nephritis and uveitis," *Current Opinion in Ophthalmology*, vol. 28, no. 6, pp. 629–635, 2017.

[3] C. Goda, S. Kotake, A. Ichiishi, K. Namba, N. Kitaichi, and S. Ohno, "Clinical features in tubulointerstitial nephritis and uveitis (TINU) syndrome," *American Journal of Ophthalmology*, vol. 140, no. 4, pp. 637–641, 2005.

[4] F. Mackensen and H. Billing, "Tubulointerstitial nephritis and uveitis syndrome," *Current Opinion in Ophthalmology*, vol. 20, no. 6, pp. 525–531, 2009.

[5] V. Saarela, M. Nuutinen, M. Ala-Houhala, P. Arikoski, K. Rönnholm, and T. Jahnukainen, "Tubulointerstitial nephritis and uveitis syndrome in children: a prospective multicenter study," *Ophthalmology*, vol. 120, no. 7, pp. 1476–1481, 2013.

[6] M. C. Aguilar, M. Lonngi, and A. de-la-Torre, "Tubulointerstitial nephritis and uveitis syndrome: case report and review of the literature," *Ocular Immunology and Inflammation*, vol. 24, no. 4, pp. 415–421, 2016.

[7] N. Ohguro, K. H. Sonoda, M. Takeuchi, M. Matsumura, and M. Mochizuki, "The 2009 prospective multi-center epidemiologic survey of uveitis in Japan," *Japanese Journal of Ophthalmology*, vol. 56, no. 5, pp. 432–435, 2012.

[8] J. T. H. Mandeville, R. D. Levinson, and G. N. Holland, "The tubulointerstitial nephritis and uveitis syndrome," *Survey of Ophthalmology*, vol. 46, no. 3, pp. 195–208, 2001.

[9] J. M. Han, Y. J. Lee, and S. J. Woo, "A case of tubulointerstitial nephritis and uveitis syndrome in an elderly patient," *Korean Journal of Ophthalmology*, vol. 26, no. 5, pp. 398–401, 2012.

[10] M. Legendre, H. Devilliers, L. Perard et al., "Clinicopathologic characteristics, treatment, and outcomes of tubulointerstitial nephritis and uveitis syndrome in adults: a national retrospective strobe-compliant study," *Medicine*, vol. 95, no. 26, article e3964, 2016.

[11] N. Gion, P. Stavrou, and C. S. Foster, "Immunomodulatory therapy for chronic tubulointerstitial nephritis-associated uveitis," *American Journal of Ophthalmology*, vol. 129, no. 6, pp. 764–768, 2000.

[12] B. Sobolewska, T. Bayyoud, C. Deuter, D. Doycheva, and M. Zierhut, "Long-term follow-up of patients with tubulointerstitial nephritis and uveitis (TINU) syndrome," *Ocular Immunology and Inflammation*, pp. 1–7, 2016.

[13] U. Gafter, Y. Kalechman, D. Zevin et al., "Tubulointerstitial nephritis and uveitis: association with suppressed cellular immunity," *Nephrology Dialysis Transplantation*, vol. 8, no. 9, pp. 821–826, 1993.

[14] M. B. Gorroño-Echebarría, M. A. Calvo-Arrabal, F. Albarrán, and M. Alvarez-Mon, "The tuberculointerstitial nephritis and uveitis (TINU) syndrome is associated with HLA-DR14 in Spanish patients," *The British Journal of Ophthalmology*, vol. 85, no. 8, pp. 1010-1011, 2001.

[15] R. D. Levinson, M. S. Park, S. M. Rikkers et al., "Strong associations between specific HLA-DQ and HLA-DR alleles and the tubulointerstitial nephritis and uveitis syndrome," *Investigative Ophthalmology & Visual Science*, vol. 44, no. 2, pp. 653–657, 2003.

[16] F. Mackensen, F. David, V. Schwenger et al., "HLA-DRB1* 0102 is associated with TINU syndrome and bilateral, sudden-onset anterior uveitis but not with interstitial nephritis alone," *The British Journal of Ophthalmology*, vol. 95, no. 7, pp. 971–975, 2011.

[17] K. Matsumoto, K. Fukunari, Y. Ikeda et al., "A report of an adult case of tubulointerstitial nephritis and uveitis (TINU) syndrome, with a review of 102 Japanese cases," *American Journal of Case Reports*, vol. 16, pp. 119–123, 2015.

[18] D. A. Jabs, R. B. Nussenblatt, J. T. Rosenbaum, and Standardization of Uveitis Nomenclature (SUN) Working Group, "Standardization of uveitis nomenclature for reporting clinical data. results of the first international workshop," *American Journal of Ophthalmology*, vol. 140, no. 3, pp. 509–516, 2005.

[19] T. Jahnukainen, K. Rönnholm, M. Ala-Houhala, and M. Nuutinen, "Corticosteroid therapy can be delayed but not omitted in idiopathic tubulointerstitial nephritis," *Pediatric Nephrology*, vol. 29, no. 3, p. 493, 2014.

[20] F. Mackensen, J. R. Smith, and J. T. Rosenbaum, "Enhanced recognition, treatment, and prognosis of tubulointerstitial nephritis and uveitis syndrome," *Ophthalmology*, vol. 114, no. 5, pp. 995–999.e1, 2007.

[21] Y. M. Hettinga, L. M. E. Scheerlinck, M. R. Lilien, A. Rothova, and J. H. de Boer, "The value of measuring urinary $\beta 2$-microglobulin and serum creatinine for detecting tubulointerstitial nephritis and uveitis syndrome in young patients with uveitis," *JAMA Ophthalmology*, vol. 133, no. 2, pp. 140–145, 2015.

[22] T. Takemura, M. Okada, S. Hino et al., "Course and outcome of tubulointerstitial nephritis and uveitis syndrome," *American Journal of Kidney Diseases*, vol. 34, no. 6, pp. 1016–1021, 1999.

[23] S. Savaj and M. Asgari, "Tubulointerstitial nephritis and uveitis: report of a rare syndrome," *Iranian Journal of Kidney Diseases*, vol. 5, no. 1, pp. 66–68, 2011.

[24] D. M. Hinkle and C. S. Foster, "Tubulointerstitial nephritis and uveitis syndrome," *International Ophthalmology Clinics*, vol. 48, no. 2, pp. 9–13, 2008.

[25] Y. Tan, F. Yu, Z. Qu et al., "Modified C-reactive protein might be a target autoantigen of TINU syndrome," *Clinical Journal of the American Society of Nephrology*, vol. 6, no. 1, pp. 93–100, 2011.

[26] H. Tanaka, K. Suzuki, T. Nakahata, T. Tateyama, S. Waga, and E. Ito, "Repeat renal biopsy in a girl with tubulointerstitial nephritis and uveitis syndrome," *Pediatric Nephrology*, vol. 16, no. 11, pp. 885–887, 2001.

[27] L. Abed, A. Merouani, E. Haddad, G. Benoit, L. L. Oligny, and H. Sartelet, "Presence of autoantibodies against tubular and uveal cells in a patient with tubulointerstitial nephritis and uveitis (TINU) syndrome," *Nephrology Dialysis Transplantation*, vol. 23, no. 4, pp. 1452–1455, 2007.

[28] Y. Kobayashi, M. Honda, N. Yoshikawa, and H. Ito, "Immunohistological study in sixteen children with acute tubulointerstitial nephritis," *Clinical Nephrology*, vol. 50, no. 1, pp. 14–20, 1998.

[29] Y. Shindo, S. Ohno, T. Yamamoto, S. Nakamura, and H. Inoko, "Complete association of the HLA-DRB1*04 and -DQB1*04 alleles with Vogt-Koyanagi-Harada's disease," *Human Immunology*, vol. 39, no. 3, pp. 169–176, 1994.

[30] F. M. Damico, E. Cunha-Neto, A. C. Goldberg et al., "T-cell recognition and cytokine profile induced by melanocyte epitopes in patients with HLA-DRB1*0405-positive and -negative Vogt-Koyanagi-Harada uveitis," *Investigative Ophthalmology & Visual Science*, vol. 46, no. 7, pp. 2465–2471, 2005.

6

Macular Thickness, Foveal Volume, and Choroidal Thickness in Amblyopic Eyes and their Relationships to the Treatment Outcome

Chun-Hsiu Liu,[1] Sherine Jue Ong,[2] Chung-Ying Huang,[1] Wei-Chi Wu,[1] Ling-Yuh Kao,[1] and Meng-Ling Yang[1]

[1]*Department of Ophthalmology, Chang Gung Memorial Hospital, Chang Gung University College of Medicine, No. 5, Fuhsing Street, Kweishan, Taoyuan 333, Taiwan*
[2]*Ching Ming Eye Clinic, No. 32, Zhongshan 2nd Rd., Luzhou, New Taipei 247, Taiwan*

Correspondence should be addressed to Meng-Ling Yang; menling@gmail.com

Academic Editor: Ciro Costagliola

Purpose. To assess the correlations between the retinal/choroidal structure and the treatment outcomes of amblyopic children. *Methods.* This study enrolled eyes with amblyopia resulting from strabismus, anisometropia, or ametropia. All patients underwent detailed eye examinations, including spectral domain optical coherence tomography (SD-OCT) scan. All of the subjects received amblyopic treatment and were divided into 2 groups after 6 months of follow-up: the recovered amblyopic group with a best-corrected visual acuity (BCVA) ≥0.8 and the persistent amblyopic group with a BCVA <0.8 on the Landolt C chart. *Results.* Forty-four amblyopic children were included, of which 26 were in the recovered amblyopic group after 6 months of follow-up. The patients with strabismic anisometropic amblyopia and severe amblyopia (initial VA ≤ 0.3) were significantly predisposed to developing persistent amblyopia ($P = 0.049$ and $P < 0.001$, respectively). After correcting with Littmann's formula, the thickness and volume of the parafoveal and perifoveal retinal regions in the persistent amblyopia group did not show significant differences with the recovered amblyopia group. *Conclusions.* The initial severity of amblyopia and the type of amblyopia were the risk factors related to the poor outcome of amblyopic treatment. The foveal thickness, foveal volume, and choroidal thickness were not associated with the treatment outcome.

1. Introduction

Amblyopia is the reduced best-corrected visual acuity (BCVA) of one eye or, less commonly, both eyes, which is caused by abnormal binocular interaction and the lack of adequate visual stimulation during visual development. The causes of amblyopia include strabismus, anisometropia, vision deprivation, or a combination of these factors [1]. Several morphological and functional changes have been observed in the lateral geniculate nucleus and visual cortex in subjects with various types of amblyopia [1–3].

Risk factors for the failure of amblyopia treatment have been evaluated in several reports, only a few of which discussed the correlation between the macular/choroidal biometric values and the results of treatment, and the relationship has not been clarified [4–6].

Optical coherence tomography (OCT) provides a highly qualitative, objective, and reproducible structural assessment of retinal structures. The OCT has evolved rapidly in the past few years, from time domain OCT to spectral domain OCT (SD-OCT) which allows more rapid scanning and higher resolution and permits a more detailed analysis of the optic nerve and retina. The application of OCT in amblyopia children has been demonstrated in several studies but with inconsistent results [6–9].

The purpose of this study was to evaluate the macular and choroidal thicknesses in persistent and recovered amblyopic children using SD-OCT. We sought to determine if any change in the macular or choroidal biometric values is related to the treatment outcome.

2. Materials and Methods

This study was performed at the Chang Gung Memorial Hospital between January 2012 and April 2013. The inclusion criteria included patients being older than 5 years and having a diagnosis of amblyopia, which was defined as BCVA less than 0.8. Severe amblyopia was defined as a BCVA of 0.3 or worse. The study was approved by the Ethics Committee of Chang Gung Memorial Hospital and the study's protocol adhered to the tenets of the Declaration of Helsinki.

The enrolled patients were identified according to the causes of their amblyopia. For anisometropic amblyopia, no eye deviation was noted in the cover test. Anisometropia in hyperopia, astigmatism, or myopia was defined as an interocular cycloplegic difference of 2 diopters (D) or more. Amblyopia associated with anisometropia and eye deviation was defined as strabismic anisometropic amblyopia. Patients meeting none of the criteria above were defined as strabismic amblyopia if there was eye deviation or defined as ametropic amblyopia if no eye deviation was found.

Patients were excluded if they had any organic eye disease or a history or evidence of intraocular surgery or trauma or if they were not sufficiently cooperative for an OCT examination. All of the patients underwent a comprehensive ophthalmic examination, including the BCVA, axial length measurement (Optical Biometer AL-Scan; Nidek, Japan), a slit-lamp examination, intraocular pressure assessment (Full Auto Tonometer TX-F; Canon, Japan), extraocular motility assessment, cover-uncover test, and dilated fundoscopy. All of the refraction tests were performed after instilling one drop of 1% cyclopentolate solution and 2 drops of 1% tropicamide solution at 10-minute intervals. Visual acuity testing was performed using the Landolt C chart, following the standard procedure.

Macular and choroidal thicknesses were measured using an SD-OCT system (RTVue, Optovue Inc., Fremont, CA, USA) before the amblyopia treatment. The data for the macular retinal thickness were displayed in 3 concentric circles with diameters of 1 mm (fovea), 3 mm (parafovea), and 5 mm (perifovea). To measure the choroidal thickness, we used the protocols previously described by Wang and associates [10]. Briefly, the choroid was imaged in the "choroidal mode" with the SD-OCT, and its thickness was defined as the distance between the outer border of the retinal pigment epithelium (RPE) and the hyperrefractive line behind the large vessel layers of the choroid, which is presumed to be the choroid-sclera interface (Figure 1). Only the images with a clear choroid-sclera interface were used for analysis. The choroidal thickness was measured manually beneath the fovea using the scale supplied with the system's software at 1000 μm intervals from the fovea to a distance of 3 mm in the nasal, temporal, superior, and inferior directions. The average value of the 14 choroidal thickness readings was recorded as the macular choroidal thickness. The subfoveal choroidal thickness was defined as the choroidal thickness measured at the center of the foveola. Each image was measured by two independent technicians. Data with discrepancies of 20% were reanalyzed by the author (Sherine Jue Ong).

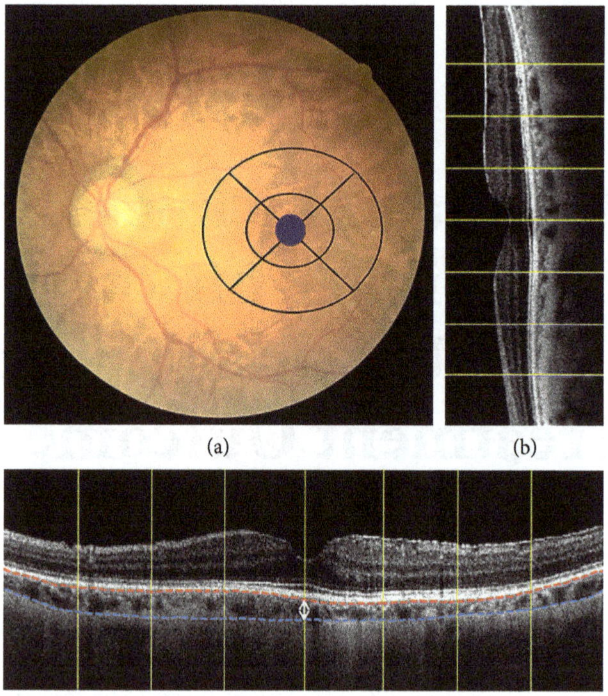

(a) (b) (c)

FIGURE 1: Measurements of the macular and choroidal thicknesses. (a) Macular retinal thickness was measured in three concentric rings, with the central ring corresponding to the fovea (1 mm diameter), the middle ring corresponding to the parafovea (3 mm diameter), and the outer ring corresponding to the perifovea (5 mm diameter). (b, c) The yellow lines indicate the locations of the 1000 μm intervals. The distance between the outer border of the retinal pigment epithelium (red dash line) and the hyperrefractive line behind the large vessel layers of the choroid (blue dash line) was defined as choroidal thickness (white arrow).

All of the patients received standard treatment including wearing spectacles for refraction correction and occlusion of the dominant fellow eye. The refraction and BCVA were rechecked every 3 months, and the final BCVA value was recorded after 6 months of follow-up. Then, the patients were divided into two groups according to the final BCVA result: those with recovered amblyopia that was defined as a final BCVA 0.8 or better and those with persistent amblyopia who had a final BCVA worse than 0.8.

The statistical analysis was performed using SPSS 20 software (IBM, Armonk, NY, USA). The OCT measurement data were corrected for the axial length-induced ocular magnification using Littmann's formula. In Littmann's formula, which is $t = p \times q \times s$ [11–13]; t is the real fundus dimension; p is the instrument-dependent magnification constant for the imaging system; q is the ocular magnification factor related to the axial length; and s is the value obtained using OCT. Logistic regression models were constructed for comparison of each related factor and the OCT data for the groups with persistent and recovered

TABLE 1: Demographic profiles of the participants with persistent amblyopia and recovered amblyopia.

	Persistent amblyopia (n = 18)	Recovered amblyopia (n = 26)	P value
Age			
Mean ± SD, years	7.46 ± 2.13	8.14 ± 3.25	0.436
Range, years	5.0–11.5	5.0–16.0	
Gender			
Male, n (%)	12 (66.67)	15 (57.70)	0.549
Female, n (%)	6 (33.33)	11 (42.31)	0.552
Severe amblyopia*, n (%)	15 (83.33)	2 (7.69)	<0.001
Type of amblyopia			
Anisometropic, n (%)	6 (33.33)	14 (53.85)	0.111
Strabismic anisometropic, n (%)	8 (44.44)	4 (15.38)	0.049
Strabismic, n (%)	3 (16.67)	2 (7.69)	0.226
Ametropic, n (%)	1 (5.56)	6 (23.08)	0.426
Spherical equivalent†			
Mean ± SD, diopters	0.47 ± 5.97	1.61 ± 4.12	0.449
Range, diopters	−12.63 to + 7.25	−10.75 to +8.5	
Axial length†			
Mean ± SD, mm	23.05 ± 1.73	22.58 ± 1.33	0.359
Range, mm	20.8–26.34	20.44–26.75	

SD: standard deviation. *Severe amblyopia was defined as visual acuity of <0.3 at the time of entering the study. †The worse eye of the children with bilateral amblyopia was used in the analysis.

amblyopia. For the children with bilateral amblyopia, the worse eye was used in the analysis. A paired t-test was used to compare the amblyopic eye and the dominant fellow eye for each of the patients. Statistical significance was defined as $P < 0.005$.

3. Results

A total of 44 patients were enrolled, and the mean age was 7.9 ± 2.9 years (mean ± standard deviation). The mean refractive error was +1.17 ± 4.98 D. Among the 44 patients, 18 patients (40.9%) had a final BCVA worse than 0.8 and were grouped into persistent amblyopia. The other 26 patients (59.1%) had a final BCVA of 0.8 or better and were grouped into recovered amblyopia. Table 1 summarizes the demographic profiles of these two groups. No significant difference in age, gender, spherical equivalent, or axial length was observed between these two groups. The patients who had severe amblyopia (initial VA of ≤0.3) were significantly predisposed to developing persistent amblyopia ($P < 0.001$). Among the included patients, 20 (45.5%) had anisometropic amblyopia, 12 (27.3%) had strabismic anisometropic amblyopia, 5 (11.3%) had strabismic amblyopia, and 7 (15.9%) had ametropic amblyopia. The rate of strabismic anisometropic amblyopia was significantly higher in the persistent amblyopic group than in the recovered group (44.4% and 15.4%, respectively, $P = 0.049$).

The macular and choroidal biometric values of the persistent amblyopic and recovered amblyopic groups are summarized in Table 2. The parafoveal retinal thicknesses, parafoveal retinal volumes, perifoveal retinal thicknesses, and perifoveal retinal volumes were significantly less in the persistent amblyopic group than in the recovered amblyopic group (P = 0.049, 0.046, 0.043, and 0.048, respectively). A significant difference was also noted in the retinal thicknesses of the parafoveal temporal quadrant ($P = 0.022$). However, the differences were no longer existent after data adjustment using Littmann's formula. Based on the quality of the images, the choroidal thickness could be analyzed in only 29 patients (9 in the persistent amblyopic group and 20 in the recovered amblyopic group). There was no significant difference in the choroidal thickness between these two groups.

We further compared the SD-OCT findings between the nondominant amblyopic eyes and the dominant fellow eyes (Table 3). However, there were no significant differences in the macular thickness, macular volume, or choroidal thickness, either before or after correction using Littmann's formula.

4. Discussion

In our study, nearly 60% of children achieved a BCVA of 0.8 or better after treatment for amblyopia. Reviewing the previous studies showed that the posttreatment VA was maintained or improved in 47–96.3% of amblyopic patients [14–17]. The risk factors for persistent amblyopia in our study were the type of amblyopia (strabismic anisometropic amblyopia) and the initial severity of the amblyopia (BCVA ≤ 0.3). This finding is compatible with those of other studies reported in the literature [14, 15, 18–20]. Levartovsky et al. reported that the patients with more profound amblyopia had a greater risk of deterioration and developing recurrent amblyopia after discontinuing treatment [14]. Therefore, closer follow-up may be needed for more profoundly amblyopic patients. Some clinicians have reported that patients at a younger age at the beginning of treatment achieved a better outcome [20, 21], although this result was inconsistent with those of other studies [14, 15, 19]. In this study, we did not observe an age difference between the persistent amblyopia and recovered amblyopia groups.

TABLE 2: Macular and choroidal thicknesses in persistent amblyopia and recovered amblyopia.

	Persistent amblyopia (n = 18)	Recovered amblyopia (n = 26)	P value	P value†
Fovea				
Thickness, μm	238.11 ± 16.27	245.12 ± 28.04	0.343	0.601
Volume, mm^3	0.19 ± 0.01	0.19 ± 0.02	0.355	0.591
Parafovea				
Thickness, μm	298.83 ± 19.91	310.28 ± 15.13	0.049	0.615
Volume, mm^3	1.88 ± 0.13	1.95 ± 0.09	0.046	0.892
Temporal thickness, μm	286.72 ± 18.59	300.2 ± 15.71	0.022	0.527
Superior thickness, μm	302.6 ± 26.27	313.88 ± 19.82	0.130	0.496
Nasal thickness, μm	308.11 ± 20.98	317.76 ± 17.2	0.113	0.894
Inferior thickness, μm	298.22 ± 19.29	308.92 ± 16.15	0.065	0.635
Perifovea				
Thickness, μm	283.17 ± 21.09	294.48 ± 11.68	0.043	0.633
Volume, mm^3	3.56 ± 0.26	3.7 ± 0.15	0.048	0.672
Temporal thickness, μm	276.67 ± 21.56	287.6 ± 14.04	0.061	0.702
Superior thickness, μm	279.17 ± 26.55	292.68 ± 23.42	0.103	0.349
Nasal thickness, μm	299.56 ± 22.72	308.56 ± 13.26	0.121	0.892
Inferior thickness, μm	277.89 ± 21.89	280.16 ± 26.46	0.761	0.734
Choroidal thickness (n = 29)*				
Macular, μm	251 ± 43.45	267.4 ± 42.87	0.343	0.108
Subfoveal, μm	283.78 ± 57.69	295.5 ± 43.87	0.538	0.188

SD: standard deviation. The worse eye of the children with bilateral amblyopia was used in the analysis. Unless otherwise indicated, data are given as the mean ± standard deviation. †P value calculated after correcting using Littmann's formula. *Images of good quality, as determined by a clear choroid-sclera interface, were used in the analysis (n = 29).

TABLE 3: Macular and choroidal thicknesses of the amblyopic eye and the fellow eye.

	Amblyopic eye (n = 44)	Fellow eye (n = 44)	P value†
Fovea			
Thickness, μm	242.19 ± 23.85	237.58 ± 24.47	0.623
Volume, mm^3	0.19 ± 0.02	0.19 ± 0.02	0.604
Parafovea			
Thickness, μm	305.49 ± 18	304.44 ± 14.63	0.800
Volume, mm^3	1.92 ± 0.11	1.91 ± 0.09	0.487
Temporal thickness, μm	294.56 ± 18.06	295.23 ± 15.12	0.407
Superior thickness, μm	309.16 ± 23.14	307.98 ± 19.45	0.951
Nasal thickness, μm	313.72 ± 19.25	311.74 ± 16.45	0.994
Inferior thickness, μm	304.44 ± 18.11	302.49 ± 15.53	0.999
Perifovea			
Thickness, μm	289.74 ± 17.03	287.14 ± 14.07	0.748
Volume, mm^3	3.64 ± 0.21	3.56 ± 0.31	0.219
Temporal thickness, μm	283.02 ± 18.18	279.72 ± 14.06	0.785
Superior thickness, μm	287.02 ± 25.37	288.02 ± 14.95	0.443
Nasal thickness, μm	304.79 ± 18.15	303.09 ± 15.22	0.925
Inferior thickness, μm	279.21 ± 24.4	275.6 ± 26.48	0.142
Choroidal thickness (n = 29)*			
Macular, μm	262.31 ± 42.97	260.3 ± 36.38	0.771
Subfoveal, μm	297.83 ± 47.83	289.59 ± 43.2	0.924

SD: standard deviation. Unless otherwise indicated, data are given as the mean ± standard deviation. †P value calculated after correcting using Littmann's formula. *Images of good quality, as determined by a clear choroid-sclera interface, were used in the analysis (n = 29). In children with bilateral amblyopia, the worse eye was considered to be the amblyopic eye and the other eye was considered to be the dominant fellow eye.

Previous studies have emphasized the differences between the OCT findings in amblyopic eyes compared with those in normal control eyes or in the fellow eyes [9, 22]. The presence of amblyopia was associated with increased foveal thickness, but the origin or significance of this finding is still uncertain. Some clinicians have suggested that differences exist only in some specific types of amblyopia [8, 23–25], but others have reported that no significant differences in the macular structures were found [6, 26]. Bruce et al. found that differences exist between the amblyopic eyes and visually normal eyes but not between the amblyopic eyes and fellow eyes [27]. The abovementioned variations may be due to the lack of control groups, differences in the OCT instruments utilized, variations in the ages of the enrolled subjects, refractive errors, or the types of amblyopia. Considering the effects of the axial lengths and refractive errors on the OCT images, Littmann's formula was used for correction in the present study [11, 12]. The result showed that the corrected macular and choroidal biometric values of the amblyopic eyes and the dominant fellow eyes were not significantly different.

We also found that the corrected macular and choroidal biometric values of the recovered amblyopic eyes and the persistent amblyopic eyes were not significantly different either. This finding is consistent with the results of previous studies [28, 29]. Tugcu et al. studied macular thickness in the persistent amblyopic and resolved amblyopic eyes and did not found significant difference between the two groups [28]. Chen et al. compared the macular thickness of the amblyopic eyes with those of fully corrected previous amblyopic eyes and nonamblyopic controls and found there was no significant difference among the three groups [29]. By contrast, Pang et al. reported that the central macular thickness in myopic anisometropic amblyopia significantly reduced after amblyopia treatment [30]. However, the measurements in their study were not adjusted for axial length and refractive error. To clarify the role of retinal alternation in the amblyopia treatment, further longitudinal and comparative studies are required.

Previous studies have reported the measurements of choroidal thickness in healthy children by different instruments [31–33]. Read et al. reported that the choroid is significantly thinner in children during early childhood than in children of older age groups [31]. The subfoveal choroidal thickness has been reported to be thicker in amblyopic eyes than in control eyes [34]. In our study, the subfoveal choroidal thickness in the amblyopic eye was relatively thinner compared with other studies. Since the choroidal thickness was reported to be greater in the hyperopia than in emmetropia and myopia children [35], one of the children in our study had high myopia of -10.75 D, in which the measured subfoveal choroidal thickness was 143 μm, which might explain the different result. Besides, an increased macular choroidal thickness was found to be related to a better BCVA, less myopia, and a shorter axial length in studies of myopia [10, 36]. Further studies related to the choroidal thickness and amblyopia are worth studying.

There are several limitations to our study. First, there was no normal control group for comparing the macular and choroidal structures. Second, the macular choroidal thickness was measured manually, and new automated software will reduce the bias involved and the time required to obtain measurements of the macular choroidal thickness. Third, a small number of patients were enrolled, precluding subgroup analysis based on the different types of amblyopia. Further long-term studies with larger samples may be needed.

In conclusion, the initial VA and the type of amblyopia play important roles in visual recovery during amblyopic treatment. No difference was found in the macular and choroidal thicknesses between the persistent and recovered amblyopic eyes. There were also no prominent interocular differences in the amblyopic patients. The thickness of the retina and choroid obtained using OCT before treatment might have limited value for predicting the treatment outcome. Further studies with a longer follow-up period are warranted to determine whether retinal or choroidal structures have any effect on the response to amblyopia therapy.

Conflicts of Interest

The authors declare that they have no conflicts of interest.

Acknowledgments

The authors thank Lin Yu Jr. of the Biostatistical Center for Clinical Research of Chang Gung Memorial Hospital, Taiwan, for assistance with the statistical analyses.

References

[1] E. Campos, "Amblyopia," *Survey of Ophthalmology*, vol. 40, no. 1, pp. 23–39, 1995.

[2] G. K. von Noorden, M. L. Crawford, and R. A. Levacy, "The lateral geniculate nucleus in human anisometropic amblyopia," *Investigative Ophthalmology & Visual Science*, vol. 24, no. 6, pp. 788–790, 1983.

[3] G. K. von Noorden and M. L. Crawford, "The lateral geniculate nucleus in human strabismic amblyopia," *Investigative Ophthalmology & Visual Science*, vol. 33, no. 9, pp. 2729–2732, 1992.

[4] S. Q. Wu, L. W. Zhu, Q. B. Xu, J. L. Xu, and Y. Zhang, "Macular and peripapillary retinal nerve fiber layer thickness in children with hyperopic anisometropic amblyopia," *International Journal of Ophthalmology*, vol. 6, no. 1, pp. 85–89, 2013.

[5] A. Miki, M. Shirakashi, K. Yaoeda et al., "Retinal nerve fiber layer thickness in recovered and persistent amblyopia," *Clinical Ophthalmology*, vol. 4, pp. 1061–1064, 2010.

[6] A. Dickmann, S. Petroni, V. Perrotta et al., "Measurement of retinal nerve fiber layer thickness, macular thickness, and foveal volume in amblyopic eyes using spectral-domain optical coherence tomography," *Journal of American Association for Pediatric Ophthalmology and Strabismus*, vol. 16, no. 1, pp. 86–88, 2012.

[7] M. X. Repka, R. T. Kraker, S. M. Tamkins, D. W. Suh, N. A. Sala, and R. W. Beck, "Retinal nerve fiber layer thickness in amblyopic eyes," *American Journal of Ophthalmology*, vol. 148, no. 1, pp. 143–147, 2009.

[8] C. E. Al-Haddad, G. M. Mollayess, C. G. Cherfan, D. F. Jaafar, and Z. F. Bashshur, "Retinal nerve fibre layer and macular thickness in amblyopia as measured by spectral-domain optical coherence tomography," *British Journal of Ophthalmology*, vol. 95, no. 12, pp. 1696–1699, 2011.

[9] S. C. Huynh, C. Samarawickrama, X. Y. Wang et al., "Macular and nerve fiber layer thickness in amblyopia," *Ophthalmology*, vol. 116, no. 9, pp. 1604–1609, 2009.

[10] N. K. Wang, C. C. Lai, H. Y. Chu et al., "Classification of early dry-type myopic maculopathy with macular choroidal thickness," *American Journal of Ophthalmology*, vol. 153, no. 4, pp. 669–677, 2012.

[11] A. G. Bennett, A. R. Rudnicka, and D. F. Edgar, "Improvements on Littmann's method of determining the size of retinal features by fundus photography," *Graefe's Archive for Clinical and Experimental Ophthalmology*, vol. 232, no. 6, pp. 361–367, 1994.

[12] V. Aykut, V. Oner, M. Tas, Y. Iscan, and A. Agachan, "Influence of axial length on peripapillary retinal nerve fiber layer thickness in children: a study by RTVue spectral-domain optical coherence tomography," *Current Eye Research*, vol. 38, no. 12, pp. 1241–1247, 2013.

[13] G. Savini, P. Barboni, V. Parisi, and M. Carbonelli, "The influence of axial length on retinal nerve fibre layer thickness and optic-disc size measurements by spectral-domain OCT," *British Journal of Ophthalmology*, vol. 96, no. 1, pp. 57–61, 2011.

[14] S. Levartovsky, M. Oliver, N. Gottesman, and M. Shimshoni, "Factors affecting long term results of successfully treated amblyopia: initial visual acuity and type of amblyopia," *British Journal of Ophthalmology*, vol. 79, no. 3, pp. 225–228, 1995.

[15] G. Woodruff, F. Hiscox, J. R. Thompson, and L. K. Smith, "Factors affecting the outcome of children treated for amblyopia," *Eye*, vol. 8, no. 6, pp. 627–631, 1994.

[16] H. Leiba, M. Shimshoni, M. Oliver, N. Gottesman, and S. Levartovsky, "Long-term follow-up of occlusion therapy in amblyopia," *Ophthalmology*, vol. 108, no. 9, pp. 1552–1555, 2001.

[17] J. Ohlsson, M. Baumann, J. Sjostrand, and M. Abrahamsson, "Long term visual outcome in amblyopia treatment," *British Journal of Ophthalmology*, vol. 86, no. 10, pp. 1148–1151, 2002.

[18] G. Arikan, A. Yaman, and A. T. Berk, "Efficacy of occlusion treatment in amblyopia and clinical risk factors affecting the results of treatment," *Strabismus*, vol. 13, no. 2, pp. 63–69, 2005.

[19] R. Beardsell, S. Clarke, and M. Hill, "Outcome of occlusion treatment for amblyopia," *Journal of Pediatric Ophthalmology and Strabismus*, vol. 36, no. 1, pp. 19–24, 1999.

[20] M. A. Hussein, D. K. Coats, A. Muthialu, E. Cohen, and E. A. Paysse, "Risk factors for treatment failure of anisometropic amblyopia," *Journal of American Association for Pediatric Ophthalmology and Strabismus*, vol. 8, no. 5, pp. 429–434, 2004.

[21] W. E. Scott, P. J. Kutschke, R. V. Keech, W. L. Pfeifer, B. Nichols, and L. Zhang, "Amblyopia treatment outcomes," *Journal of American Association for Pediatric Ophthalmology and Strabismus*, vol. 9, no. 2, pp. 107 111, 2005.

[22] F. Aguirre, E. Mengual, J. R. Hueso, and M. Moya, "Comparison of normal and amblyopic retinas by optical coherence tomography in children," *European Journal of Ophthalmology*, vol. 20, no. 2, pp. 410–418, 2010.

[23] S. Y. Kee, S. Y. Lee, and Y. C. Lee, "Thicknesses of the fovea and retinal nerve fiber layer in amblyopic and normal eyes in children," *Korean Journal of Ophthalmology*, vol. 20, no. 3, pp. 177–181, 2006.

[24] A. Dickmann, S. Petroni, A. Salerni, R. Dell'Omo, and E. Balestrazzi, "Unilateral amblyopia: an optical coherence tomography study," *Journal of American Association for Pediatric Ophthalmology and Strabismus*, vol. 13, no. 2, pp. 148–150, 2009.

[25] A. Dickmann, S. Petroni, V. Perrotta et al., "A morphofunctional study of amblyopic eyes with the use of optical coherence tomography and microperimetry," *Journal of American Association for Pediatric Ophthalmology and Strabismus*, vol. 15, no. 4, pp. 338–341, 2011.

[26] O. Altintas, N. Yuksel, B. Ozkan, and Y. Caglar, "Thickness of the retinal nerve fiber layer, macular thickness, and macular volume in patients with strabismic amblyopia," *Journal of Pediatric Ophthalmology and Strabismus*, vol. 42, no. 4, pp. 216–221, 2005.

[27] A. Bruce, I. E. Pacey, J. A. Bradbury, A. J. Scally, and B. T. Barrett, "Bilateral changes in foveal structure in individuals with amblyopia," *Ophthalmology*, vol. 120, no. 2, pp. 395–403, 2013.

[28] B. Tugcu, B. Araz-Ersan, E. T. Erdogan et al., "Structural and functional comparison of the persistent and resolved amblyopia," *Documenta Ophthalmologica*, vol. 128, no. 2, pp. 101–109, 2014.

[29] W. Chen, J. Chen, F. Zhang, X. Zhu, and F. Lu, "Visual outcome in isoametropic amblyopic children with high hyperopia and the effect of therapy on retinal thickness," *American Journal of Ophthalmology*, vol. 155, no. 3, pp. 536–543.e1, 2013.

[30] Y. Pang, K. A. Frantz, S. Block, G. W. Goodfellow, and C. Allison, "Effect of amblyopia treatment on macular thickness in eyes with myopic anisometropic amblyopia," *Investigative Ophthalmology & Visual Science*, vol. 56, no. 4, pp. 2677–2683, 2015.

[31] S. A. Read, M. J. Collins, S. J. Vincent, and D. Alonso-Caneiro, "Choroidal thickness in childhood," *Investigative Ophthalmology & Visual Science*, vol. 54, no. 5, pp. 3586–3593, 2013.

[32] A. Fujiwara, C. Shiragami, Y. Shirakata, S. Manabe, S. Izumibata, and F. Shiraga, "Enhanced depth imaging spectral-domain optical coherence tomography of subfoveal choroidal thickness in normal Japanese eyes," *Japanese Journal of Ophthalmology*, vol. 56, no. 3, pp. 230–235, 2012.

[33] J. M. Ruiz-Moreno, I. Flores-Moreno, F. Lugo, J. Ruiz-Medrano, J. A. Montero, and M. Akiba, "Macular choroidal thickness in normal pediatric population measured by swept-source optical coherence tomography," *Investigative Ophthalmology & Visual Science*, vol. 54, no. 1, pp. 353–359, 2013.

[34] O. Kara, O. Altintas, S. Karaman, E. Emre, and Y. Caglar, "Analysis of choroidal thickness using spectral-domain OCT in children with unilateral amblyopia," *Journal of Pediatric Ophthalmology and Strabismus*, vol. 52, no. 3, pp. 159–166, 2015.

[35] G. Y. Lee, S. Yu, H. G. Kang, J. S. Kim, K. W. Lee, and J. H. Lee, "Choroidal thickness variation according to refractive error measured by spectral domain-optical coherence tomography in Korean children," *Korean Journal of Ophthalmology*, vol. 31, no. 2, pp. 151–158, 2017.

[36] K. Hayashi, K. Ohno-Matsui, N. Shimada et al., "Long-term pattern of progression of myopic maculopathy: a natural history study," *Ophthalmology*, vol. 117, no. 8, pp. e1595–e1611, 2010.

7

HMBG1 as a Driver of Inflammatory and Immune Processes in the Pathogenesis of Ocular Diseases

Yi Liu,[1] Guo-Bin Zhuang,[2] and Xue-Zhi Zhou[3]

[1]*Department of Ophthalmology, Nanjing Hospital of Chinese Medicine, The Third Affiliated Hospital of Nanjing University of Chinese Medicine, Nanjing, Jiangsu 210001, China*
[2]*Department of Ophthalmology, Quanzhou First Hospital, Quanzhou, Fujian 362000, China*
[3]*Department of Ophthalmology, Xiangya Hospital, Central South University, Changsha, Hunan 410078, China*

Correspondence should be addressed to Xue-Zhi Zhou; heisezhixiang@163.com

Academic Editor: Masaru Takeuchi

High-mobility group box 1 (HMGB1) is a nuclear protein that can also act as an extracellular trigger of inflammation, proliferation, and migration in eye diseases. It induces signaling pathways by binding to the receptor for advanced glycation end products (RAGE) and Toll-like receptors (TLRs) 2, 4, and 9. This proinflammatory activity is considered to be important in the pathogenesis of a wide range of ocular diseases resulting from hemodynamic changes, presence of neovascular endothelial cells, secretion of intraocular immune factors or inflammation, and apoptosis of retinal cell layers. Further work is needed to elucidate in detail how HMGB1 contributes to ocular disease and how its damaging activity can be modulated. In this review, we summarize current knowledge on HMGB1 as a ligand that can evoke inflammation and immune responses in ocular diseases.

1. Introduction

The eye is a relatively independent and closed system in which various tissues and cells interact in complex ways [1]. Many eye diseases have been described, such as glaucoma, keratitis, diabetic retinopathy, and age-related macular degeneration, and these diseases often arise as a result of pathogenic immune responses against eye autoantigens or as a local manifestation of a systemic autoimmune response. Although development of new drugs and innovations in surgical methods has led to effective treatment of ocular diseases, how these diseases occur and progress remains poorly understood. Several studies indicate that ocular diseases have a close relationship with autoimmune reactions and inflammatory responses [2–5], and a key protein in such processes is high-mobility group box 1 (HMGB1) [6–8]. The present review examines the role of HMGB1 in eye diseases.

HMGB1 is a DNA-binding nuclear protein discovered over 30 years ago [9–11]. Normally, this protein exists in the cell nucleus; when it is released outside the cell, it becomes an immune-inflammatory factor [12–14]. It can be released from damaged cells or secreted by activated immune cells such as macrophages, dendritic cells (DCs), and natural killer cells [15–18]. It may induce signaling pathways by binding to the receptor for advanced glycation end products (RAGE) and Toll-like receptors (TLRs) 2, 4, and 9 [19, 20].

HMGB1 is closely related to many inflammatory diseases, such as ischemia of liver and kidney, hepatitis, arthritis, stroke, ischemia of liver and kidney, sepsis, and systemic lupus erythematosus [21–25]. In this review, our focus is the important role of HMGB1 in inflammatory immune eye diseases, including keratitis, uveitis, dry eye, diabetic retinopathy, and retinal degeneration. Inhibition of this protein may be an effective new treatment for patients with immune-inflammatory eye disease. We suggest that more research with both animal and human models is needed to confirm that HMGB1 has the therapeutic potential suggested by initial studies.

2. HMGB1 Structure

HMGB1 was identified as a nonhistone chromatin-binding protein about 30 years ago [9–11]. This protein is abundantly expressed in nearly all eukaryotic cells [26]. It acts as a damage-associated molecular pattern (DAMP) molecule [27]. HMGB1 is a member of the high-mobility group (HMG) chromosomal protein family [28]. HMG chromosomal proteins are divided into the three superfamilies HMGB, HMGN, and HMGA [29]. Human HMGB1 is an alarmin encoded by a single gene that is located on chromosome 13q12 [30]. In most cell types, HMGB1 is mainly located in the nucleus under physiological conditions. When cells are stimulated or suffer injury or death, HMGB1 translocates from inside to outside the cell [31, 32]. HMGB1 contains 215 amino acids arranged into two DNA-binding domains (HMG A box and HMG B box) and one C-terminal acidic tail, which contains a stretch of approximately 30 glutamic and aspartic acid residues [27, 33]. The HMG A and B boxes can bind to DNA and participate in DNA folding and twisting [34–36]. The HMG B box causes macrophages to secrete additional proinflammatory cytokines; in fact, the B box on its own can trigger the same processes as full-length HMGB1 [27, 37]. The A box can antagonize cytokine activity [38, 39]. The spatial arrangement of A and B boxes was regulated by C-terminal acidic tail. [10, 40, 41].

Each HMGB1 domain interacts with different receptors, and these interactions regulate the biological activity of extracellar HMGB1. TLR4 is binding with residues 89–108 of HMGB1 [42, 43], while RAGE is binding with residues 150–184 of HMGB1 [44]. Within the C-terminal acidic tail (residues 186–215), residues 201–205 exert anti-inflammatory activity [45]. Two nuclear localization sequences in HMGB1 may stabilize the chromatin structure and regulate gene transcription.

3. Expression of HMGB1 in Eye Disease

Numerous studies suggest that HMGB1 may contribute to eye disease by acting as an inflammatory cytokine. In a model of retinal ischemia reperfusion injury and inflammation, HMGB1 expression is upregulated in retinal pigment epithelium, retinal endothelial cells, ganglion cells, Müller cells, astrocytes, and photoreceptors [46]. Chronic epithelial cell damage to the cornea or lacrimal glands triggers HMGB1 secretion, which initiates an inflammatory cycle [47]. HMGB1 levels are elevated in the cytoplasm and extracellular space in eye disease. All these studies indicate that HMGB1 is abundantly expressed in ocular diseases, which reflects its role in contributing to these disorders.

4. HMGB1 and Diabetic Retinopathy

Dysfunction of retinal endothelial cells, damage to the blood-retinal barrier, ischemia, and retinal neovascularization are the characters of diabetic retinopathy at different stages [48]. Inflammation factor-mediated damage to the retina and optic nerve are key factors in the pathogenesis of diabetic retinopathy, which appears to involve continuous, low-level inflammation [49]. HMGB1 helps drive this process by acting as a late inflammatory factor [50].

In patients with proliferative diabetic retinopathy (PDR), HMGB1 levels in vitreous humor increased significantly [51]. The expression level of HMGB1 in vitreous body of patients with active PDR is significantly higher than that of inactive PDR patients [52]. HMGB1 may interact with vascular adhesion protein 1 (VAP-1), 8-hydroxy-2'-deoxyguanosine (8-OHdG), and heme oxygenase-1 (HO-1) in contributing to the pathogenesis of inflammation and angiogenesis in PDR [53].

HMGB1 is involved in the pathogenesis of diabetic retinopathy through the combination of RAGE and TLR9 [53]. In BV2 cells, a signaling pathway mediated by HMGB1, RAGE, TLR4, p38, and nuclear factor kappa light chain enhancer of activated B cells (NF-κB) activates matrix metalloprotease-9 in response to high glucose levels [54]. In RGC-5 cells, short interfering RNA against HMGB1 obviously downregulates expression of TLR4 and NF-κB mRNA in response to high glucose [55]. Treating human retinal endothelial cells with high glucose activates HMGB1 to trigger signaling by ERK1/2 and NF-κB, which in turn induces inflammatory responses and break vascular barrier of retinal [56].

The presence of diabetes in rats or intravitreal injection of HMGB1 in normal rats significantly upregulates the levels of mRNAs encoding SDF-1/CXCL12 receptor CXCR4, as well as levels of HIF-1, EGR-1, TK-2, and CXCL12/CXCR4 proteins in the chemokine axis [57]. In diabetic retinopathy, HMGB1 is closely related not only to the apoptosis of nerve cells but also to neovascularization; the latter involves STAT-3 as a downstream effector of HMGB1 to drive angiogenesis [58]. In human retinal microvascular endothelial cells, HMGB1 significantly upregulates levels of IL-1β and reactive oxygen species, as well as expression of NADPH oxidase 2 (Nox2), caspase-3, and PARP-1 [59]. HMGB1 exerts these proinflammatory and angiogenic effects via TNFα and VEGF [57].

Together, these studies demonstrate that HMGB1 helps to drive diabetic retinopathy in two ways. HMGB1 binds to TLR4 and RAGE to trigger nerve cell death. At the same time, HMGB1 triggers release of proangiogenic factors to induce pathological neovascularization (Figure 1).

5. HMGB1 and Uveitis

Inflammation of the iris, ciliary body, vitreous body, retina, or choroid is a typical feature of uveitis. It refers to a group of intraocular inflammatory diseases that arise without a clear infectious trigger and is a leading cause of visual impairment and legal blindness, particularly in the younger population. It contributes to 10–15% of all cases of blindness (defined as central visual acuity of 1/10 or less in the better eye) in developed countries. Such blindness arises mainly as a result of macular edema, ocular hypertonia, or retinal ischemia.

Topical and systemic anti-inflammatory and immunosuppressive medications can completely eliminate inflammatory signs such as keratic precipitates, aqueous flare, miosis, cortical (equatorial) cataracts, vitreal opacification, and lesions of the fundus or optic nerve head. Inflammation can recur after such therapy.

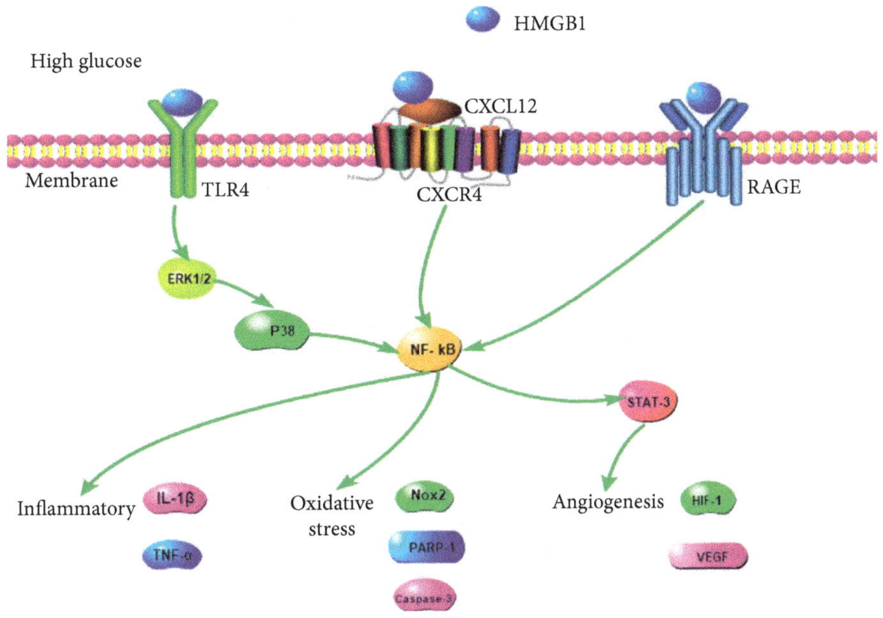

Figure 1: HMGB1 signal by binding to TLR4, CXCR4, and RAGE to moderate BV2 cells, RGC cells, retinal endothelial cells, and retinal microvascular endothelial cells function in PDR. In these cells, HMGB1 binds TLR4 and activates ERK1/2-P38-NF-κB signal pathway. HMGB1 also binds RAGE and upregulated the expression of NF-κB. In human retinal microvascular endothelial cells, HMGB1 binds CXCR4 to activate NF-κB/STAT-3 signal pathway. These three signaling has been implicated in cell inflammatory, oxidative stress, and angiogenesis.

Uveitis is closely related to the immune response associated with T cells. Indeed, experimental autoimmune uveitis is induced by autogenous reactive T-cell injection in rodents [60].

In models of experimental autoimmune uveoretinitis, RAGE is upregulated in inflammatory cells, including macrophages infiltrating the anterior chamber, vitreous cavity, retina, subretinal space, and choroid [61]. HMGB1 activates RAGE, promoting the release of TNF-α, ICAM-1, VCAM-1, and IL-6. HMGB1 also induces CXCL12 release by infiltrating effector T cells [62]. Release of intraocular HMGB1 and CXCL12 at one day after cell transfer may attract inflammatory T cells [63]. Elevated HMGB1 levels may subsequently be associated with the participation of T cells and the retina lesion [62]. Autoimmune uveitis is activated by IRBP-specific T cells [64]. These kinds of T cells were interacted with substantive cells including Müller cells, DCs, astrocytes, and microglia. These cells produce HMGB1 via Fas/FasL-mediated signaling. RIP2 is also involved in HMGB1 release which is deeply related with Fas in uveitis [65]. This suggests the active involvement of the HMGB1-Fas-RIP2 axis in uveitis.

HMGB1 plays an important role in Behcet's disease, one of the forms of uveitis. Although this disease involves elevated HMGB1 levels in serum, these serum levels do not appear to be associated with disease activity or specific organ damage [66]. Neutrophils help drive Behcet's disease, and expression of proinflammatory cytokines such as TNF-α, IFN-γ, and IL-6 in neutrophils is enhanced by extracellular HMGB1, which acts via the NF-κB pathway [6]. These findings suggest that pathogenesis of Behcet's disease is linked to the ability of HMGB1 to activate the NF-κB signaling pathway and thereby stimulate the secretion of inflammatory cytokines (Figure 2).

6. HMGB1 and AMD

AMD is a disease of macular degeneration, which is the main cause of irreversible central vision loss in the elderly in developed countries [67]. This vision loss is thought to involve degeneration of retinal pigment epithelial cells and the overlying photoreceptors, which rely on the retinal pigment epithelium for trophic support.

In a culture model of AMD in which retinal pigment epithelial cells are treated with $NaIO_3$, HMGB1 is released from the nucleus [68]. HMGB1 is also released from the nucleus and secreted by retinal pigment epithelial cells in response to oxidative stress [69]. Depleting HMGB1 from the culture medium inhibits the induction of TNF-α production by retinal pigment epithelial cells [70]. Treating wild-type retinal pigment epithelial cells with poly(I:C) and Z-VAD induces the secretion of substantial amounts of HMGB1, which is completely blocked by deleting the *Rip3* gene from the epithelial cells [70]. The release of HMGB1 from necrotic retinal pigment epithelial cells can increase the generation of IL-6 and TNF-α in macrophages and release of these cytokines from retinal pigment epithelial cells; the cytokine release is inhibited by deleting the *Rip3* gene [71]. In another culture model of AMD in which retinal pigment epithelial cells are treated with poly(I:C) and Z-VAD, NF-κB signaling is directly modulated by HMGB1 and receptor-interacting protein kinase 3 (Rip3) [72].

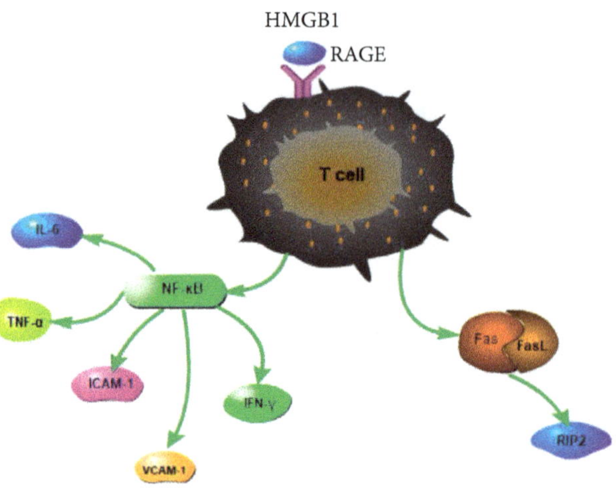

Figure 2: HMGB1 signals by binding to RAGE to activate T-cell cytokine release and Fas/FasL signal pathway in uveitis. In uveoretinitis, HMGB1 binds RAGE and activates NF-κB, promoting the release of TNF-α, IL-6, ICAM-1, and VCAM-1. HMGB1 also can activate Fas/FasL-mediated signaling. In Behcet's disease, expression of proinflammatory cytokines such as TNF-α, IL-6, and IFN-γ in neutrophils is enhanced by extracellular HMGB1, which acts via the NF-κB pathway.

7. HMGB1 and Glaucoma

Acute glaucoma is an ophthalmic emergency that progresses to blindness if untreated. Obstruction of the drainage of the aqueous humour as a result of narrowing or closure of the anterior chamber angle causes high intraocular pressure, which damages the optic nerve and triggers retinal ischemic reperfusion injury and retinal ganglion cell death. In rats, HMGB1 has been linked to glaucoma induced by elevated intraocular pressure [73]. Treating cocultures of retinal ganglion cells and glia with HMGB1 causes ganglion cell death [74].

HMGB1 significantly upregulates cleaved caspase-8 and activates the canonical NLRP3-inflammasome, which induces the processing of IL-1β via pathways dependent on caspase-1 and caspase-8 and leads to retinal ganglion cell death and retinal damage [75]. In a model of retinal IR, HMGB1 appears to upregulate expression of the p65 subunit of p-NF-κB and activate the NF-κB pathway [75]. RAGE and TLR4 mediate the ability of HMGB1 to activate proinflammatory pathways and enhance retinal damage. Treating ganglion cell layer neurons with anti-HMGB1 antibody improves their survival more than knocking out either RAGE or TLR4 expression [73].

8. HMGB1 and Corneal Diseases

One of the most general reasons of microbial keratitis is *pseudomonas aeruginosa* which is widespread in patients with prolonged contact lenses and impaired immunity. Impaired healing of corneal wounds resulting from alkaline burn is also a major cause of impaired vision, and strategies for treatment should be improved in order to avoid keratoplasty. These two kinds of corneal diseases are refractory: so far, there is no effective treatment to cure them. HMGB1 is involved in the pathogenesis of both diseases, and it may have potential as a therapeutic target [76].

In *P. aeruginosa*-induced keratitis, elevated levels of extracellular HMGB1 exacerbate inflammation by stimulating neutrophils via RAGE and TLR pathways [77]. Attenuating HMGB1-mediated disease progression can help treat keratitis. In an animal model of bacterial keratitis, silencing HMBG1 reduces expression of IL-1β, MIP-2, and TNF-α by inhibition of NF-κB as well as the receptors TLR4 and RAGE [78]. Silencing HMGB1 also downregulates CXCL12 and CXCR4 expression. Silencing HMGB1 in a mouse model of *P. aeruginosa*-induced keratitis increases levels of anti-inflammatory cytokines, reduces levels of inflammatory cytokines and neutrophil infiltration, and improves prognosis [79].

HMGB1 also plays an important role in corneal healing and corneal neovascularization. There are two neovascularization processes. One of these processes is the production of endothelial cells from existing blood vessels. The other process is initiated by bone-derived progenitor cells, which then drive endothelial progenitor cells to target sites and into the vascular endothelium. Endothelial cells are also bone-derived progenitor cells. Then, the progenitor cells differentiate into endothelial cells and support the construction of new blood vessels. HMGB1 accelerates corneal neovascularization via TLR4- and RAGE-mediated signaling pathways by activating macrophages, stimulating the secretion of proangiogenic factors and promoting TLR4-induced recruitment of endothelial progenitor cells [80]. Of the three HMBG1 receptors (TLR2, TLR4, and RAGE), HMBG1 appears to act via TLR4 to drive corneal neovascularization. Nuclear HMGB1 interacts with TLR2, which is present in human and rat corneal epithelial cells, but this receptor has no effect on secreted HMGB1 [81]. Silencing TLR2 does not significantly affect corneal neovascularization [81]. Alkaline burns upregulating RAGE and TLR4 in mouse cornea with similar kinetics, but the upregulation of RAGE is small [47] (Figure 3).

9. Conclusion and Perspectives

Although tremendous advances have been made in the study of the structure, release patterns, and receptors of HMGB1, the intracellular signaling pathways that it modulates are still poorly understood, especially its interaction with TLRs and RAGE. This is important to understand in order to clarify how HMGB1 contributes to ocular diseases and develop better therapeutic strategies. HMGB1 antagonists have shown significant therapeutic effects in animal models, but more extensive trials are needed in animals and ultimately in humans. Future studies should also address whether post-translational modifications affect HMGB1-mediated signaling and whether other carrier or binding proteins assist HMGB1 in modulating cytokine activity in ocular diseases.

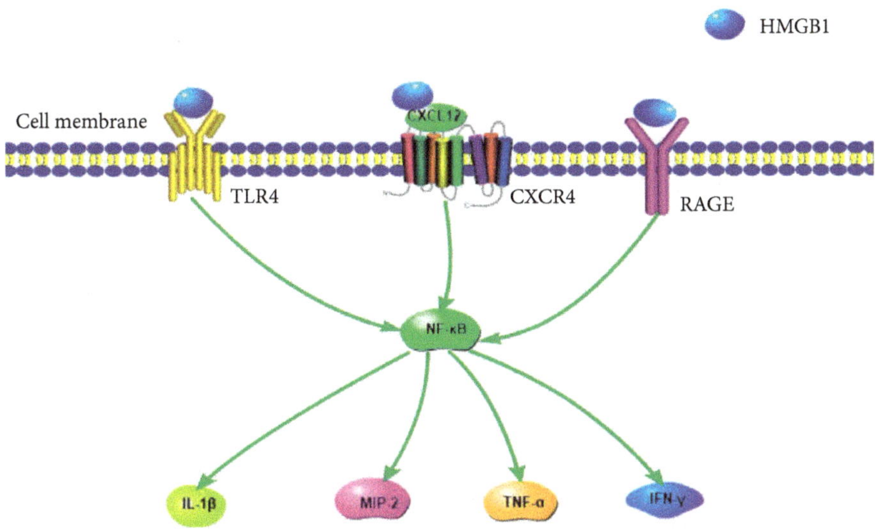

Figure 3: Signaling pathways downstream of RAGE, TLR4, and CXCR4 mediate the effects of HMGB1 in corneal diseases. RAGE signals, TLR4 signals, and CXCR4 signals promote the activation of NF-κB. After the activation of NF-κB, the inflammatory cytokines such as IL-1β, MIP-2, TNF-α, and IFN-γ are released.

This work may solidify HMGB1 as a novel therapeutic approach.

Disclosure

Yi Liu and Guo-Bin Zhuang are co-first authors, and they contributed equally to this work.

Conflicts of Interest

The authors declare that there are no conflicts of interest regarding the publication of this article.

Authors' Contributions

Xuezhi Zhou and Yi Liu conceived and designed the study. Yi Liu and Guo-bin Zhuang wrote this paper. Xuezhi Zhou reviewed and edited the manuscript. All authors read and approved the manuscript.

References

[1] R. Barea, L. Boquete, M. Mazo, and E. Lopez, "System for assisted mobility using eye movements based on electrooculography," *IEEE Transactions on Neural Systems and Rehabilitation Engineering*, vol. 10, no. 4, pp. 209–218, 2002.

[2] D. A. Jabs and J. T. Rosenbaum, "Guidelines for the use of immunosuppressive drugs in patients with ocular inflammatory disorders: recommendations of an expert panel," *American Journal of Ophthalmology*, vol. 131, no. 5, p. 679, 2001.

[3] M. A. Toscano, A. G. Commodaro, J. M. Ilarregui et al., "Galectin-1 suppresses autoimmune retinal disease by promoting concomitant Th2- and T regulatory-mediated anti-inflammatory responses," *Journal of Immunology*, vol. 176, no. 10, pp. 6323–6332, 2006.

[4] V. L. Perez and R. R. Caspi, "Immune mechanisms in inflammatory and degenerative eye disease," *Trends in Immunology*, vol. 36, no. 6, pp. 354–363, 2015.

[5] E. J. Lee, B. R. Brown, E. E. Vance et al., "Mincle activation and the syk/card9 signaling axis Are central to the development of autoimmune disease of the eye," *Journal of Immunology*, vol. 196, no. 7, pp. 3148–3158, 2016.

[6] M. Magna and D. S. Pisetsky, "The role of HMGB1 in the pathogenesis of inflammatory and autoimmune diseases," *Molecular Medicine*, vol. 20, pp. 138–146, 2014.

[7] H. Yang, H. Wang, S. S. Chavan, and U. Andersson, "High mobility group box protein 1 (HMGB1): the prototypical endogenous danger molecule," *Molecular Medicine*, vol. 21, no. 1, pp. S6–S12, 2015.

[8] S. Martinotti, M. Patrone, and E. Ranzato, "Emerging roles for HMGB1 protein in immunity, inflammation, and cancer," *ImmunoTargets and Therapy*, vol. 4, pp. 101–109, 2015.

[9] N. M. Agalave and C. I. Svensson, "Extracellular high-mobility group box 1 protein (HMGB1) as a mediator of persistent pain," *Molecular Medicine*, vol. 20, pp. 569–578, 2015.

[10] D. Musumeci, G. N. Roviello, and D. Montesarchio, "An overview on HMGB1 inhibitors as potential therapeutic agents in HMGB1-related pathologies," *Pharmacology & Therapeutics*, vol. 141, no. 3, pp. 347–357, 2014.

[11] Q. Chen, X. Guan, X. Zuo, J. Wang, and W. Yin, "The role of high mobility group box 1 (HMGB1) in the pathogenesis of kidney diseases," *Acta Pharmaceutica Sinica B*, vol. 6, no. 3, pp. 183–188, 2016.

[12] F. C. Wang, J. X. Pei, J. Zhu et al., "Overexpression of HMGB1 A-box reduced lipopolysaccharide-induced intestinal inflammation via HMGB1/TLR4 signaling in vitro," *World Journal of Gastroenterology*, vol. 21, no. 25, pp. 7764–7776, 2015.

[13] S. Tancharoen, T. Tengrungsun, T. Suddhasthira et al., "Overexpression of receptor for advanced glycation end products and high-mobility group box 1 in human dental pulp inflammation," *Mediators of Inflammation*, vol. 2014, Article ID 754069, 13 pages, 2014.

[14] W. Wan, L. Cao, R. Khanabdali, B. Kalionis, X. Tai, and S. Xia, "The emerging role of HMGB1 in neuropathic pain: a potential therapeutic target for neuroinflammation," *Journal of Immunology Research*, vol. 2016, Article ID 6430423, 9 pages, 2016.

[15] H. Saidi, M. Bras, P. Formaglio et al., "HMGB1 is involved in IFN-alpha production and TRAIL expression by HIV-1-exposed plasmacytoid dendritic cells: impact of the cross-talk with NK cells," *PLoS Pathogens*, vol. 12, no. 2, Article ID e1005407, 2016.

[16] C. Semino, G. Angelini, A. Poggi, and A. Rubartelli, "NK/iDC interaction results in IL-18 secretion by DCs at the synaptic cleft followed by NK cell activation and release of the DC maturation factor HMGB1," *Blood*, vol. 106, no. 2, pp. 609–616, 2005.

[17] L. Ulloa and D. Messmer, "High-mobility group box 1 (HMGB1) protein: friend and foe," *Cytokine & Growth Factor Reviews*, vol. 17, no. 3, pp. 189–201, 2006.

[18] S. Zhang, J. Zhong, P. Yang, F. Gong, and C. Y. Wang, "HMGB1, an innate alarmin, in the pathogenesis of type 1 diabetes," *International Journal of Clinical and Experimental Pathology*, vol. 3, no. 1, pp. 24–38, 2009.

[19] H. E. Harris, U. Andersson, and D. S. Pisetsky, "HMGB1: a multifunctional alarmin driving autoimmune and inflammatory disease," *Nature Reviews Rheumatology*, vol. 8, no. 4, pp. 195–202, 2012.

[20] U. Andersson and H. E. Harris, "The role of HMGB1 in the pathogenesis of rheumatic disease," *Biochimica et Biophysica Acta (BBA)—Gene Regulatory Mechanisms*, vol. 1799, no. 1-2, pp. 141–148, 2010.

[21] S. L. Yu, C. K. Wong, and L. S. Tam, "The alarmin functions of high-mobility group box-1 and IL-33 in the pathogenesis of systemic lupus erythematosus," *Expert Review of Clinical Immunology*, vol. 9, no. 8, pp. 739–749, 2013.

[22] L. M. Bellussi, S. Cocca, L. Chen, F. M. Passali, C. Sarafoleanu, and D. Passali, "Rhinosinusal inflammation and high mobility group box 1 protein: a new target for therapy," *ORL*, vol. 78, no. 2, pp. 77–85, 2016.

[23] H. Wang, O. Bloom, M. Zhang et al., "HMG-1 as a late mediator of endotoxin lethality in mice," *Science*, vol. 285, no. 5425, pp. 248–251, 1999.

[24] B. Wittemann, G. Neuer, H. Michels, H. Truckenbrodt, and F. A. Bautz, "Autoantibodies to nonhistone chromosomal proteins HMG-1 and HMG-2 in sera of patients with juvenile rheumatoid arthritis," *Arthritis & Rheumatism*, vol. 33, no. 9, pp. 1378–1383, 1990.

[25] L. M. Ayer, R. L. Rubin, G. H. Dixon, and M. J. Fritzler, "Antibodies to HMG proteins in patients with drug-induced autoimmunity," *Arthritis & Rheumatism*, vol. 37, no. 1, pp. 98–103, 1994.

[26] L. Campana, L. Bosurgi, and P. Rovere-Querini, "HMGB1: a two-headed signal regulating tumor progression and immunity," *Current Opinion in Immunology*, vol. 20, no. 5, pp. 518–523, 2008.

[27] M. E. Bianchi and A. A. Manfredi, "High-mobility group box 1 (HMGB1) protein at the crossroads between innate and adaptive immunity," *Immunological Reviews*, vol. 220, no. 1, pp. 35–46, 2007.

[28] J. R. Klune, R. Dhupar, J. Cardinal, T. R. Billiar, and A. Tsung, "HMGB1: endogenous danger signaling," *Molecular Medicine*, vol. 14, no. 7-8, pp. 476–484, 2008.

[29] W. Huang, Y. Tang, and L. Li, "HMGB1, a potent proinflammatory cytokine in sepsis," *Cytokine*, vol. 51, no. 2, pp. 119–126, 2010.

[30] N. K. Sun and C. C. Chao, "The cytokine activity of HMGB1--extracellular escape of the nuclear protein," *Chang Gung Medical Journal*, vol. 28, no. 10, pp. 673–682, 2005.

[31] H. Schierbeck, P. Lundback, K. Palmblad et al., "Monoclonal anti-HMGB1 (high mobility group box chromosomal protein 1) antibody protection in two experimental arthritis models," *Molecular Medicine*, vol. 17, no. 9-10, pp. 1039–1044, 2011.

[32] A. Tsung, S. Tohme, and T. R. Billiar, "High-mobility group box-1 in sterile inflammation," *Journal of Internal Medicine*, vol. 276, no. 5, pp. 425–443, 2014.

[33] I. E. Dumitriu, P. Baruah, A. A. Manfredi, M. E. Bianchi, and P. Rovere-Querini, "HMGB1: guiding immunity from within," *Trends in Immunology*, vol. 26, no. 7, pp. 381–387, 2005.

[34] N. T. Sebastian, E. M. Bystry, N. A. Becker, and L. J. Maher III, "Enhancement of DNA flexibility in vitro and in vivo by HMGB box A proteins carrying box B residues," *Biochemistry*, vol. 48, no. 10, pp. 2125–2134, 2009.

[35] K. T. Bauerle, E. Kamau, and A. Grove, "Interactions between N- and C-terminal domains of the Saccharomyces cerevisiae high-mobility group protein HMO1 are required for DNA bending," *Biochemistry*, vol. 45, no. 11, pp. 3635–3645, 2006.

[36] M. E. Churchill, J. Klass, and D. L. Zoetewey, "Structural analysis of HMGD-DNA complexes reveals influence of intercalation on sequence selectivity and DNA bending," *Journal of Molecular Biology*, vol. 403, no. 1, pp. 88–102, 2010.

[37] D. S. Pisetsky, H. Erlandsson-Harris, and U. Andersson, "High-mobility group box protein 1 (HMGB1): an alarmin mediating the pathogenesis of rheumatic disease," *Arthritis Research & Therapy*, vol. 10, no. 3, p. 209, 2008.

[38] H. Yang, M. Ochani, J. Li et al., "Reversing established sepsis with antagonists of endogenous high-mobility group box 1," *Proceedings of the National Academy of Sciences*, vol. 101, no. 1, pp. 296–301, 2004.

[39] J. P. Bidwell, J. Yang, and A. G. Robling, "Is HMGB1 an osteocyte alarmin?," *Journal of Cellular Biochemistry*, vol. 103, no. 6, pp. 1671–1680, 2008.

[40] H. Wang, T. Lei, J. Liu, M. Li, H. Nan, and Q. Liu, "A nuclear factor of high mobility group box protein in Toxoplasma gondii," *PLoS One*, vol. 9, no. 11, Article ID e111993, 2014.

[41] Q. Wang, M. Zeng, W. Wang, and J. Tang, "The HMGB1 acidic tail regulates HMGB1 DNA binding specificity by a unique mechanism," *Biochemical and Biophysical Research Communications*, vol. 360, no. 1, pp. 14–19, 2007.

[42] R. Chen, W. Hou, Q. Zhang, R. Kang, X. G. Fan, and D. Tang, "Emerging role of high-mobility group box 1 (HMGB1) in liver diseases," *Molecular Medicine*, vol. 19, no. 1, pp. 357–366, 2013.

[43] S. A. Lee, M. S. Kwak, S. Kim, and J. S. Shin, "The role of high mobility group box 1 in innate immunity," *Yonsei Medical Journal*, vol. 55, no. 5, pp. 1165–1176, 2014.

[44] H. Rauvala and A. Rouhiainen, "RAGE as a receptor of HMGB1 (Amphoterin): roles in health and disease," *Current Molecular Medicine*, vol. 7, no. 8, pp. 725–734, 2007.

[45] G. P. Sims, D. C. Rowe, S. T. Rietdijk, R. Herbst, and A. J. Coyle, "HMGB1 and RAGE in inflammation and cancer," *Annual Review of Immunology*, vol. 28, no. 1, pp. 367–388, 2010.

[46] G. Dvoriantchikova, E. Hernandez, J. Grant, A. R. Santos, H. Yang, and D. Ivanov, "The high-mobility group box-1 nuclear factor mediates retinal injury after ischemia reperfusion," *Investigative Opthalmology & Visual Science*, vol. 52, no. 10, pp. 7187–7194, 2011.

[47] S. Yang, T. S. Yang, F. Wang, and S. B. Su, "High-mobility group box-1-Toll-Like receptor 4 axis mediates the recruitment of endothelial progenitor cells in alkali-induced corneal neovascularization," *International Immunopharmacology*, vol. 28, no. 1, pp. 450–458, 2015.

[48] T. A. Ciulla, A. G. Amador, and B. Zinman, "Diabetic retinopathy and diabetic macular edema: pathophysiology, screening, and novel therapies," *Diabetes Care*, vol. 26, no. 9, pp. 2653–2664, 2003.
[49] A. P. Adamis and A. J. Berman, "Immunological mechanisms in the pathogenesis of diabetic retinopathy," *Seminars in Immunopathology*, vol. 30, no. 2, pp. 65–84, 2008.
[50] S. Gardella, C. Andrei, D. Ferrera et al., "The nuclear protein HMGB1 is secreted by monocytes via a non-classical, vesicle-mediated secretory pathway," *EMBO Reports*, vol. 3, no. 10, pp. 995–1001, 2002.
[51] A. M. El-Asrar, M. I. Nawaz, D. Kangave et al., "High-mobility group box-1 and biomarkers of inflammation in the vitreous from patients with proliferative diabetic retinopathy," *Molecular Vision*, vol. 17, pp. 1829–1838, 2011.
[52] A. M. El-Asrar, L. Missotten, and K. Geboes, "Expression of high-mobility groups box-1/receptor for advanced glycation end products/osteopontin/early growth response-1 pathway in proliferative vitreoretinal epiretinal membranes," *Molecular Vision*, vol. 17, pp. 508–518, 2011.
[53] A. M. Abu El-Asrar, K. Alam, M. Garcia-Ramirez et al., "Association of HMGB1 with oxidative stress markers and regulators in PDR," *Molecular Vision*, vol. 23, pp. 853–871, 2017.
[54] S. H. Zhu, B. Q. Liu, M. J. Hao et al., "Paeoniflorin suppressed high glucose-induced retinal microglia MMP-9 expression and inflammatory response via inhibition of TLR4/NF-kappaB pathway through upregulation of SOCS3 in diabetic retinopathy," *Inflammation*, vol. 40, no. 5, pp. 1475–1486, 2017.
[55] J. J. Lee, C. C. Hsiao, I. H. Yang et al., "High-mobility group box 1 protein is implicated in advanced glycation end products-induced vascular endothelial growth factor A production in the rat retinal ganglion cell line RGC-5," *Molecular Vision*, vol. 18, pp. 838–850, 2012.
[56] S. Jiang and X. Chen, "HMGB1 siRNA can reduce damage to retinal cells induced by high glucose in vitro and in vivo," *Drug Design, Development and Therapy*, vol. 11, pp. 783–795, 2017.
[57] A. M. Abu El-Asrar, G. Mohammad, M. I. Nawaz, and M. M. Siddiquei, "High-mobility group box-1 modulates the expression of inflammatory and angiogenic signaling pathways in diabetic retina," *Current Eye Research*, vol. 40, no. 11, pp. 1141–1152, 2015.
[58] G. Mohammad, D. Jomar, M. M. Siddiquei, K. Alam, and A. M. Abu El-Asrar, "High-mobility group box-1 protein mediates the regulation of signal transducer and activator of transcription-3 in the diabetic retina and in human retinal muller cells," *Ophthalmic Research*, vol. 57, no. 3, pp. 150–160, 2017.
[59] G. Mohammad, K. Alam, M. I. Nawaz, M. M. Siddiquei, A. Mousa, and A. M. Abu El-Asrar, "Mutual enhancement between high-mobility group box-1 and NADPH oxidase-derived reactive oxygen species mediates diabetes-induced upregulation of retinal apoptotic markers," *Journal of Physiology and Biochemistry*, vol. 71, no. 3, pp. 359–372, 2015.
[60] H. Shao, H. J. Kaplan, and D. Sun, "Major histocompatibility complex molecules on parenchymal cells of the target organ protect against autoimmune disease," *Chemical Immunology and Allergy*, vol. 92, pp. 94–104, 2007.
[61] T. Watanabe, H. Keino, Y. Sato, A. Kudo, H. Kawakami, and A. A. Okada, "High mobility group box protein-1 in experimental autoimmune uveoretinitis," *Investigative Opthalmology & Visual Science*, vol. 50, no. 5, pp. 2283–2290, 2009.
[62] J. Yun, G. Jiang, Y. Wang et al., "The HMGB1-CXCL12 complex promotes inflammatory cell infiltration in uveitogenic T cell-induced chronic experimental autoimmune uveitis," *Frontiers in Immunology*, vol. 8, p. 142, 2017.
[63] G. Jiang, D. Sun, H. Yang, Q. Lu, H. J. Kaplan, and H. Shao, "HMGB1 is an early and critical mediator in an animal model of uveitis induced by IRBP-specific T cells," *Journal of Leukocyte Biology*, vol. 95, no. 4, pp. 599–607, 2014.
[64] G. Jiang, Y. Ke, D. Sun, G. Han, H. J. Kaplan, and H. Shao, "Reactivation of uveitogenic T cells by retinal astrocytes derived from experimental autoimmune uveitis-prone B10RIII mice," *Investigative Opthalmology & Visual Science*, vol. 49, no. 1, pp. 282–289, 2008.
[65] G. Jiang, Y. Wang, J. Yun et al., "HMGB1 release triggered by the interaction of live retinal cells and uveitogenic T cells is Fas/FasL activation-dependent," *Journal of Neuroinflammation*, vol. 12, no. 1, p. 179, 2015.
[66] A. W. de Souza, S. F. Perazzio, N. R. de Franca et al., "High mobility group box 1 serum levels are increased in Behcet's disease, but not associated with disease activity or disease manifestations," *Rheumatology (Oxford)*, vol. 54, no. 12, pp. 2151–2155, 2015.
[67] D. S. Friedman, B. J. O'Colmain, B. Munoz et al., "Prevalence of age-related macular degeneration in the United States," *Archives of ophthalmology*, vol. 122, no. 4, pp. 564–572, 2004.
[68] J. Hanus, C. Anderson, D. Sarraf, J. Ma, and S. Wang, "Retinal pigment epithelial cell necroptosis in response to sodium iodate," *Cell Death Discovery*, vol. 2, no. 1, article 16054, 2016.
[69] J. Hanus, C. Anderson, and S. Wang, "RPE necroptosis in response to oxidative stress and in AMD," *Ageing Research Reviews*, vol. 24, pp. 286–298, 2015.
[70] J. Hanus, H. Zhang, Z. Wang, Q. Liu, Q. Zhou, and S. Wang, "Induction of necrotic cell death by oxidative stress in retinal pigment epithelial cells," *Cell Death & Disease*, vol. 4, no. 12, p. e965, 2013.
[71] A. Kaczmarek, P. Vandenabeele, and D. V. Krysko, "Necroptosis: the release of damage-associated molecular patterns and its physiological relevance," *Immunity*, vol. 38, no. 2, pp. 209–223, 2013.
[72] Y. Murakami, H. Matsumoto, M. Roh et al., "Programmed necrosis, not apoptosis, is a key mediator of cell loss and DAMP-mediated inflammation in dsRNA-induced retinal degeneration," *Cell Death & Differentiation*, vol. 21, no. 2, pp. 270–277, 2014.
[73] U. Andersson and K. J. Tracey, "HMGB1 is a therapeutic target for sterile inflammation and infection," *Annual Review of Immunology*, vol. 29, no. 1, pp. 139–162, 2011.
[74] M. Schallenberg, V. Prokosch, and S. Thanos, "Regulation of retinal proteome by topical antiglaucomatous eye drops in an inherited glaucoma rat model," *PLoS One*, vol. 7, no. 7, Article ID e33593, 2012.
[75] W. Chi, H. Chen, F. Li, Y. Zhu, W. Yin, and Y. Zhuo, "HMGB1 promotes the activation of NLRP3 and caspase-8 inflammasomes via NF-kappaB pathway in acute glaucoma," *Journal of Neuroinflammation*, vol. 12, no. 1, p. 137, 2015.
[76] S. A. Ekanayaka, S. A. McClellan, R. P. Barrett, and L. D. Hazlett, "Topical glycyrrhizin is therapeutic for *Pseudomonas aeruginosa* keratitis," *Journal of Ocular Pharmacology and Therapeutics*, vol. 34, no. 3, pp. 239–249, 2018.
[77] S. A. Ekanayaka, S. A. McClellan, R. P. Barrett, S. Kharotia, and L. D. Hazlett, "Glycyrrhizin reduces HMGB1 and bacterial load in *Pseudomonas aeruginosa* keratitis," *Investigative Opthalmology & Visual Science*, vol. 57, no. 13, pp. 5799–5809, 2016.

[78] S. McClellan, X. Jiang, R. Barrett, and L. D. Hazlett, "High-mobility group box 1: a novel target for treatment of *Pseudomonas aeruginosa* keratitis," *Journal of Immunology*, vol. 194, no. 4, pp. 1776–1787, 2015.

[79] L. D. Hazlett, S. A. McClellan, and S. A. Ekanayaka, "Decreasing HMGB1 levels improves outcome of *Pseudomonas aeruginosa* keratitis in mice," *Journal of Rare Diseases Research & Treatment*, vol. 1, no. 1, pp. 36–39, 2016.

[80] S. Yang, L. Xu, T. Yang, and F. Wang, "High-mobility group box-1 and its role in angiogenesis," *Journal of Leukocyte Biology*, vol. 95, no. 4, pp. 563–574, 2014.

[81] Q. Lin, X. P. Yang, D. Fang et al., "High-mobility group box-1 mediates toll-like receptor 4-dependent angiogenesis," *Arteriosclerosis, Thrombosis, and Vascular Biology*, vol. 31, no. 5, pp. 1024–1032, 2011.

8

Mineralocorticoid Receptor Antagonist Treatment for Steroid-Induced Central Serous Chorioretinopathy Patients with Continuous Systemic Steroid Treatment

Jin Young Kim,[1] Ju Byung Chae,[2] Jisoo Kim,[2] and Dong Yoon Kim[2]

[1] *Department of Ophthalmology, Jeju National University Hospital, Jeju National University School of Medicine, Jeju, Republic of Korea*
[2] *Department of Ophthalmology, Chungbuk National University Hospital, College of Medicine, Chungbuk National University, Cheongju, Republic of Korea*

Correspondence should be addressed to Dong Yoon Kim; umlover9@gmail.com

Jin Young Kim and Ju Byung Chae contributed equally to this work.

Academic Editor: Lawrence S. Morse

Purpose. To investigate the effectiveness of mineralocorticoid receptor (MR) antagonist in patients with steroid-induced central serous chorioretinopathy (CSC). *Methods.* A retrospective review was conducted of steroid-induced CSC patients who were treated with the MR antagonist spironolactone 50 mg once per day for at least 1 month. The primary outcome measure was complete resolution rate of subretinal fluid (SRF) after spironolactone treatment. Secondary outcomes included central subfield thickness (CST), subfoveal choroidal thickness (SFCT), and best-corrected visual acuity (BCVA) changes after spironolactone treatment. *Results.* Seventeen eyes from 15 patients were included in this study. Conditions warranting chronic systemic steroid use were myasthenia gravis (6/15, 40%), glomerulonephritis (5/15, 33.3%), and organ transplantation (4/15, 26.7%). Mean symptom duration of CSC was 4.00 ± 3.04 months. After spironolactone treatment, 14 eyes (82.4%) showed complete resolution of SRF ($P < 0.001$) without discontinuation of systemic steroid. CST and BCVA were significantly improved after spironolactone treatment. SFCT was significantly decreased after spironolactone treatment. No patients experienced electrolyte imbalance after spironolactone treatment. *Conclusion.* MR antagonist treatment may be a therapeutic option for steroid-induced CSC patients. This treatment modality may be especially beneficial for steroid-induced CSC patients who cannot discontinue steroid medication due to systemic conditions.

1. Introduction

Central serous chorioretinopathy (CSC) is characterized by neurosensory retinal detachment; it is a self-limiting disease that usually has a good visual prognosis. Male sex, type A personality, abnormal coagulation and platelet aggregation, and infection with *Helicobacter pylori* are considered relevant risk factors for CSC [1–7].

Endogenous or exogenous steroid therapy is a significant risk factor for CSC [8]. Elevated serum glucocorticoid hormone levels are caused by systemic or endogenous steroids that act by binding to the glucocorticoid receptor (GR) and to the mineralocorticoid receptor (MR). MR activation by steroids leads to the expression of proteins regulating ion and water transport, resulting in the reabsorption of sodium [9, 10]. MRs are also present in retinal pigment epithelium (RPE) cells and in endothelial cells of the retinal and choroidal vessels [11]. Activation of MRs in the choroidal vessel by steroids causes choroid vessel dilation and leakage, resulting in choroidal hyperpermeability, which is known to be a major pathogenic factor in CSC [11]. Experimental studies have shown that intravitreal injection of glucocorticoid in rat eyes induces choroidal enlargement. Increased choroidal hyperpermeability due to MR activation by steroids can be blocked by MR antagonists. Therefore, MR antagonists are attracting interest as therapeutic agents for CSC; several experimental studies on the effects of MR antagonists have recently been published and have demonstrated favorable therapeutic effects of MR antagonists in CSC [12–18].

We speculate that the therapeutic effect of MR antagonists on CSC may be exaggerated in the case of steroid-induced CSC. However, there have been no studies on the therapeutic effects of MR antagonists on steroid-induced CSC. Therefore, we investigated the effectiveness of MR antagonist therapy in patients with steroid-induced CSC.

2. Methods

The medical records of steroid-induced CSC patients who were diagnosed and treated at Chungbuk National University Hospital, Cheongju, Korea, from March 2015 through December 2017 were reviewed. This study was approved by the Institutional Review Board of Chungbuk National University Hospital and followed the tenets of the Declaration of Helsinki. The inclusion criteria were as follows: (1) definite presence of subretinal fluid (SRF) in the fovea on spectral domain optical coherence tomography (SD-OCT) at baseline; (2) patients taking systemic steroids for more than 1 month; (3) evidence of diffuse and/or focal leakage on fluorescein angiography (FA); (4) CSC treatment by MR antagonist; and (5) no prior treatment, such as intravitreal bevacizumab injection (IVB) or half-fluence photodynamic therapy (H-PDT) for CSC. Patients with choroidal neovascularization or other macular disease, other ophthalmologic diseases that can affect vision, and active intraocular inflammation or infection were excluded.

2.1. Ophthalmic Examination. A complete ophthalmologic examination was performed at baseline. Best-corrected visual acuity (BCVA) was measured with a Snellen chart and converted to a logMAR scale. Medical histories, including symptom duration, concomitant medication, and other medical illness, were also collected from the medical records. Every patient underwent fundus photography, FA, and SD-OCT. A Heidelberg Retina Angiograph 2 (Heidelberg Engineering, Heidelberg, Germany) was used to obtain FA and indocyanine green angiographs (ICGA). ICGAs were used to assess choroidal hyperpermeability and to rule out choroidal neovascularization or polypoidal choroidal vasculopathy. A Spectralis ophthalmic imaging platform (Heidelberg Engineering, Heidelberg, Germany) was used to acquire SD-OCT images, and a custom $20^\circ \times 20^\circ$ volume acquisition protocol was employed to obtain a set of high-speed scans from each eye. The integrated follow-up mode of the device was used to acquire scans of the same retinal areas at each visit. Central subfield thickness (CST) was automatically calculated as the average retinal thickness within a central circle having a 500 μm radius. We also manually measured the subfoveal choroid thickness (SFCT) by using the enhanced depth image (EDI) OCT image [19].

During each visit, ophthalmic examinations were performed, including the BCVA measurement, applanation tonometry, slit-lamp examination, dilated fundus examination, fundus photography, and SD-OCT.

Table 1: Demographics of included patients.

Number of patients (eyes)	15 (17)
Age (years)	49.24 ± 7.70
Sex (male/female)	10/5
Symptom duration (months)	4.00 ± 3.04
Follow-up duration (months)	17.09 ± 6.40
Steroid dose (mg)	15.59 ± 5.58
Steroid use duration (months)	8.94 ± 9.03
Spironolactone dose (mg)	50
Spironolactone use duration (months)	2.59 ± 1.19
Underlying disease	
Myasthenia gravis (%)	8 (47.1)
Glomerular nephritis (%)	5 (29.4)
After organ transplantation (%)	4 (23.5)

2.2. Mineralocorticoid Antagonist Treatment. Steroid-induced CSC patients were treated with systemic spironolactone 50 mg once per day until SRF resolved. Considering the possible side effects that may occur after the use of the drug, if the SRF did not decrease despite use of spironolactone for 1 month, the patient was regarded as a nonresponder, and drug use was discontinued. Spironolactone is a potassium-preserving diuretic and may cause medical side effects such as electrolyte abnormality [20]. We performed serum electrolyte examination before treatment and every month during treatment. If an imbalance occurred in serum electrolyte levels, spironolactone treatment was discontinued.

2.3. Statistical Analysis. The SPSS version 21.0 statistical software package (SPSS, Inc., Chicago, IL, USA) was used for statistical analysis. The paired t-test was used to compare BCVA, retinal thickness, and SFCT changes after spironolactone treatment. The McNemar test was used to compare eyes with SRF before and after spironolactone treatment. In all analyses, a value of $P < 0.05$ was considered statistically significant.

3. Results

3.1. Clinical Characteristics. Seventeen steroid-induced CSC eyes from 15 patients were included in this study. The participants comprised 10 males and 5 females with a mean age of 49.24 ± 7.70 years. Symptom duration prior to treatment and mean follow-up duration were 4.00 ± 3.04 months and 17.09 ± 6.40 months, respectively. Conditions warranting chronic systemic steroid use were myasthenia gravis (6/15, 40%), glomerulonephritis (5/15, 33.3%), and organ transplantation (4/15, 26.7%). The mean daily dose of systemic prednisolone and mean steroid use duration were 15.59 ± 5.58 mg and 8.94 ± 9.03 months, respectively (Table 1). The spironolactone dose was 50 mg per day and the mean duration of spironolactone treatment was 2.59 ± 1.19 months.

3.2. Optical Coherence Tomographic Findings Change after Spironolactone Treatment. Figure 1 shows the percentage of eyes with SRF before and after spironolactone treatment.

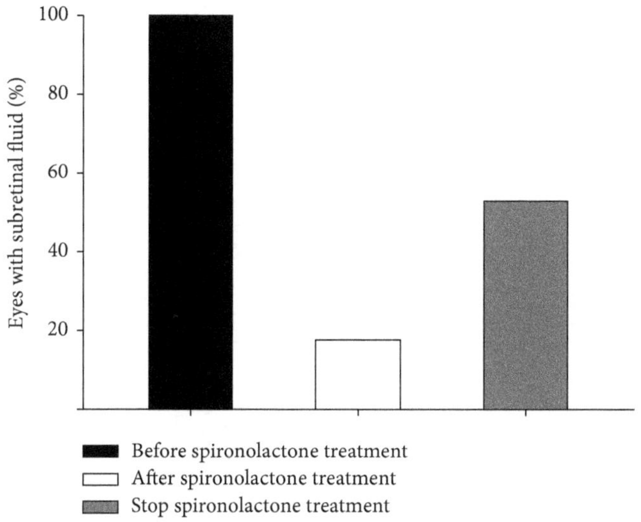

FIGURE 1: Eyes with subretinal fluid (SRF) before and after spironolactone treatment. After spironolactone treatment, 14 eyes (82.4%) showed complete resolution of the SRF ($P < 0.001$). However, among 14 eyes with complete resolution of SRF, SRF reappeared after discontinuation of spironolactone treatment in 9 eyes (64.3%, $P < 0.001$).

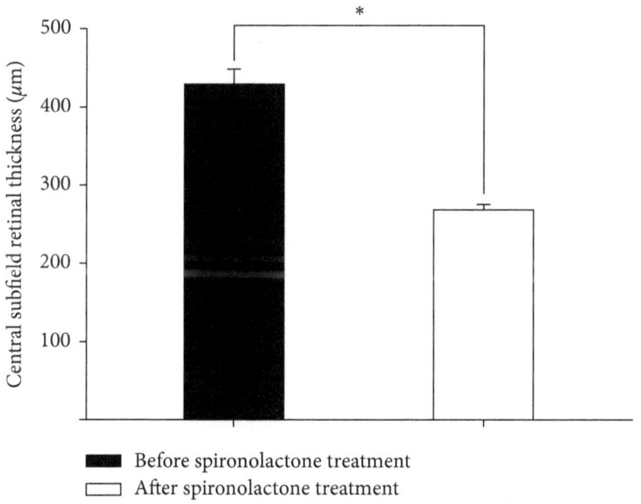

FIGURE 2: Central subfield thickness (CST) changes after spironolactone treatment. The mean CST was significantly decreased after spironolactone treatment ($428.94 \pm 77.70\,\mu$m versus $268.47 \pm 28.53\,\mu$m, $^*P < 0.001$).

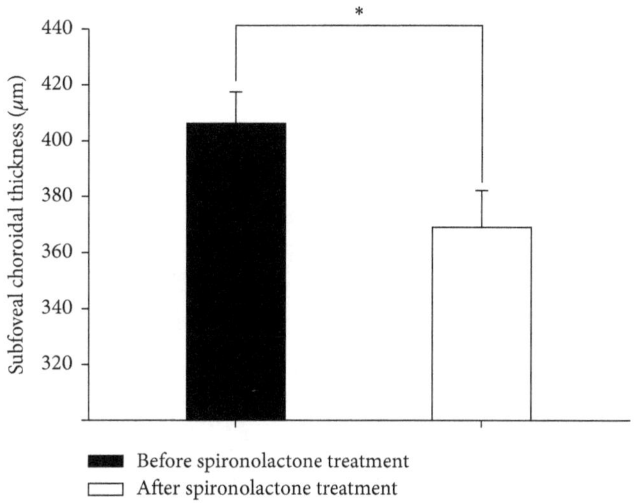

FIGURE 3: Subfoveal choroidal thickness (SFCT) changes after spironolactone treatment. The mean SFCT was significantly decreased after spironolactone treatment ($406.06 \pm 47.08\,\mu$m versus $368.94 \pm 54.29\,\mu$m, $^*P < 0.005$).

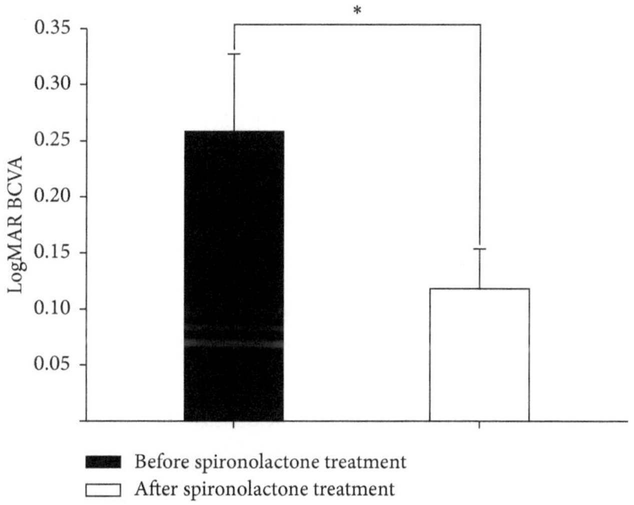

FIGURE 4: Best-corrected visual acuity (BCVA) changes after spironolactone treatment. LogMAR BCVA was significantly improved after spironolactone treatment (before, 0.280 ± 0.068; after, 0.146 ± 0.035, $^*P = 0.021$).

After spironolactone treatment, 14 eyes (82.4%) showed complete resolution of the SRF ($P < 0.001$). However, after discontinuation of spironolactone treatment, SRF reappeared in nine eyes (64.3%, $P < 0.001$). Mean time interval between discontinuation of spironolactone and recurrence was 1.55 ± 0.72 months. And, among eyes with recurrence, 6 eyes were retreated with spironolactone. After retreatment of spironolactone, SRF of 5 eyes (83.3%) was completely resolved.

The mean CST decreased significantly after spironolactone treatment ($428.94 \pm 77.70\,\mu$m versus $268.47 \pm 28.53\,\mu$m, $P < 0.001$) (Figure 2). The mean SFCT also decreased significantly after spironolactone treatment ($406.06 \pm 47.08\,\mu$m versus $368.94 \pm 54.29\,\mu$m, $P = 0.034$) (Figure 3).

Among 17 eyes, three eyes still showed subretinal fluid at the fovea. However, after spironolactone treatment, CST ($410.00 \pm 46.89\,\mu$m versus $312.00 \pm 14.42\,\mu$m, $P = 0.035$) of these 3 eyes was decreased, while the BCVA was not improved significantly (0.27 ± 0.15 versus 0.21 ± 0.20; $P = 0.188$). Considering CST decrease, these three eyes could be regarded as spironolactone responder.

3.3. Changes in BCVA after Spironolactone Treatment. Figure 4 shows the BCVA changes after resolution of CSC. LogMAR BCVA significantly improved after spironolactone

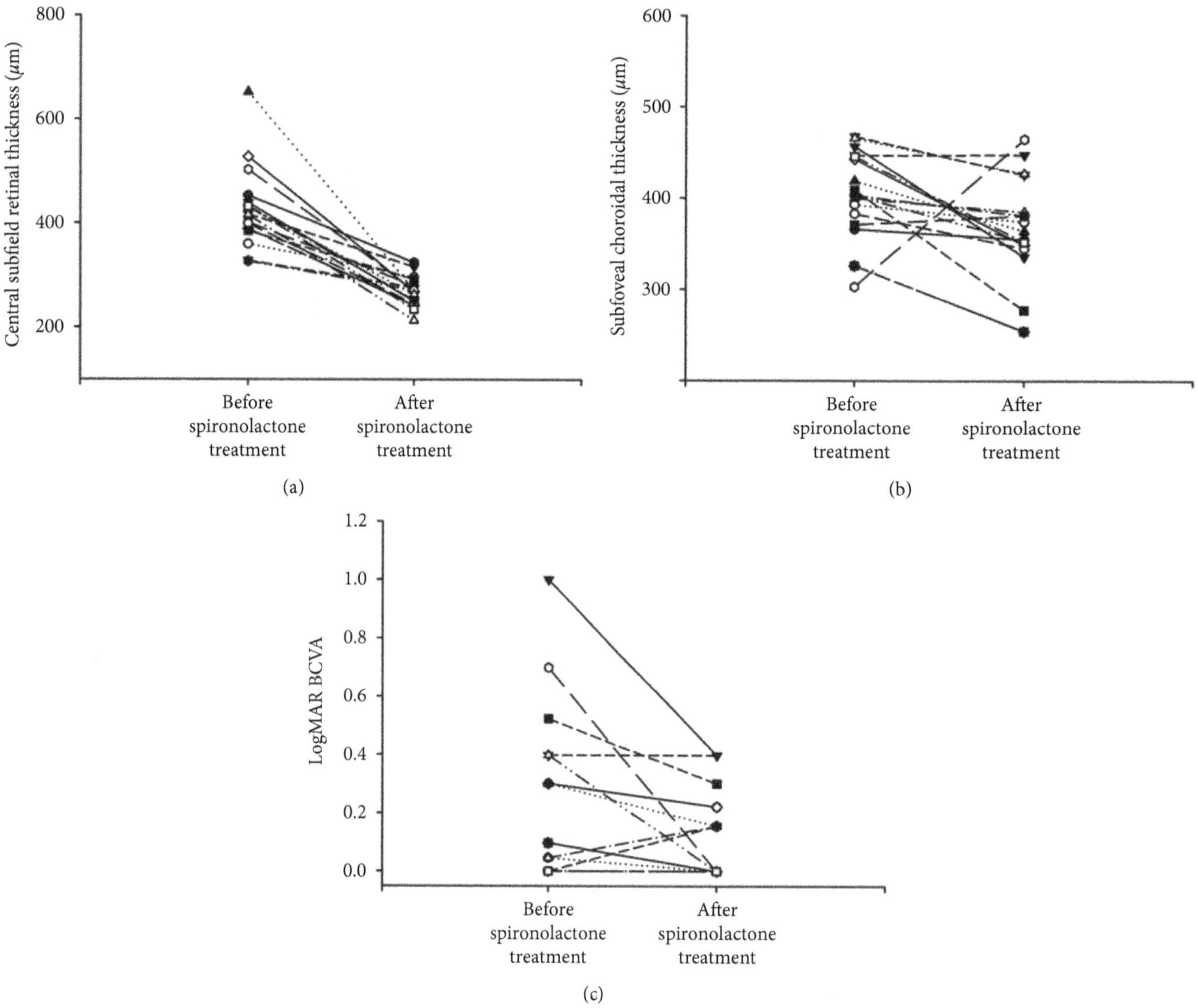

Figure 5: (a) Central subfield thickness (CST), (b) subfoveal choroidal thickness (SFCT), and (c) best-corrected visual acuity (BCVA) changes in each spironolactone-treated eye.

treatment (before, 0.280 ± 0.068; after, 0.146 ± 0.035; $P = 0.021$).

Figure 5 shows CST, SFCT, and BCVA change in each spironolactone-treated eye. And Figure 6 shows a representative case of steroid-induced CSC. The patient, a 59-year-old man, underwent kidney transplantation. Three months after transplantation, he was referred to the ophthalmologic clinic for visual disturbance of his right eye. Visual acuity of his right eye was 0.4, and SD-OCT examination revealed a bullous SRF (Figure 6(a)). At that time, steroid 20 mg was used to prevent graft rejection. We diagnosed steroid-induced CSC and started spironolactone treatment. Two months after spironolactone treatment, the SRF was completely resolved in the patient's right eye, and the visual acuity of his right eye improved from 0.4 to 1.0 without discontinuation of systemic steroid use (Figure 6(b)). No spironolactone treatment-related electrolyte imbalance was observed.

3.4. Serum Level Changes of Potassium and Creatinine after Spironolactone Treatment. Table 2 presents serum level changes in potassium and creatinine after spironolactone treatment. There were no significant changes in serum potassium or creatinine levels after spironolactone treatment. Moreover, there were no cases in which drug therapy had to be discontinued because of an electrolyte imbalance or spironolactone-related side effect.

4. Discussion

The primary finding of this study is that CST and BCVA significantly improved after spironolactone treatment in patients with steroid-induced CSC. In most patients, SRF was completely resolved after spironolactone treatment. However, resolved SRF recurred after discontinuation of spironolactone treatment. No patients experienced electrolyte imbalances after spironolactone treatment.

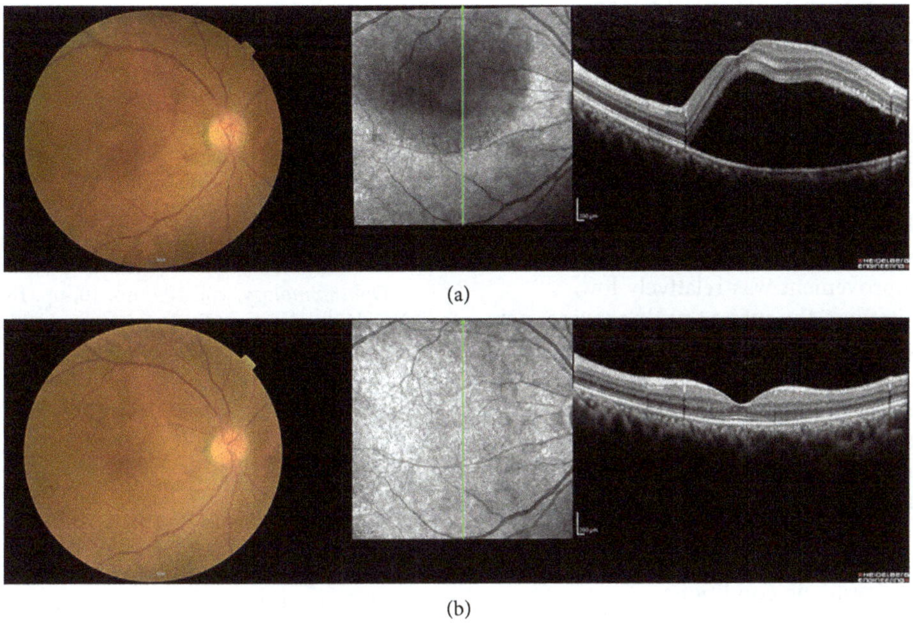

FIGURE 6: Representative case of steroid-induced CSC patient.

The most conventional therapeutic approach for steroid-induced CSC patients is discontinuation of regional or systemic steroids. After discontinuation of steroid use, most cases of CSC resolve without additional treatment. However, in certain patients who have received organ transplants or others requiring chronic immunosuppression, continued use of corticosteroids may be necessary, despite the presence of CSC. In these patients, recurrent or chronic CSC due to systemic steroid use can be difficult to manage and may possibly result in irreversible vision loss [8]. Argon laser photocoagulation, transpupillary thermotherapy, intravitreal injection of antivascular endothelial growth factors (VEGF), micropulse diode laser photocoagulation, and photodynamic therapy have all been used to manage steroid-induced CSC patients who cannot discontinue steroid therapy [8, 21–26]. However, to date, there has been no established treatment for steroid-induced CSC patients who cannot discontinue systemic steroid use.

Endogenous or exogenous steroid therapy is a risk factor for CSC [8]. Glucocorticoids bind to the GR and to the MR. Both GR and MR are expressed in the retina and in the choroid vessels, demonstrating that the retina and the choroid are novel targets for steroid therapy [11]. Activation of the MR in the choroid by steroids causes choroid vessel dilation and leakage, leading to choroidal hyperpermeability that is known to be a major pathogenic factor in CSC [11]. This steroid-induced choroidal hyperpermeability can be blocked by MR antagonists [11]. Therefore, MR blockers are expected to have a therapeutic effect on CSC, and many studies have already shown good therapeutic efficacy of these drugs in treating CSC [12–18].

CSC may be caused by a variety of factors, but steroid-induced CSC is directly caused by steroids; we expected that MR antagonists may be more effective against this condition.

TABLE 2: Serum level changes of potassium and creatinine after spironolactone treatment.

	Before spironolactone	After spironolactone	P value*
Serum potassium	4.85 ± 0.47	4.91 ± 0.45	0.153
Serum creatinine	1.21 ± 0.35	1.30 ± 0.41	0.468

*Paired t-test.

In this current study, as expected, the MR antagonist showed good therapeutic effect in patients with steroid-induced CSC. Therefore, we considered that MR antagonists could be an important therapeutic option for patients with steroid-induced CSC who cannot discontinue steroid use. However, as seen in the present study result, when the MR antagonist was discontinued, SRF recurred. Continuous use of an MR antagonist should be considered during systemic steroid therapy in patients with steroid-induced CSC to prevent recurrence. Further studies are required on the efficacy and safety of long-term use of MR antagonists in steroid-induced CSC patients.

One of the major hurdles in using spironolactone for CSC treatment is systemic side effects. Spironolactone is a potassium-preserving diuretic and may cause medical side effects such as electrolyte abnormality [20]. To assess the presence of systemic side effects, we performed serum electrolyte examinations before treatment and every month during treatment. We found no significant changes in serum potassium or creatinine levels after spironolactone treatment (Table 2). There were no cases in which the drug had to be discontinued because of an electrolyte imbalance or spironolactone-related side effect. Therefore, this study showed that spironolactone used for CSC treatment produced fewer systemic side effects.

Our present study had several limitations due to its retrospective design. The sample size was also relatively small, which may have limited the statistical strength of the analysis. And, symptom duration of included patients was relatively short (4.00 ± 3.04 months). Therefore, it is possible that some of the improvement that was documented would have happened spontaneously. However, since the patients included in the study were not idiopathic CSC patients but CSC patients who were taking steroids, we thought that the probability of self-improvement was relatively low.

Despite these limitations, the current study provides new insights into the therapeutic effects of a MR antagonist in treating steroid-induced CSC. This study demonstrated that MR antagonist treatment, which blocks steroids from binding to the MR, was effective in treating steroid-induced CSC. In conclusion, MR antagonist treatment may be a therapeutic option for steroid-induced CSC patients. This treatment modality may be especially beneficial for steroid-induced CSC patients who cannot discontinue steroid medication because of systemic conditions.

Conflicts of Interest

The authors declare that they have no conflicts of interest.

Authors' Contributions

Jin Young Kim, Ju Byung Chae, and Dong Yoon Kim were involved in the design of the study; Jin Young Kim, Ju Byung Chae, and Dong Yoon Kim were responsible for collection and management of the data; Jin Young Kim, Ju Byung Chae, Jisoo Kim, and Dong Yoon Kim analyzed and interpreted the data; Jin Young Kim, Ju Byung Chae, Jisoo Kim, and Dong Yoon Kim were responsible for preparation of the manuscript, statistical analysis, and interpretation; Jin Young Kim, Ju Byung Chae, Jisoo Kim, and Dong Yoon Kim were responsible for review and approval of the manuscript.

References

[1] E. K. de Jong, M. B. Breukink, R. L. Schellevis et al., "Chronic central serous chorioretinopathy is associated with genetic variants implicated in age-related macular degeneration," *Ophthalmology*, vol. 122, no. 3, pp. 562–570, 2015.

[2] A. Miki, N. Kondo, S. Yanagisawa, H. Bessho, S. Honda, and A. Negi, "Common variants in the complement factor H gene confer genetic susceptibility to central serous chorioretinopathy," *Ophthalmology*, vol. 121, no. 5, pp. 1067–1072, 2014.

[3] L. A. Yannuzzi, "Type A behavior and central serous chorioretinopathy," *Retina*, vol. 32, no. 1, p. 709, 2012.

[4] A. Mateo-Montoya and M. Mauget-Fayse, "Helicobacter pylori as a risk factor for central serous chorioretinopathy: literature review," *World Journal of Gastrointestinal Pathophysiology*, vol. 5, no. 3, pp. 355–358, 2014.

[5] G. Liew, G. Quin, M. Gillies, and S. Fraser-Bell, "Central serous chorioretinopathy: a review of epidemiology and pathophysiology," *Clinical and Experimental Ophthalmology*, vol. 41, no. 2, pp. 201–214, 2013.

[6] B. Nicholson, J. Noble, F. Forooghian, and C. Meyerle, "Central serous chorioretinopathy: update on pathophysiology and treatment," *Survey of Ophthalmology*, vol. 58, no. 2, pp. 103–126, 2013.

[7] Y. J. Park, K. H. Park, and S. J. Woo, "Clinical features of pregnancy-associated retinal and choroidal diseases causing acute visual disturbance," *Korean Journal of Ophthalmology: KJO*, vol. 31, no. 4, pp. 320–327, 2017.

[8] C. A. Carvalho-Recchia, L. A. Yannuzzi, S. Negrao et al., "Corticosteroids and central serous chorioretinopathy," *Ophthalmology*, vol. 109, no. 10, pp. 1834–1837, 2002.

[9] S. Viengchareun, D. Le Menuet, L. Martinerie, M. Munier, L. Pascual-Le Tallec, and M. Lombes, "The mineralocorticoid receptor: insights into its molecular and (patho)physiological biology," *Nuclear Receptor Signaling*, vol. 4, p. e012, 2007.

[10] N. Farman and M. E. Rafestin-Oblin, "Multiple aspects of mineralocorticoid selectivity," *American Journal of physiology-Renal Physiology*, vol. 280, no. 2, pp. F181–F192, 2001.

[11] F. Behar-Cohen and M. Zhao, "Corticosteroids and the retina: a role for the mineralocorticoid receptor," *Current Opinion in Neurology*, vol. 29, no. 1, pp. 49–54, 2016.

[12] M. Zhao, I. Celerier, E. Bousquet et al., "Mineralocorticoid receptor is involved in rat and human ocular chorioretinopathy," *Journal of Clinical Investigation*, vol. 122, no. 7, pp. 2672–2679, 2012.

[13] I. Chatziralli, S. A. Kabanarou, E. Parikakis, A. Chatzirallis, T. Xirou, and P. Mitropoulos, "Risk factors for central serous chorioretinopathy: multivariate approach in a case-control study," *Current Eye Research*, vol. 42, no. 7, pp. 1069–1073, 2017.

[14] A. Gruszka, "Potential involvement of mineralocorticoid receptor activation in the pathogenesis of central serous chorioretinopathy: case report," *European Review for Medical and Pharmacological Sciences*, vol. 17, no. 10, pp. 1369–1373, 2013.

[15] A. Daruich, A. Matet, A. Dirani et al., "Oral mineralocorticoid-receptor antagonists: real-life experience in clinical subtypes of nonresolving central serous chorioretinopathy with chronic epitheliopathy," *Translational Vision Science and Technology*, vol. 5, no. 2, p. 2, 2016.

[16] R. P. Singh, J. E. Sears, R. Bedi, A. P. Schachat, J. P. Ehlers, and P. K. Kaiser, "Oral eplerenone for the management of chronic central serous chorioretinopathy," *International Journal of Ophthalmology*, vol. 8, no. 2, pp. 310–314, 2015.

[17] R. Gergely, I. Kovacs, M. Schneider et al., "Mineralocorticoid receptor antagonist treatment in bilateral chronic central serous chorioretinopathy: a comparative study of exudative and nonexudative fellow eyes," *Retina*, vol. 37, no. 6, pp. 1084–1091, 2017.

[18] T. R. Herold, K. Rist, S. G. Priglinger, M. W. Ulbig, and A. Wolf, "Long-term results and recurrence rates after spironolactone treatment in non-resolving central serous chorio-retinopathy (CSCR)," *Graefe's Archive for Clinical and Experimental Ophthalmology*, vol. 255, no. 2, pp. 221–229, 2017.

[19] R. F. Spaide, H. Koizumi, and M. C. Pozzoni, "Enhanced depth imaging spectral-domain optical coherence tomography," *American Journal of Ophthalmology*, vol. 146, no. 4, pp. 496–500, 2008.

[20] P. Kolkhof and L. Barfacker, "30 YEARS OF THE MINERALOCORTICOID RECEPTOR: mineralocorticoid receptor antagonists: 60 years of research and development," *Journal of Endocrinology*, vol. 234, no. 1, pp. T125–T140, 2017.

[21] M. Gemenetzi, G. De Salvo, and A. J. Lotery, "Central serous chorioretinopathy: an update on pathogenesis and treatment," *Eye*, vol. 24, no. 12, pp. 1743–1756, 2010.

[22] A. Katsanos and M. Stefaniotou, "Central serous chorioretinopathy in patients who cannot discontinue steroids," *Journal of Crohn's and Colitis*, vol. 7, no. 1, p. e25, 2013.

[23] T. G. Lee and J. E. Kim, "Photodynamic therapy for steroid-associated central serous chorioretinopathy," *British Journal of Ophthalmology*, vol. 95, no. 4, pp. 518–523, 2011.

[24] M. P. Ruiz-Del-Tiempo, P. Calvo, A. Ferreras, J. Lecinena, L. Pablo, and O. Ruiz-Moreno, "Anatomical retinal changes after photodynamic therapy in chronic central serous chorioretinopathy," *Journal of Ophthalmology*, vol. 2018, Article ID 4081874, 4 pages, 2018.

[25] E. Ozmert, S. Demirel, O. Yanik, and F. Batioglu, "Low-fluence photodynamic therapy versus subthreshold micropulse yellow wavelength laser in the treatment of chronic central serous chorioretinopathy," *Journal of Ophthalmology*, vol. 2016, Article ID 3513794, 8 pages, 2016.

[26] Y. J. Kim, Y. G. Lee, D. W. Lee, and J. H. Kim, "Selective retina therapy with real-time feedback-controlled dosimetry for treating acute idiopathic central serous chorioretinopathy in korean patients," *Journal of Ophthalmology*, vol. 2018, Article ID 6027871, 9 pages, 2018.

9

Analysis of Morphologic and Functional Outcomes in Macular Edema due to Central Retinal Vein Occlusion Treated with Intravitreal Dexamethasone Implant

Alfredo Niro, Giancarlo Sborgia, Alessandra Sborgia, Luigi Sborgia, Claudio Furino, Nicola Recchimurzo, and Giovanni Alessio

Department of Medical Science, Neuroscience and Sense Organs, Eye Clinic, University of Bari "A. Moro", Bari, Italy

Correspondence should be addressed to Alfredo Niro; alfred.nir@tiscali.it

Academic Editor: Dirk Sandner

Purpose. To analyze anatomic and functional retinal changes and their correlation after intravitreal dexamethasone implant (DEX implant) in patients with central retinal vein occlusion- (CRVO-) related macular edema (ME) using optical coherence tomography and microperimetry. *Methods.* Fifteen treatment-naïve patients with functional impairment due to CRVO-related ME were enrolled in this prospective interventional case series. Main outcomes were best-corrected visual acuity (BCVA), retinal sensitivity (RS), and central retinal thickness (CRT). Secondary outcomes were ellipsoid zone (EZ) status and fixation behaviour. All patients underwent DEX implant and were retreated according to predefined criteria. Data were prospectively recorded at baseline and at month 1, 3, 6, 9, and 12. Correlation between main outcomes was analyzed. *Results.* Fifteen eyes of 15 patients (9 men, 6 women; mean age 61.8 ± 10.9 years) were included. BCVA and CRT significantly improved at all follow-up visits, while RS significantly improved at 3, 6, 9, and 12 months. EZ status and fixation behaviour did not change significantly. Baseline CRT had a significant negative correlation with BCVA and RS at different follow-up visits ($r = -0.52$ to -0.63, $p \leq 0.04$; $r = -0.52$, $p = 0.04$; resp.). At all time points, there was not a significant correlation between CRT and BCVA and RS, while RS and BCVA showed a significant correlation, increasing over time ($r = -0.72$ to -0.89; $p < 0.001$). *Conclusion.* DEX implant led to a significant morphofunctional improvement. Baseline CRT is predictive of changes of functional outcomes whose correlation increases over time after treatment.

1. Introduction

Macular edema (ME) is a common complication of central retinal vein occlusion (CRVO) causing vision loss [1]. The pathogenesis of ME in retinal vein occlusion is not completely understood but may result from a variety of factors, including hydrostatic effects from increased venous pressure, the presence of inflammatory cytokines, the dysregulation of endothelial tight junction proteins [2], or increased amounts of vascular permeability factors, such as vascular endothelial growth factor (VEGF) [3]. Treatment options include intravitreal corticosteroids and antagonists of VEGF (anti-VEGF) [4–12]. The slow-release intravitreal dexamethasone implant 0.7 mg (DEX implant; Ozurdex®, Allergan plc, Dublin, Ireland) has proved very effective improving visual acuity and reducing macular thickness in patients with CRVO-related ME [13, 14]. Best-corrected visual acuity (BCVA) and central retinal thickness (CRT) assessed by optical coherence tomography (OCT), reflecting foveal status, are widely used as efficacy outcomes of DEX implant in clinical trials and clinical practice. However, visual acuity and its relationship with CRT could not be comprehensive in monitoring the morphologic and functional recovery of a larger retinal area beyond the fovea after DEX implant. Retinal sensitivity (RS), assessed by microperimetry, as a reproducible point-to-point measure of macular function was used as a biomarker of functional changes in retinal vein occlusion [15, 16] and recovery after

DEX implant [17–22]. However, the correlation between morphologic and functional parameters and their predictive role for recovery after DEX implant over a long follow-up remains unclear. So we analyzed both CRT and visual function parameters, as BCVA and RS, and their correlation in CRVO-related ME patients after DEX implant over 12-months follow-up.

2. Methods

This was a prospective interventional case series of intravitreal dexamethasone implant (Ozurdex) in consecutive naive patients with visual impairment and clinical and/or instrumental diagnosis of ME following CRVO within previous three months before enrollment. The main exclusion criteria were a BCVA worse than 1.5 logMAR, previous intravitreal implant or injection, previous vitreoretinal surgery, manifest glaucoma, presence of diabetic macular edema, epiretinal membrane, retinal neovascularization, previous central or branch retinal vein occlusion, retinal dystrophies, severe cataract, and other diseases affecting visual acuity in the affected eye. All subjects underwent DEX implant and were followed at month 1, 3, 6, 9, and 12. All subjects underwent a complete examination including BCVA evaluation, slit-lamp biomicroscopy, dilated fundus examination, intraocular pressure (IOP) measurement, optical coherence tomography (OCT; Cirrus HD-OCT Zeiss, Carl Zeiss Meditec, Germany), and microperimetry (MP1; Navis Software, version 1.7.6; Nidek Technologies, Padova, Italy). Fluorescein angiography was performed at baseline, 4 and 12 months. Primary outcome measures were BCVA, CRT measured by OCT, and RS measured by MP1. BCVA was evaluated using a standardized Early Treatment Diabetic Retinopathy Study (ETDRS) protocol. We used a macular thickness map protocol with a macular cube 512 × 128 combo to measure CRT as the mean thickness in the central 1000-μm diameter area, considering the distance between the internal limiting membrane and outer border of the photoreceptor cells [23]. RS was considered as the mean sensitivity measured across a 45-point grid centered on the central 12 degrees using pattern Macula 12°–0 dB. At each point in the grid, sensitivity was measured for a white stimulus 0.438 in diameter (Goldmann size III) presented for 200 msec against a mesopic background (1.27 cd/m^2). Threshold at each point was determined by using a 4-2 staircase. When the automatic localization of the foveal area was difficult, that site has been manually located at a distance of two papillary disc temporally and a disc-third lower than the center of the optic disc. The "follow-up" feature of the MP1 was used to perform sensitivity measurements at the same retinal locations across all visits. Secondary outcomes were the integrity of the ellipsoid zone (EZ) at the foveal site revealed by the continuity of hypereflective band of photoreceptor inner/outer segment junction at horizontal OCT high-resolution linear scans (HD 5-lines) and classified as absent or present and fixation stability revealed by plotting the position of each fixation point on Cartesian axes and calculating the percent of the points falling within 2° and 4° circle by using MP-1 software as recommended by Fujii et al. [24]. All patients were retreated from month 4 according to an open pro re nata (PRN) regime (if either a significant decline in the BCVA, as demonstrated by a loss of at least one line, or an increased CRT of ≥100 μm was noticed from the previous visit), provided the patient had not experienced raised IOP above 30 mm Hg following their first injection. Additionally, supplementing sectorial or panretinal laser photocoagulation was considered on the individual retinal perfusion. Ocular and systemic complications were recorded. The treatment described adhered to the tenets of the Declaration of Helsinki. Written informed consent for implant for one eye each and research aim was requested.

2.1. Statistical Analysis. Statistical analysis was based on all patients included in the study. No formal sample size calculation was performed. Baseline was defined as the day before implant. A *t*-test was performed on the change from baseline in CRT, BCVA, and RS. The statistical analysis for the evaluation of the correlation between primary outcomes was based on the observed data collected during the 12-month study period and examined by Pearson correlation coefficient. All statistical tests were 2-sided and performed at the *p*0.05 significance level. Data processing, summaries, and analysis were performed using the statistical software package SAS version 9.1 or higher (SAS Institute Inc, Cary, NC).

3. Results

The baseline characteristics of the study population are summarized in Table 1. Only 15 consecutive patients out of 21 CRVO-related ME patients who underwent dexamethasone slow-release implant were included in this study because 6 patients refused consent for research. Mean age of the 9 men and 6 women included was 61.8 ± 10.9 years (range: 46–80 years). Due to the recurrence of ME, a second DEX implant was performed in two and two eyes at 6 and 9 months, respectively. Six eyes underwent laser treatment during follow-up. The mean CRT significantly decreased from 577 ± 170.2 μm at baseline to 287.7 ± 44.2 μm ($p < 0.0001$) at 1 month, to 271.87 ± 43.8 μm ($p < 0.0001$) at 3 months, to 316.3 ± 123 μm ($p = 0.0002$) at 6 months, to 318.4 ± 90.2 μm ($p = 0.0002$) at 9 months, and to 294.1 ± 60.6 μm ($p < 0.0001$) at 12 months (Figure 1). Respect to baseline CRT, the largest mean thickness reductions were observed at 3 (289.3 ± 126.5 μm) and 12 months (282.8 ± 109.6 μm) after implant. At 6 and 9 months, an increase of 44.73 ± 120.7 μm and 47.33 ± 98.06 μm of the mean CRT, respectively, respect to the earliest 3 months, occurred. The analysis of the EZ integrity at the foveal site was realized from the first follow-up visit at 1 month because at baseline large intraretinal cystic spaces masked the reflectivity of the outer layers at OCT scans. Two patients had a discontinuity of the reflectivity of the EZ at months 1 and 12 after implant. OCT scans highlighted occurrence of a discontinuity in the EZ in only one patient at last follow-up (Table 2). At baseline, OCT scans revealed subretinal fluid in 5 patients. The mean BCVA significantly improved from 0.76 ± 0.54 logMAR at

TABLE 1: Patient characteristics.

Patient, *n*	15
Age (years ± SD)	61.8 ± 10.9
Sex (men/women), *n*	9/6
Retreated eyes, *n*	4/15
Eyes underwent laser, *n*	6/15

SD, standard deviation.

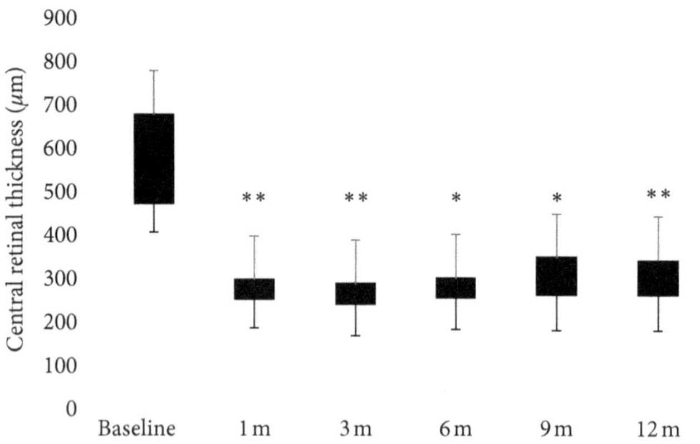

FIGURE 1: Central retinal thickness (CRT) improvement over time (μm: micronmeters; m: month(s)). $^{*}p$ 0.002; $^{**}p < 0.0001$.

TABLE 2: Secondary outcomes.

EZ status at 1 month (absent/present), *n*	2/13	
EZ status at 12 months (absent/present), *n*	3/12	
Fixation stability within 4 degrees, *n*	Baseline	12 months
Stable	11/15	8/15
Relatively stable	—	2/15
Relatively unstable	—	4/15
unstable	4/15	1/15

EZ: ellipsoid zone.

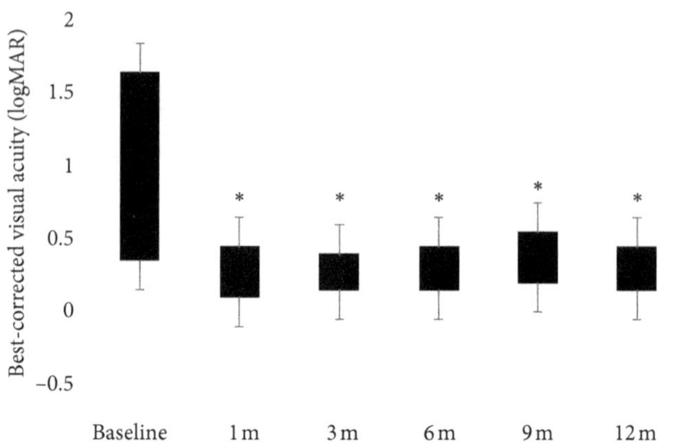

FIGURE 2: Best-corrected visual acuity improvement over time (logMAR: logarithm of the minimum angle of resolution; m: month(s)). $^{*}p < 0.001$.

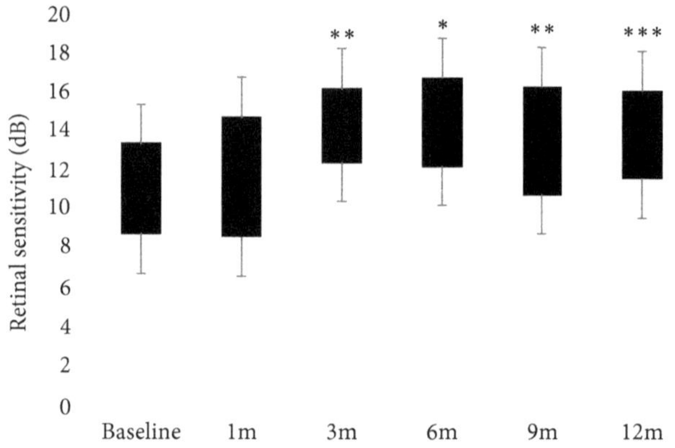

FIGURE 3: Retinal sensitivity improvement over time (dB: decibels; m: month(s)). $^{*}p < 0.01$; $^{**}p < 0.001$; $^{***}p < 0.0001$.

baseline to 0.37 ± 0.33 logMAR at 1 month ($p < 0.001$), 0.34 ± 0.33 logMAR at 3 months ($p < 0.001$), 0.37 ± 0.34 logMAR at 6 months ($p < 0.001$), 0.38 ± 0.31 logMAR at 9 months ($p < 0.001$), and 0.35 ± 0.32 logMAR at 12 months ($p < 0.001$) (Figure 2). Respect to baseline BCVA, the largest mean visual improvements of 0.42 ± 0.38 logMAR and 0.41 ± 0.36 logMAR were seen at 3 and 12 months, respectively. At 6 and 9 months, a mean visual impairment of 0.05 ± 0.08 LogMAR and 0.12 ± 0.10 logMAR, respectively, respect to the earliest 3 months, occurred. The mean RS improved from 10.39 ± 5.03 dB at baseline to 11.86 ± 5.91 dB at 1 month ($p > 0.05$), 13.03 ± 6.09 dB at 3 months ($p < 0.001$), 12.92 ± 7.1 dB at 6 months ($p < 0.01$), 13.03 ± 5.86 dB at 9 months ($p < 0.001$), and 13.14 ± 5.6 dB at 12 months ($p < 0.0001$). (Figure 3) Respect to baseline sensitivity, the largest mean sensitivity improvements of 2.77 ± 2.28 dB and 2.89 ± 2.29 dB were seen at 3 and 12 months, respectively. At 6 months, a mean sensitivity impairment of 0.53 ± 0.4 dB from earliest 3 months occurred. In the four eyes retreated, the second implant gave a mean CRT (170 ± 93.5 μm) and functional improvement (0.2 ± 0.3 LogMAR; 0.5 ± 1.1 dB). In regard to the fixation behaviour, comparing baseline and last follow-up data, three patients revealed a mild improvement (unstable to relatively stable) while two patients suffered a mild impairment (stable to relatively unstable) in the fixation stability within central 4° (Table 2). The baseline CRT was significantly correlated with BCVA at months 1, 3, 6, and 12 ($r = -0.52$ to -0.63, $p \leq 0.04$) (Table 3). At each follow-up visit, BCVA and CRT showed a weak correlation ($r = -0.07$ to -0.26) never statistically significant ($p > 0.05$). The baseline CRT was significantly correlated with RS at 9 months ($r = -0.52$ $p = 0.04$) after treatment (Table 3). At each follow-up visit RS and CRT showed a weak correlation ($r = -0.40$ to -0.46) never statistically significant ($p > 0.05$). At each time point, BCVA and RS showed a strong negative correlation ($r = -0.72$ to -0.96, $p < 0.01$), increasing over time (Table 4). At 6 and 9 months after a single implant, OCT scans revealed vitreomacular interfaces disorders (VID), not present at baseline, in a total of 6 patients. In one patient, a significant cataract progression occurred after two implants, so he underwent surgery during follow-up. In two patients, IOP elevation (<30 mmHg) was successfully managed with antihypertensive topical therapy, suspended after 1 month from implant.

TABLE 3: Correlation between baseline CRT and main functional outcomes.

	Baseline CRT				
	1 month	3 months	6 months	9 months	12 months
BCVA	$r = -0.55$ $p =$ **0.03**	$r = -0.63$ $p =$ **0.01**	$r = -0.55$ $p =$ **0.03**	$r = -0.40$ $p = 0.13$	$r = -0.52$ $p =$ **0.04**
RS	$r = -0.45$ $p = 0.09$	$r = -0.46$ $p = 0.07$	$r = -0.45$ $p = 0.09$	$r = -0.52$ $p =$ **0.04**	$r = -0.40$ $p = 0.13$

Note. p values indicate statistical significance. BCVA: best-corrected visual acuity; RS: retinal sensitivity; CRT: central retinal thickness.

4. Discussion

Ozurdex may offer patients with CRVO-related ME a long-lasting relief from visual symptoms and edema with a limited number of treatments and follow-up visits [25–27]. In our study, DEX implant significantly improved primary outcomes, such as CRT and BCVA at all follow-up visits. By analyzing our results and comparing with results of GENEVA, OCTOME (Report 1), and SOLO studies, albeit with a nonoverlapping follow-up, we found a similar trend in morphologic and functional recovery. A significant mean visual improvement (0.42 ± 0.38 logMAR) and CRT reduction ($289.3 \pm 126.5\,\mu$m) occurred over early three months, followed by a mild functional impairment and increase in mean CRT at the sixth and ninth month compared to previous time points, due to edema recurrence and/or VID or cataract occurrence, and a new mean morphofunctional recovery, lower than the previous, after the second implant, as reported by the literature [13, 22]. With regard to RS, we found the same trend with an early improvement of 2.77 ± 2.28 dB at 3 months, followed by a mild impairment at the sixth and ninth month compared to previous visits. At 12 months, a new mean sensitivity improvement (2.89 ± 2.29 dB) was recorded. The ME recurrence at the sixth and ninth month justified an additional implant in overall 4 (26.6 %) patients, really lower than 50% of patient retreated in GENEVA Study. All these results might suggest a correlation between macular sensitivity, visual acuity, and retinal thickness. In this study, we evaluated the correlation between morphologic and functional parameters as outcomes of intravitreal DEX implant administered on a PRN regime for CRVO-related ME. Noma et al. found that BCVA was significantly correlated with macular thickness in eyes with CRVO-related ME [15]. Querques et al. reported that macular thickness was positively correlated with BCVA at months 1 and 3 after DEX implant [18]. Bulut et al. observed a moderate correlation between macular thickness and BCVA only at 3 months after DEX implant. No correlation was detected between BCVA and macular thickness at baseline and 6 months [28]. We found that baseline CRT had a significant negative correlation with visual acuity at different follow-up visits (at months 1, 3, 6, and 12) after implant, but conversely, CRT had a weak correlation with simultaneous visual acuity at each time points. That data suggest that baseline CRT could be considered a predictive factor for visual acuity changes after treatment, but the weak correlation at each time point could reveal that anatomical degenerative changes caused by vein occlusion influence functional parameters over time, regardless of macular thickness. Furthermore, baseline CRT showed no significant relationship with BCVA at 9 months. CRT could have only a time-limited predictive role and not have an explanatory role on visual acuity recovery over follow-up, probably due to later neuroretinal modifications occurring beyond the period of efficacy of DEX implant. So, it should not be the only morphologic finding recorded. In the same way, the functional changes cannot be completely assessed by visual acuity. Visual acuity primarily reflects foveal function, but retinal sensitivity studied by using microperimetry, creating a map of macular sensitivity, records the central and paracentral retinal function that visual acuity is not able to assess. OCTOME study (Report 1) reported a sensitivity improvement of 4 dB in a population affected by different retinal vascular diseases at 6 months after DEX implant [22]. Several papers reported a mean sensitivity improvement ranging from 1.1 dB to 3.9 dB over a variable follow-up period (3 to 12 months) after DEX implant [17–21]. In our study, including only patients with CRVO-related ME over a 12-month follow-up, a RS mean recovery of 2.75 dB was recorded with a slower trend than visual acuity. Noma et al. reported a significant correlation between baseline CRT and RS [15]. Querques et al. found a negative significant correlation between macular thickness and retinal sensitivity over 3 months after DEX implant [17, 18]. We found a negative significant correlation between baseline CRT and RS only at nine months after implant. This finding supports the complex interaction between morphologic and functional parameters. Not only the retinal thickness but also the compartmentalization of edema involving neurosensory layers and subretinal space was found to contribute differently to the reduction and recovery of visual function [29, 30]. A relationship between ganglion cell layer thinning and a decrease in local visual field sensitivity and visual acuity has been found in several studies [31]. Inner retinal layers displacement, dysfunction, and loss affecting a greater area than foveal site due to fluid accumulation may explain decreased retinal sensitivity out of the fovea [32]. The sensitivity recovery is influenced by the reconstitution of neuroretinal architecture after retinal edema resolution. But these changes could occur over a long time justifying the slow recovery trend of retinal sensitivity. Furthermore, the reduction of retinal thickness does not imply an immediate functional recovery. With worsening ischemia, the increased interstitial pressure causing compromised perfusion and the tissue reperfusion might lead to irreversible damage of the neuroretina influencing functional recovery, so BCVA and RS, differently, can remain poor even though the ME is resolved. Previous papers revealed a reduction of foveal and parafoveal retinal superficial and deep vascular density and choriocapillaris density in eyes with vein occlusion-related ME [33–35]. Although Mastropasqua et al. found that retinal vessel plexi density did not change significantly after DEX implant and there was no correlation between vessel density and functional parameters such as visual acuity and retinal sensitivity [36], it has been demonstrated that intravitreal steroid, in

Table 4: Correlation between BCVA and RS.

	BCVA					
	Baseline	1 month	3 months	6 months	9 months	12 months
RS	$r = -0.72$ $p =$ **0.002**	$r = -0.82$ $p =$ **0.0001**	$r = -0.91$ $p <$ **0.00001**	$r = -0.93$ $p <$ **0.00001**	$r = -0.96$ $p <$ **0.00001**	$r = -0.90$ $p <$ **0.00001**

BCVA: best-corrected visual acuity; RS: retinal sensitivity.

eyes with macular edema due to retinal vein occlusion or diabetic retinopathy, causes a reduction of vessel diameter probably due to the blockage of VEGF [37, 38]. Vessel occlusion may lead to functional damage of photoreceptor cells that influence visual acuity and retinal sensitivity. This effect on photoreceptor cells could explain the significant negative correlation between visual acuity and retinal sensitivity and its progressive increase over follow-up. In our study, five patients had subretinal fluid at baseline, and three of those showed an EZ discontinuity at last follow-up. These three patients had worst baseline BCVA (range, 1.3–1.5 logMAR) and RS (range, 1.2–2 dB) and worst final visual outcomes (range, 0.7–1 logMAR; 5.8–2 dB). SCORE study (Report 13) highlighted the correlation between functional parameters and outer retinal layer integrity [39]. In retinal vein occlusion [40, 41] or diabetic macular edema [42], as well as in age-related macular degeneration [43], a significant association between changes of EZ and BCVA was reported, on the other hand, they did not find a statistically significant correlation between photoreceptor layer feature and CRT. OMAR study revealed that visual acuity was better for BRVO, although CRT showed no significant difference between central and branch vein occlusion groups [44]. Altunel et al. found that outer nuclear layer thickness and photoreceptor layer thickness were more closely related to visual acuity improvement than CRT decrement [45]. The CRT before the treatment and the presence of an intact EZ at the time of the ME resolution were significantly correlated with the BCVA and RS at 6 months after anti-VEGF therapy for retinal vein occlusion [46]. RS has been shown to be significantly correlated not only with the BCVA but also with morphologic findings, such as EZ status, and it can thus be used to monitor the effectiveness of treatments [47–49] CRT reflects the status of the edema not revealing outer retina integrity at the foveal site. Histologic studies have shown that severe ME leads to photoreceptor dysfunction and photoreceptor cell loss [50]. However, OCT scans show neuroretinal swelling due to edema, masking the EZ that could be preserved or interrupted. We evaluated outer retinal layers at 1 month after treatment because the pretreatment status of the EZ could be masked by the edema. A significant visual gain was achieved only in eyes showing preserved outer retinal layers at baseline regardless of the CRVO types, whereas eyes with absent layers at baseline were unable to attain any visual improvement [51]. With regard to the fixation behaviour, it did not show significant changes from baseline to 12-month follow-up. It was stable or partially stable in the majority of patients. However, fixation stability was not related to visual acuity, and the compensation of fixation instability does not improve visual acuity in patients with macular disease [52]. In the present study, multivariate analysis was not performed because the statistical model was unsuitable due to the small number of patients. This study also had some other limitations: the eyes were not categorized according to ischemic or nonischemic feature of CRVO; study visits were not scheduled between months 1, 3, and 6, therefore not revealing the exact time point of drug peak efficacy, its corresponding duration, and possible need for early retreatment. It must be said for completeness of analysis which is inherent connotation of each psychophysical test and as such also the microperimetry, the measurement error, or intrinsic variability. Factors acting on test variability are related to patients' compliance and their anatomical and functional condition and to the examiner and/or instrument used. An important patient-related factor influencing test execution is the "learning factor" which can justify a certain degree of improvement during follow-up. With regards to the instrument, it should be mentioned the eye-tracker system, not able to ensure the same accuracy of analysis between the posterior pole and peripheral retina; the "point to point" overlapping error (0.5° to 2°) when "follow-up" program is used; the "4-2 strategy" which can extend the duration of the test; the "ceiling effect" of MP-1, meaning the tendency to accumulate responses at the highest limit of the sensitivity threshold; the size of the given stimulus (Goldmann III, 4 mm^2 area, 26 min diameter of arc, or 0.4°) that, because of "spatial summation," involves more photoreceptors which converge centrally on a single ganglion cell; the wider extension of tested area (central 20°) respect to central 4° and 8° which would result in a more reliable parameter for spatial localization of functional defect. Further investigations will be needed to clarify the relations between macular function and morphology in CRVO patients with macular edema. In conclusion, beyond the efficacy of DEX implant, our analysis suggests that baseline CRT might have a prognostic role on functional changes and that mutual behaviour of functional parameters over time might be related to the restoration of the integrity of photoreceptor cells after macular edema resolution. So, comprehensive evaluation of both visual acuity and macular sensitivity might be important when assessing retinal function in CRVO patients with macular edema before and after DEX implant and their correlation could reveal the added value of microperimetry as a diagnostic tool.

Conflicts of Interest

The authors declare that they have no conflicts of interest.

References

[1] M. Rehak and P. Wiedemann, "Retinal vein thrombosis: pathogenesis and management," *Journal of Thrombosis and Haemostasis*, vol. 8, no. 9, pp. 1886–1894, 2010.

[2] D. A. Antonetti, A. J. Barber, S. Khin, E. Lieth, J. M. Tarbell, and T. W. Gardner, "Penn state retina research group. Vascular permeability in experimental diabetes is associated with reduced endothelial occludin content: vascular endothelial growth factor decreases occludin in retinal endothelial cells," *Diabetes*, vol. 47, pp. 1953–1959, 1998.

[3] P. A. Campochiaro, G. Hafiz, S. M. Shah et al., "Ranibizumab for macular edema due to retinal vein occlusions: implication of VEGF as a critical stimulator," *Molecular Therapy*, vol. 16, no. 4, pp. 791–799, 2008.

[4] R. A. Adelman, A. J. Parnes, S. Bopp, I. S. Othman, and D. Ducournau, "Strategy for the management of macular edema in retinal vein occlusion: the European VitreoRetinal Society macular edema study," *BioMed Research International*, vol. 2015, Article ID 870987, 8 pages, 2015.

[5] N. Feltgen, A. Pielen, L. Hansen et al., "Intravitreal drug therapy for retinal vein occlusion–pathophysiological mechanisms and routinely used drugs," *Klinische Monatsblatter fur Augenheilkunde*, vol. 227, no. 9, pp. 681–693, 2010.

[6] M. J. Koss, H. Naser, A. Sener et al., "Combination therapy in diabetic macular oedema and retinal vein occlusion–past and present," *Acta Ophthalmologica*, vol. 90, no. 6, pp. 580–589, 2012.

[7] M. S. Ip, I. U. Scott, P. C. VanVeldhuisen et al., "A randomized trial comparing the efficacy and safety of intravitreal triamcinolone with observation to treat vision loss associated with macular edema secondary to central retinal vein occlusion: the Standard Care vs Corticosteroid for Retinal Vein Occlusion (SCORE) study report 5," *Acta Ophthalmologica*, vol. 127, no. 9, pp. 1101–1114, 2009.

[8] I. U. Scott, M. S. Ip, P. C. VanVeldhuisen et al., "SCORE study report 6-A randomized trial comparing the efficacy and safety of intravitreal triamcinolone with standard care to treat vision loss associated with macular Edema secondary to branch retinal vein occlusion: the Standard Care vs Corticosteroid for Retinal Vein Occlusion (SCORE) study report 6," *Acta Ophthalmologica*, vol. 127, no. 9, pp. 1115–1128, 2009.

[9] A. P. Ciardella, M. Morara, F. Pichi, M. Alkabes, S. Romano, and P. Nucci, "Management of macular edema secondary to retinal vein occlusions," *Expert Review of Ophthalmology*, vol. 6, no. 5, pp. 557–564, 2011.

[10] C. Campa, G. Alivernini, E. Bolletta, M. B. Parodi, and P. Perri, "Anti-VEGF therapy for retinal vein occlusions," *Current Drug Targets*, vol. 17, no. 3, pp. 328–336, 2016.

[11] T. Braithwaite, A. A. Nanji, K. Lindsley, and P. B. Greenberg, "Anti-vascular endothelial growth factor for macular oedema secondary to central retinal vein occlusion," *Cochrane Database of Systematic Reviews*, vol. 1, no. 5, article CD007325, 2014.

[12] T. Higashiyama, O. Sawada, M. Kakinoki, T. Sawada, H. Kawamura, and M. Ohji, "Prospective comparisons of intravitreal injections of triamcinolone acetonide and bevacizumab for macular oedema due to branch retinal vein occlusion," *Acta Ophthalmologica*, vol. 91, no. 4, pp. 318–324, 2013.

[13] J. A. Haller, F. Bandello, R. Belfort Jr. et al., "Randomized, sham-controlled trial of dexamethasone intravitreal implant in patients with macular edema due to retinal vein occlusion," *Ophthalmology*, vol. 117, no. 6, pp. 1134e3–1146e3, 2010.

[14] A. Bezatis, G. Spital, F. Höhn et al., "Functional and anatomical results after a single intravitreal Ozurdex injection in retinal vein occlusion: a 6-month follow-up–the SOLO study," *Acta Ophthalmologica*, vol. 91, no. 5, pp. 340–347, 2013.

[15] H. Noma, T. Mimura, and K. Shimada, "Retinal function and morphology in central retinal vein occlusion with macular oedema," *Current Eye Research*, vol. 38, no. 1, pp. 143–149, 2013.

[16] S. Winterhalter, A. Lux, A. K. Maier et al., "Microperimetry as a routine diagnostic test in the follow-up of retinal vein occlusion?," *Graefe's Archive for Clinical and Experimental Ophthalmology*, vol. 250, no. 2, pp. 175–183, 2012.

[17] G. Querques, M. L. Cascavilla, E. Cavallero et al., "Changes in macular function after Ozurdex for retinal vein occlusion," *Optometry and Vision Science*, vol. 91, no. 7, pp. 760–768, 2014.

[18] G. Querques, R. Lattanzio, L. Querques et al., "Impact of intravitreal dexamethasone implant (Ozurdex) on macular morphology and function," *Retina*, vol. 34, no. 2, pp. 330–341, 2014.

[19] M. Parravano, F. Oddone, B. Boccassini et al., "Exploring the morphological and functional retinal changes after dexamethasone intravitreal implant (Ozurdex®) in macular edema due to retinal vein occlusion," *Ophthalmic Research*, vol. 51, no. 3, pp. 153–160, 2014.

[20] F. Bandello, M. Parravano, E. Cavallero et al., "Prospective evaluation of morphological and functional changes after repeated intravitreal dexamethasone implant (Ozurdex®) for retinal vein occlusion," *Ophthalmic Research*, vol. 53, no. 4, pp. 207–216, 2015.

[21] S. Winterhalter, G. A. vom Brocke, and M. K. Klamann, "Monthly microperimetry (MP1) measurement of macular sensitivity after dexamethasone implantation (Ozurdex) in retinal vein occlusions," *Graefe's Archive for Clinical and Experimental Ophthalmology*, vol. 253, no. 11, pp. 1873–1882, 2015.

[22] R. Mathew, E. Pearce, R. Muniraju et al., "Monthly OCT monitoring of Ozurdex for macular oedema related to retinal vascular diseases: re-treatment strategy (OCTOME Report 1)," *Eye*, vol. 28, no. 3, pp. 318–326, 2014.

[23] U. E. K. Wolf-Schnurrbusch, L. Ceklic, C. K. Brinkmann et al., "Macular thickness measurements in healthy eyes using six different optical coherence tomography instruments," *Investigative Ophthalmology and Visual Science*, vol. 50, pp. 3432–3437, 2009.

[24] G. Y. Fujii, E. de Juan Jr., J. Sunness et al., "Patient selection for macular translocation surgery using the scanning laser ophthalmoscope," *Ophthalmology*, vol. 109, no. 9, pp. 1737–1744, 2002.

[25] A. Chan, L. S. Leung, and M. S. Blumenkranz, "Critical appraisal of the clinical utility of the dexamethasone intravitreal implant (Ozurdex) for the treatment of macular edema related to branch retinal vein occlusion or central retinal vein occlusion," *Clinical Ophthalmology*, vol. 5, pp. 1043–1049, 2011.

[26] M. B. Parodi, P. Iacono, M. Cascavilla, I. Zucchiatti, and F. Bandello, "Compassionate use of dexamethasone implant for the treatment of macular edema secondary to central retinal vein occlusion in a clinical setting," *Acta Ophthalmologica*, vol. 90, no. 4, pp. 322–333, 2012.

[27] T. Bertelmann, N. Kičová, A. Messerschmidt-Roth et al., "The vitreomacular interface in retinal vein occlusion," *Acta Ophthalmologica*, vol. 89, no. 4, pp. 327–331, 2011.

[28] M. N. Bulut, U. Çallı, G. Akçay et al., "Effects of dexamethasone implant on multifocal electroretinography in central retinal vein occlusion," *Journal of Ophthalmic and Vision Research*, vol. 13, no. 1, pp. 23–28, 2018.

[29] M. R. Munk, C. G. Kiss, W. Huf et al., "Visual acuity and microperimetric mapping of lesion area in eyes with inflammatory cystoid macular oedema," *Acta Ophthalmologica*, vol. 92, no. 4, pp. 332–338, 2014.

[30] I. Y. Wong, L. P. Iu, H. Koizumi, and W. W. Lai, "The inner segment/outer segment junction: what have we learnt so far?," *Current Opinion in Ophthalmology*, vol. 23, no. 3, pp. 210–218, 2012.

[31] A. S. Raza, J. Cho, C. G. de Moraes et al., "Retinal ganglion cell layer thickness and local visual field sensitivity in glaucoma," *Archives of Ophthalmology*, vol. 129, no. 12, pp. 1529–1536, 2011.

[32] L. Pelosini, C. C. Hull, J. F. Boyce et al., "Optical coherence tomography may be used to predict visual acuity in patients with macular edema," *Investigative Opthalmology and Visual Science*, vol. 52, no. 5, pp. 2741–2748, 2011.

[33] J. Nobre Cardoso, P. A. Keane, D. A. Sim et al., "Systematic evaluation of optical coherence tomography angiography in retinal vein occlusion," *American Journal of Ophthalmology*, vol. 163, pp. 93.e6–107.e6, 2016.

[34] F. Coscas, A. Glacet-Bernard, A. Miere et al., "Optical coherence tomography angiography in retinal vein occlusion: evaluation of superficial and deep capillary plexa," *American Journal of Ophthalmology*, vol. 161, pp. 160.e2–171.e2, 2016.

[35] W. A. Samara, A. Shahlaee, J. Sridhar et al., "Quantitative optical coherence tomography angiography features and visual function in eyes with branch retinal vein occlusion," *American Journal of Ophthalmology*, vol. 166, pp. 76–83, 2016.

[36] R. Mastropasqua, L. Toto, L. Di Antonio et al., "Optical coherence tomography angiography microvascular findings in macular edema due to central and branch retinal vein occlusions," *Scientific Reports*, vol. 18, no. 7, article 40763, 2017.

[37] F. Semeraro, A. Russo, D. Rizzoni et al., "Diameters and wall-to-lumen ratio of retinal arterioles in patients with retinal vein occlusion before and after treatment with dexamethasone intravitreal implants," *Journal of Ocular Pharmacology and Therapeutics*, vol. 30, no. 7, pp. 573–579, 2014.

[38] S. S. Wickremasinghe, S. L. Rogers, M. C. Gillies, M. Zhu, and T. Y. Wong, "Retinal vascular caliber changes after intravitreal triamcinolone treatment for diabetic macular edema," *Investigative Opthalmology and Visual Science*, vol. 49, no. 11, pp. 4707–4711, 2008.

[39] A. Domalpally, Q. Peng, R. Danis et al., "Association of outer retinal layer morphology with visual acuity in patients with retinal vein occlusion: SCORE Study Report 13," *Eye*, vol. 26, no. 7, pp. 919–924, 2012.

[40] M. Ota, A. Tsujikawa, M. Kita et al., "Integrity of foveal photoreceptor layer in central retinal vein occlusion," *Retina*, vol. 28, no. 10, pp. 1502–1508, 2008.

[41] M. Ota, A. Tsujikawa, T. Murakami et al., "Foveal photoreceptor layer in eyes with persistent cystoid macular edema associated with branch retinal vein occlusion," *American Journal of Ophthalmology*, vol. 145, no. 2, pp. 273.e1–280.e1, 2008.

[42] A. S. Maheshwary, S. F. Oster, R. M. Yuson et al., "The association between percent disruption of the photoreceptor inner segment-outer segment junction and visual acuity in diabetic macular edema," *American Journal of Ophthalmology*, vol. 150, no. 1, pp. 63.e1–67.e1, 2010.

[43] H. Hayashi, K. Yamashiro, A. Tsujikawa et al., "Association between foveal photoreceptor integrity and visual outcome in neovascular age-related macular degeneration," *American Journal of Ophthalmology*, vol. 148, pp. 83–90, 2009.

[44] A. Ozkok, O. A. Saleh, D. K. Sigford et al., "THE OMAR STUDY: comparison of Ozurdex and triamcinolone acetonide for refractory cystoid macular edema in retinal vein occlusion," *Retina*, vol. 35, no. 7, pp. 1393–1400, 2015.

[45] O. Altunel, N. Duru, A. Goktas, A. Ozkose, E. Goktas, and M. Atas, "Evaluation of foveal photoreceptor layer in eyes with macular edema associated with branch vein occlusion after Ozurdex treatment," *International Ophthalmology*, vol. 37, no. 2, pp. 333–339, 2017.

[46] Y. Mitamura, A. Fujihara-Mino, N. Inomoto, H. Sano, K. Akaiwa, and K. Semba, "Optical coherence tomography parameters predictive of visual outcome after anti-VEGF therapy for retinal vein occlusion," *Clinical Ophthalmology*, vol. 10, pp. 1305–1313, 2016.

[47] S. Richter-Mueksch, P. V. Vecsei-Marlovits, S. G. Sacu et al., "Functional macular mapping in patients with vitreomacular pathologic features before and after surgery," *American Journal of Ophthalmology*, vol. 144, no. 1, pp. 23.e1–31.e1, 2007.

[48] W. C. Chen, Y. Wang, and X. X. Li, "Morphologic and functional evaluation before and after successful macular hole surgery using spectral-domain optical coherence tomography combined with microperimetry," *Retina*, vol. 32, no. 9, pp. 1733–1742, 2012.

[49] A. Fujiwara, C. Shiragami, S. Manabe, S. Izumibata, A. Murata, and F. Shiraga, "Normal values of retinal sensitivity determined by macular integrity assessment," *Nippon Ganka Gakkai Zasshi*, vol. 118, no. 1, pp. 15–21, 2014.

[50] M. O. Tso, "Pathology of cystoid macular edema," *Ophthalmology*, vol. 89, no. 8, pp. 902–915, 1982.

[51] M. Battaglia Parodi, P. Iacono, M. Scaramuzzi et al., "Outer retinal layer changes after dexamethasone implant for central retinal vein occlusion," *Retina*, vol. 37, no. 10, pp. 1888–1895, 2017.

[52] A. F. Macedo, M. D. Crossland, and G. S. Rubin, "Investigating unstable fixation in patients with macular disease," *Investigative Ophthalmology and Visual Science*, vol. 52, no. 3, pp. 1275–1280, 2011.

10

Clinical Efficacy of Platelet-Rich Plasma in the Treatment of Neurotrophic Corneal Ulcer

Dominika Wróbel-Dudzińska,[1] Jorge Alio,[2,3] Alejandra Rodriguez,[3] Ewa Suchodoła-Ratajewicz,[4] Ewa Kosior-Jarecka,[1] Beata Rymgayłło-Jankowska,[1] Agnieszka Ćwiklińska-Haszcz,[1] and Tomasz Żarnowski[1]

[1]*Department of Diagnostics and Microsurgery of Glaucoma, Medical University of Lublin, Lublin, Poland*
[2]*Department of Cornea and Refractive Surgery, Vissum Corporation, Alicante, Spain*
[3]*Research and Development Department, Vissum Corporation, Alicante, Spain*
[4]*Department of General Ophthalmology, Medical University of Lublin, Lublin, Poland*

Correspondence should be addressed to Dominika Wróbel-Dudzińska; ddudzinska@interia.pl

Academic Editor: Sotiria Palioura

Purpose. Platelet-rich plasma (PRP) is an autologous blood product without preservatives and rich in proteins and growth factors which make it possible for cells to differentiate, proliferate, and migrate, thus stimulating healing and regeneration of tissues. The aim of this study was to evaluate the efficiency of autologous platelet-rich plasma in the treatment of neurotrophic keratopathy. *Methods.* The study group consists of 25 patients with nonhealing corneal ulcers due to herpes simplex or herpes zoster infection and facial nerve or trigeminal nerve paralysis as a result of a neurosurgical operation caused by a tumour or stroke. The patients were given autologous platelet-rich plasma drops five times a day and additionally preservative-free artificial tears and a vitamin A ointment at night for maximum 3 months. The following were evaluated: best corrected visual acuity (BCVA), healing of corneal surface, subjective symptoms, and changes in corneal thickness with the use of anterior segment optical coherent tomography (AS-OCT). *Results.* BCVA before the treatment was 0.10 ± 0.14, and after the treatment it was -0.3 ± 0.27 ($p = 0.001$). Improved visual acuity and less subjective symptoms were observed in all patients. Complete healing of the ulceration was observed in 20 patients (80%). Four patients (16%) experienced considerable improvement of their clinical condition (reduced size and depth of the ulceration and inflammatory state: smaller conjunctival injection and swelling, improved visual acuity, and less subjective symptoms). In one of the patients, an amniotic membrane was transplanted due to the lack of improvement of his local condition. In all patients, the progression of corneal thinning was stopped. An average corneal thickness in its thinnest point was 322.3 ± 125.8 m before the treatment, and 404.5 ± 118.7 m ($p < 0.05$) after the treatment. None of the patients reported general or local side effects of the treatment. *Conclusions.* Autologous platelet-rich plasma is a blood-based product which seems efficient in the treatment of neurotrophic keratopathy.

1. Introduction

Neurotrophic keratitis (NK) is a rare degenerative disease characterized by reduction or absence of corneal sensitivity and consequently dysfunction of corneal healing process (reduction in the lacrimation reflex, corneal epithelium disruption, healing impairment, development of corneal opacification and stromal ulcers, and melting and perforation), followed by irreversible visual deficit [1, 2]. The most common causes of neurotrophic keratitis are presented in Table 1 [3, 4].

Diagnosis of NK is challenging, and the success may be achieved by acquired extremely detailed medical history to consider all potential risk factors and conducted comprehensive examination of the ocular surface. Unfortunately, most often NK is diagnosed in its advanced stages when visual acuity has worsened as a result of damage to the

Table 1: Etiopathogenesis of neurotrophic keratitis.

Infectious factors	Herpes simplex Herpes zoster *Acanthamoeba* Leprosy
Corneal diseases	Chemical burns Foreign body Corneal dystrophies Refractive corneal surgery Corneal damage caused by contact lenses
Topical drugs	Chronic use of anesthetics, glucocorticoids, or β-blockers
Medicines used generally	Antihistamines Neuroleptics
V nerve palsy	Intracranial tumours Intracranial aneurysms Craniofacial injuries Neurosurgical procedures Stroke
Systemic diseases	Diabetes mellitus Multiple sclerosis Autoimmune diseases Sjögren syndrome Vitamin A deficiency
Other	Transscleral cyclophotocoagulation Pars plana vitrectomy with panretinal endophotocoagulation
Congenital	Riley–Day syndrome Möbius syndrome Goldenhar syndrome Ectodermal dysplasia Hereditary sensory neuropathy

Table 2: Clinical classification of neurotrophic keratopathy based on the Mackie classification.

Stage	Clinical findings
I	Corneal epithelial irregularity Gaule spots Superficial punctuate keratopathy Increase viscosity of tear mucus Decrease break-up time Superficial corneal neovascularization Stromal scarring Dellen
II	Persistent corneal epithelial defect with smooth and rolled epithelium edges Descemet's membrane folds Stroma swelling Anterior chamber inflammatory reaction (±hypopyon)
III	Corneal ulcer Stromal melting Corneal perforation

corneal epithelium and corneal scarring. Patients rarely complain about other ocular symptoms such as red eye, pain, discomfort, burning sensation, and the foreign body sensation, since their corneal sensory innervation has been impaired. Individuals whose palpebral fissure does not close completely complain about watery eyes. It is very important that any diagnostic procedures should include taking a complete medical history into account general diseases coexistent with NK as well as any previous surgical procedures. The NK was classified as an orphan disease and divided into three stages according to the Mackie classification (Table 2) [5].

In the case of neurotrophic keratopathy, both diagnostic process and treatment are extremely difficult. There is no one efficient course of treatment whose aim would be to improve the condition of corneal epithelium and at the same time to prevent the development of corneal ulcers and their subsequent perforation. Taking into consideration pathophysiology of the disease, the role of neurotransmitters and growth factors, cytokines, a search for agents which would regenerate damaged epithelium continues. In the light of the enormous interest in regenerative medicine, blood-based products have started to receive more attention. One of them is platelet-rich plasma (PRP), commonly used in many areas of medicine such as oral and maxillofacial surgery, plastic and reconstructive surgery, orthopaedics, cardiovascular surgery, and esthetic medicine. Therapy of NK is based on promoting corneal healing; thus, such grate reservoir of growth factors and cytokines seems to be desirable option. The purpose of this work was to evaluate the efficiency and safety of using autologous platelet-rich plasma in the treatment of neurotrophic keratopathy.

2. Material and Methods

This is a prospective, nonrandomized, observational consecutive pilot study that followed the tenets of the Declaration of Helsinki. After approval by the local Ethical Committee, informed consent of the patients was obtained before the initiation of the study and patient recruitment.

We studied 25 subjects (14 females and 11 males) recruited from the Department of Diagnostic and Microsurgery of Glaucoma, University of Lublin, Poland, from January 2016 to September 2017.

2.1. Inclusion Criteria. Patients older than 18 years with neurotrophic corneal ulcers due to herpes infection or cranial nerve V or VII palsy in the stages II or III according to the Mackie classification, not responding to conventional treatment, were recruited.

All patients underwent a comprehensive ophthalmological examination and responded to the survey questionnaire, which concerned subjective symptoms such as photophobia, lacrimation, pain, and discomfort (*Questions* required either *Yes/No* response). Microbiological examination of corneal scrape was performed to exclude bacterial and fungal infection.

2.2. Exclusion Criteria. Patients with a history of corneal surgery, trauma, chemical burns, contact lens abuse, topical anesthetic abuse, corneal dystrophies, or neurotrophic corneal ulcers stages I according to the Mackie classification were excluded.

2.3. Treatment. The patients were treated with eye platelet-rich plasma drops five times a day, preservative-free artificial tears five times a day, and vitamin A ointment once at night for maximum 3 months. Some patients with NK due to herpes simplex or herpes zoster infection received additional general (orally acyclovir 400 mg four times a day) and/or topical antiviral treatment (with acyclovir 5 times a day). Those with infectious keratitis with/without hypopyon were given topical antibiotics treatment (with tobramycin and ciprofloxacin four times a day), cycloplegics treatment (with atropine once a day), and a treatment with the use of a bandage contact lens.

2.4. Patient Follow-Up. Patients attended follow-up consultations on days 1, 7, 14, and 21 and at 1, 2, and 3 months after the treatment initiation. The treatment was stopped after 3 months or when the corneal healing was achieved.

2.5. Main Outcome Measures. The following were assessed: best corrected visual acuity (BCVA) for the distance measured on the Snellen chart (decimal scale); anterior segment evaluation, healing of the corneal surface (size of the epithelial defect/ulcer: width and height measured by calipers) with fluorescein staining; corneal sensitivity in the central and peripheral cornea measured by cotton wisp test; condition of the conjunctiva (oedema and hyperemia) and the presence of any pathological discharge; subjective symptoms (pain, discomfort, lacrimation, photophobia, and foreign body sensation) given by the patients; and the results of the anterior segment optical coherence tomography (AS-OCT) (size and depth of the epithelial defect/ulcer, corneal thickness at the thinnest location) conducted with a Casia I (Tomey) photographic assessment.

In the ophthalmologic examination, special attention was paid to the size and depth of the epithelial defect and ulceration. The size (width and height) of the corneal epithelial defect was measured by calipers and classified as large when it exceeded 4.0 mm, medium when it was between 2.0 and 4.0 mm, and small when it was smaller or equal to 2.0 mm.

Subjective symptoms were evaluated based on the self-administered questionnaire, which was completed once at the time of enrollment in the study (baseline) and again after treatment with eye platelet-rich plasma (E-PRP). Patients were asked to report any change in their perception of pain, discomfort, foreign body sensation, photophobia, and lacrimation, giving yes or no answer.

2.6. Autologous PRP Preparation. Platelet-rich plasma drops were prepared according to the previous description [6, 7]. The strict sterility conditions using sterile and disposable materials and operating inside a laminar flow hood were needed to prepare PRP. Autologous drops were produced from 40 to 80 ml of whole blood, obtained from patients by venipuncture and collected into 10 ml sterile tubes containing 1 ml of sodium citrate. The tubes including blood were spun at room temperature 1400 rpm for 10 minutes. 90% of obtained plasma was used as the final product, and then three to four millilitres were placed into new, sterilized 10 ml bottles with eye drop applicators. Patients were given the instruction to wash their hands prior to the application of the product, to keep the area of application clean and not to touch the eyedropper. The bottle in use should be kept at +4°C and the rest at −20°C.

2.7. Statistical Analysis. Statistical analysis was conducted using Excel and Statistica 12 programs. The Shapiro–Wilk test was used to test the normality of the distribution of the evaluated qualities. The value of $p < 0.05$ was considered to be statistically significant. Depending on the level of measurement of variables, different statistical tests and coefficients were employed: *t*-Student and ANOVA.

3. Results

The patients' characteristics are shown in Table 3. Average patient age was 66.08 ± 16.45. In 15 patients, the persistence epithelial defect or ulceration was caused by a herpes zoster or simplex infection, and in 10 patients it was the result of an injury to the trigeminal nerve and/or facial nerve incurred during a neurosurgical procedure. Eight patients presented with inadequate closing of the palpebral fissure as well as weakened Bell's reflex.

Improved visual acuity was observed in almost all the patients. Best corrected visual acuity before the treatment was 0.11 ± 0.14, and after the treatment it considerably improved to 0.3 ± 0.27 ($p = 0.001$).

Mean time of the treatment was 9.2 ± 2.85 weeks. An average size of epithelial defect/ulceration before the treatment was 3.7 ± 1.1 x 2.8 ± 0.9 mm. After the treatment, complete reepithelialization of the persistence epithelial defect or ulcer was observed in 20 patients (80%), and 4 patients (16%) experienced considerable improvement, defined as at least 0.5 mm changes in the area of the epithelial defect/ulcer. Moreover, in almost all patients, reduction of the inflammatory state was observed: smaller conjunctival injection and swelling. Two of the participants had hypopyon, which disappeared after basic and additional treatment. The lack of corneal sensitivity was observed in 19 patients, the rest had it weakened. The corneal sensation did not change during the treatment. Unfortunately, in one of the patients an amniotic membrane was transplanted due to the lack of improvement of the local condition and high risk of corneal perforation.

A change in subjective symptoms was reported by the patients after the treatment. Lack of discomfort and photophobia was observed in 96% of participants. 6 patients declared (100%) reduction of foreign body sensation.

In all cases, the progression of corneal thinning was stopped. An average corneal thickness in its thinnest point was $322.3 \pm 125.83\,\mu$m before the treatment, and $404.53 \pm 118.68\,\mu$m ($p < 0.05$) after the treatment.

None of the patients reported general or local side effects of the treatment. Moreover, no recurrence of the corneal ulcer was observed within 10 months, which was our follow-up time.

Figures 1–3 show the clinical condition of patients, both before and after the treatment.

Table 3: Characteristics of the study group.

Patient number	Age	Gender	Etiology	Mackie classification	Ulcer size	Additional treatment	Additional surgical procedures	Corneal sensation
1	79	F	Herpes zoster	3	Big	Y	N	Lack
2	66	M	Herpes simplex	2	Big	Y	N	Weakened
3	60	F	Cranial nerve palsy	3	Big	Y	N	Lack
4	82	M	Cranial nerve palsy	2	Medium	N	N	Lack
5	89	M	Herpes simplex	3	Medium	Y	N	Lack
6	59	M	Cranial nerve palsy	3	Big	N	N	Lack
7	58	M	Herpes zoster	2	Big	Y	N	Lack
8	46	M	Cranial nerve palsy	2	Medium	N	N	Weakened
9	82	F	Herpes simplex	3	Big	Y	N	Lack
10	74	F	Cranial nerve palsy	2	Big	N	N	Weakened
11	43	F	Herpes simplex	3	Big	Y	Y	Lack
12	74	M	Cranial nerve palsy	3	Big	Y	N	Lack
13	83	M	Herpes simplex	3	Medium	Y	N	Lack
14	70	M	Herpes simplex	2	Small	Y	N	Weakened
15	80	M	Herpes simplex	2	Small	Y	N	Weakened
16	41	F	Cranial nerve palsy	2	Small	N	N	Lack
17	60	F	Herpes simplex	2	Small	Y	N	Lack
18	60	F	Cranial nerve palsy	3	Small	N	N	Lack
19	69	F	Cranial nerve palsy	2	Small	N	N	Lack
20	52	F	Herpes simplex	3	Medium	Y	N	Lack
21	74	F	Cranial nerve palsy	3	Medium	N	N	Lack
22	59	F	Cranial nerve palsy	3	Big	Y	N	Lack
23	81	F	Cranial nerve palsy	3	Big	Y	N	Lack
24	82	F	Herpes simplex	2	Medium	Y	N	Weakened
25	23	M	Cranial nerve palsy	2	Medium	N	N	Lack

F: female; M: male. Mackie classification stage 2: persistent epithelial defects with thickened and rolled edges, oedematous stroma, stage 3: corneal ulcer, stromal melting, impending perforation. Ulcer size (width and height): small: smaller or equal to 2 mm; medium: between 2 and 4 mm; big: greater than 4 mm. Y: yes; N: no.

4. Discussion

Standard NK therapy depends on the stage in the Mackie classification [5]. The main target is to treat according to the etiopathogenesis and enhancing corneal healing to prevent corneal perforation. It is crucial to cure concomitant ocular disorders such as dry eye, exposure keratitis, or limbal stem cells deficiency. Usually, all topical medications which have been administered so far are stopped and the patient is given artificial tears without preservatives, and in severe cases in order to prevent secondary infection, topical antibiotics and bandage contact lenses are introduced [2, 8]. Topical glucocorticosteroids (GCs) are contraindicated in the case of a viral infection, as they increase viral replication, lengthen the time it takes for the stroma to heal and increase the risk of corneal perforation. However, they might prove useful when it comes to reducing inflammation. When treating NK, nonsteroidal anti-inflammatory drugs (NSAIDs) should be avoided, as well as eye drops with cyclosporine which has an adverse effect on the regeneration of corneal nerve fibres [2, 9].

To prevent melting and perforation of the cornea, some surgical procedures can be carried out, such as temporary or permanent tarsorrhaphy, injecting botulinum toxin A into the elevating muscle of upper eyelid, amniotic membrane or conjunctival patch graft, sympathectomy, transplanting mucuous membrane from the nose, Tutopatch with platelet-rich plasma, and transplanting a fragment of the sural nerve to restore corneal innervation [8, 10–13]. To improve the condition of epithelium and speed up the healing process, new unconventional methods of treatment have been introduced, including eye drops with autologous serum,

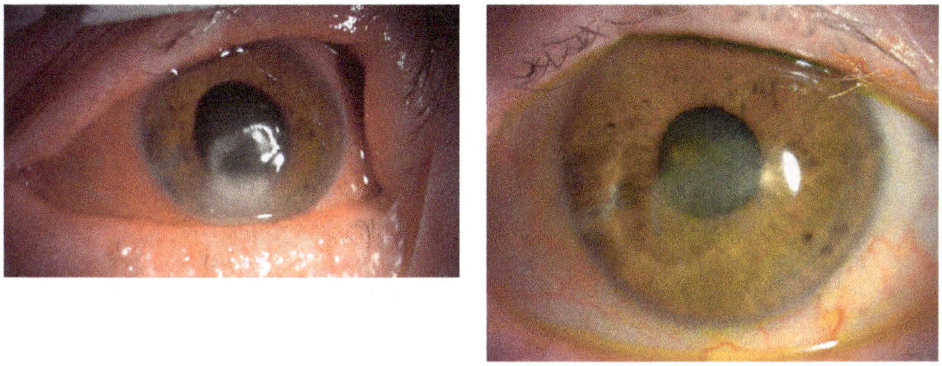

(a) (b)

FIGURE 1: (a) Representative case of the patient (number 1) with stage 3 NK: large deep corneal ulcer with rolled edges of the epithelium, mix conjunctiva injection—hyperemia, stromal melting with hypopyon. (b) Picture of the patient number 1 after the treatment showing significant improvement: corneal scar.

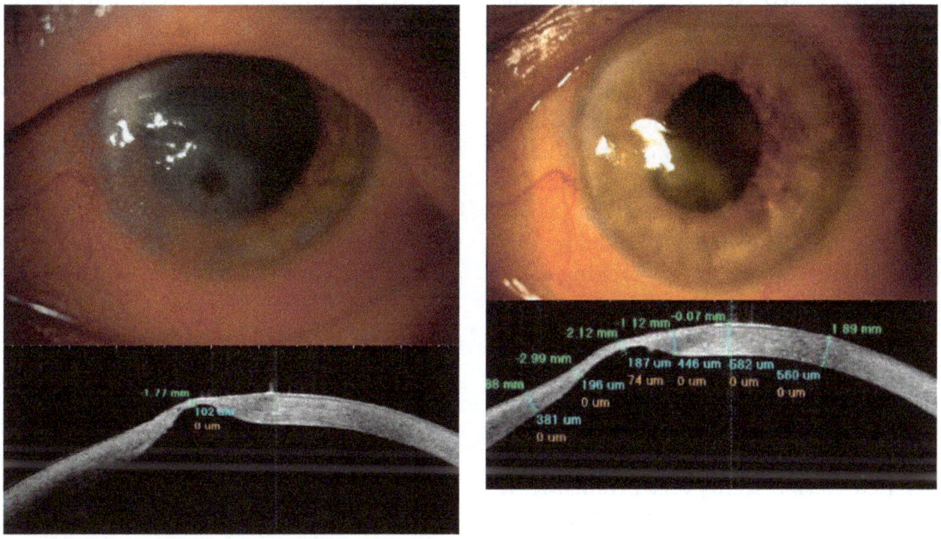

(a) (b)

FIGURE 2: (a) Representative case of the patient (number 6) with stage 3 NK: large deep corneal ulcer, impending perforation, neovascularization, conjunctival, and iris hyperemia. The corneal thickness at the thinnest point was 102 μm. (b) Clinical improvement of the patient number 6 after the treatment: large scar with superficial neovascularization. The corneal thickness improved to 187 μm.

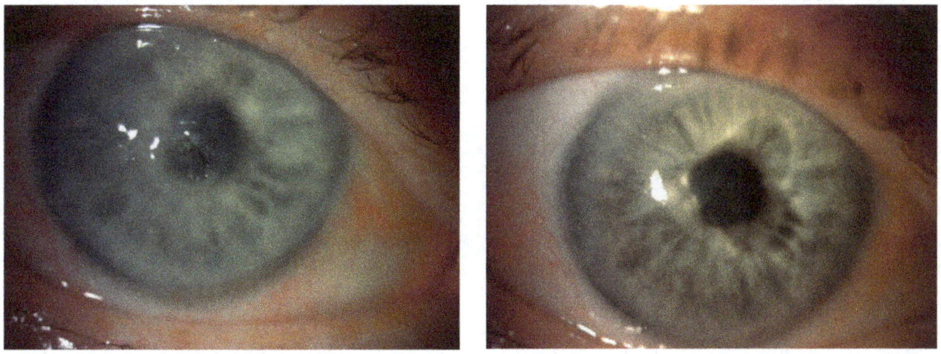

(a) (b)

FIGURE 3: (a) Representative case of the patient (number 14) with stage 3 NK: small deep corneal ulcer with rolled edges of the epithelium, mix conjunctiva injection—hyperemia, stromal melting. (b) Clinical improvement of the patient number 14 after the treatment: complete healing of the ulcer with slight corneal haze.

umbilical cord serum, platelet-rich plasma, plasma rich in growth factors, neurotrophin, neuropeptides, and growth factors, for example, nerve growth factor (NGF), substance P (SP), and thymosin beta-4 [14–18].

According to the previous encouraging reports about promising therapeutic agent as matrix regeneration therapy in NK [17], Arvola et al. conducted their own study of neurotrophic ulcer treatment with RGTA®, where the outcomes were not so much satisfying from the efficacy point of view. They observed 2 patients with complete corneal healing, 4 patients with failure to heal, and in 1 case of perforation, no visual acuity improvement [19].

Currently, clinical trials are being conducted on the use of heparin sulphate and recombinant human nerve growth factor (rhNGF) in the treatment of NK [20, 21]. The group of scientists treated more than 45 eyes with moderate and severe neurotrophic ulcers with nerve growth factor eye drops observing healing in almost 100% of the cases [16]. Regrettably, genetically engineered NGF eye drops are still not available on the market in Poland.

The interest in blood hemoderivatives is constantly growing. According to Matsumoto's study, autologous serum helped heal epithelial disorders in 11 cases of NK. This clear acellular liquid fraction has properties comparable to natural tears as far as pH and osmolarity is concerned, thus this product is more effective in dry eye treatment. López-Plandolit et al. used plasma rich in growth factors for persistent corneal epithelial defects treatment reaching quite good results: epithelial defects healed in 17 of 20 cases. The main problem of this hemoderivative application is the preparation based on especially designed devices and double centrifugation technique with platelet activation [22].

In the light of the growing interest in blood-derived products and the lack of effective treatment for neurotrophic corneal ulcer, platelet-rich plasma seems very promising. It is an autologous product without any preservatives, extremely abundant in platelets, presenting a high concentration of cell adhesion molecules and growth factors. It is a known fact that an injury to the trigeminal nerve leads to the deficiency of neuropeptides, neurotransmitters, and growth factors maintaining homeostasis of ocular surface. That is why this mixture of growth factors and cytokines plays an essential role in regeneration process. It has been proven that platelet-rich plasma contains cytokines (e.g., PF4 and CD4OL) as well as growth factors such as PDGF (platelet-derived growth factor), TGF- (transforming growth factor-) ß1 and ß2, IGF- (insulin-like growth factor-) 1, VEGF, EGF, FGF-2, and IGF [13, 23]. Most of its efficiency PRP owes to PDGF factor which is the first growth factor to appear in a wound, stimulating revascularisation, collagen synthesis, and regeneration. Its role in healing process is to increase the number of repair cells, stimulate angiogenesis, support the development of new blood vessels, and activate macrophages responsible for cleaning the wound. TGF, secreted during platelet degranulation or actively produced by macrophages, acts as paracrine growth factor, in charge of chemotaxis and epithelium proliferation. Another important protein contained in alpha granules of platelets is EGF (endothelial growth factor). It speeds up corneal epithelium proliferation and has an antiapoptotic function. PF4 and CD4OL are proteins which control antibody-mediated immunity and cell-mediated immunity [24]. VEGF (vascular epithelial growth factor) and FGF- (fibroblast growth factor-) 2 take part in angiogenesis, as a result of which nutrients and progenitor cells are delivered to the wound by new vessels. Their mechanism is based on the function of blood platelets whose role is to prevent sudden blood loss as well as to repair vessel walls and surrounding tissue [25]. Interrupted endothelium is what activates blood platelets. Then, the activated alpha granules secrete numerous proteins and growth factors: cytokines; interleukins: IL-1β, IL-2, IL-4, IL-5, IL-6, IL-7, IL-8, IL-10, IL-12, IL-13, IL-15, IL-17, PF4, and CD4OL; growth factors: PDGF AA, AB, and BB; TGF-β1 i-β3; IGF-1; EGF; INF-α (interferon alpha); FGF; and fibronectins. As we know, most molecules are secreted in the first hour, then platelets synthesize and secrete cytokines and growth factors for another 7 days (it is related to the average life span of blood platelets which is 7 to 10 days) [26]. Growth factors bind to their transmembrane receptors in the damaged tissue, triggering a cascade of reactions: activation of endogenous signalling protein, expression of genes responsible for cell proliferation, formation of cell matrixes, and the synthesis of collagen. All these mediators set off the processes of cell differentiation, proliferation and migration, angiogenesis, and, by the same token, the process of regeneration of the damaged tissue. Furthermore, platelets secrete antibacterial proteins which have an antibiotic effect [27]. Since many questions concerning the detailed mechanism in which PRP works have still not been answered, further molecular study is necessary.

The results of the studies on the product's efficiency, both ours and the ones conducted by other researchers, are promising. Alio et al. used different varieties of platelet-rich plasma in 40 patients with nonhealing corneal ulcers. They observed complete healing of the ulceration in 23 patients, considerable improvement in 15 patients, and in 2 patients, the treatment did not bring any results. In majority of the cases, reduction of the inflammation and pain was observed. Moreover, visual acuity improved in about 60% of cases. The product was well tolerated and no adverse side effects were reported [6, 7].

The recurrent corneal erosions (RCE) treatment with platelet-rich plasma (PRP) eye drops was also evaluated. Lee et al. reported that the mean frequency of recurrence of corneal erosion was 0.06 ± 0.08 per month in the PRP eye drops treated group and 0.39 ± 0.24 per month in the conventional treatment group ($p = 0.003$) [28].

The platelet-rich plasma is widely used in ophthalmology, other indications might be: macular hole and pterygium, after chemical burns [29–31].

5. Conclusion

Autologous platelet-rich plasma has been demonstrated to be effective in corneal neurotrophic ulcer treatment. The lack of preservatives, autologous quality, relative ease of its preparation, safety, and beneficial effects make PRP a promising therapeutic tool for future regenerative medicine. Despite the fact that recombinant synthetic products are available for neurotrophic ulcer treatment, those high-priced goods contain only a single growth factor.

Conflicts of Interest

The authors declare that they have no conflicts of interest.

References

[1] S. Bonini, P. Rama, D. Olzi, and A. Lambiase, "Neurotrophic keratitis," *Eye*, vol. 17, no. 8, pp. 989–995, 2003.

[2] M. Sacchetti and A. Lambiase, "Diagnosis and management of neurotrophic keratitis," *Clinical Ophthalmology*, vol. 8, pp. 571–579, 2014.

[3] C. Auchère Lavayssiere, A. Lux, A. Degoumois, M. Stchepinsky Launay, and E. Denion, "Neurotrophic keratitis after vitrectomy and circumferential endophotocoagulation for retinal detachment," *Journal Français d'Ophtalmologie*, vol. 39, no. 2, pp. 195–201, 2016.

[4] A. Fernández-Vega González, R. Barraquer Compte, A. Cárcamo Martínez, M. Torrico Delgadillo, and M. de la Paz, "Neurotrophic keratitis after transscleral diode laser cyclophotocoagulation," *Archivos de la Sociedad Española de Oftalmología*, vol. 91, no. 7, pp. 320–326, 2016.

[5] I. A. Mackie, "Neuroparalytic keratitis," in *Current Ocular Therapy*, F. Fraunfelder, F. H. Roy, and S. M. Meyer, Eds., WB Saunders, Philadelphia, PA, USA, 1995.

[6] J. L. Alio, M. Abad, A. Artola, J. L. Rodriguez-Prats, S. Pastor, and J. Ruiz-Colecha, "Use of autologous platelet-rich plasma in the treatment of dormant corneal ulcers," *Ophthalmology*, vol. 114, no. 7, pp. 1286–1293, 2007.

[7] J. L. Alio, A. E. Rodriguez, and D. WróbelDudzińska, "Eye platelet-rich plasma in the treatment of ocular surface disorders," *Current Opinion in Ophthalmology*, vol. 26, no. 4, pp. 325–332, 2015.

[8] F. Semeraro, E. Forbice, V. Romano et al., "Neurotrophic keratitis," *Ophthalmologica*, vol. 231, no. 4, pp. 191–197, 2014.

[9] A. Namavari, S. Chaudhary, J. Chang et al., "Cyclosporine immunomodulation retards regeneration of surgically transected corneal nerves," *Investigative Opthalmology and Visual Science*, vol. 53, no. 2, pp. 732–740, 2012.

[10] V. Ortuno-Prado and J. Alio, "Tratamiento de úlcera corneal neurotrófica con plasma rico en plaquetasy Tutopatch®," *Archivos De La Sociedad Espanola De Oftalmologia*, vol. 86, pp. 121–123, 2011.

[11] J. Alio, A. Rodriguez, L. Martinez, and A. Rio, "Autologous fibrin membrane combined with solid platelet-rich plasma in the management of perforated corneal ulcers: a pilot study," *JAMA Ophthalmolgy*, vol. 131, no. 6, pp. 745–751, 2013.

[12] J. Alio, A. Rodriguez, and L. Martinez, "Bovine pericardium membrane (Tutopatch) combined with solid platelet-rich plasma for the management of perforated corneal ulcers," *Cornea*, vol. 32, no. 5, pp. 619–624, 2013.

[13] J. Alio, F. Arnalich-Montiel, and A. Rodriguez, "The role of "eye platelet rich plasma" (E-PRP) for wound healing in ophthalmology," *Current Pharmaceutical Biotechnology*, vol. 13, no. 7, pp. 1257–1265, 2012.

[14] T. Chikama, K. Fukuda, N. Morishige, and T. Nishida, "Treatment of neurotrophic keratopathy with substance-P-derived peptide (FGLM) and insulin growth factor 1," *The Lancet*, vol. 351, no. 9118, pp. 1783-1784, 1998.

[15] S. Dunn, D. Heidemann, C. Chow et al., "Treatment of chronic nonhealing neurotrophic corneal epithelial defects with thymosin β4," *Annals of the New York Academy of Sciences*, vol. 1194, no. 1, pp. 199–206, 2010.

[16] S. Bonini, A. Lambiase, P. Rama, G. Caprioglio, and L. Aloe, "Topical treatment with nerve growth factor for neurotrophic keratitis," *Ophthalmology*, vol. 107, no. 7, pp. 1347–1352, 2000.

[17] A. Aifa, J. Gueudry, A. Portmann, A. Delcampe, and M. Muraine, "Topical treatment with a new matrix therapy agent (RGTA) for the treatment of corneal neurotrophic ulcers," *Investigative Opthalmology and Visual Science*, vol. 53, no. 13, pp. 8181–8185, 2012.

[18] Y. Matsumoto, M. Dogru, E. Goto et al., "Autologous serum application in the treatment of neurotrophic keratopathy," *Ophthalmology*, vol. 111, no. 6, pp. 1115–1120, 2004.

[19] R. P. Arvola, A. Robciuc, and J. M. Holopainen, "Matrix regeneration therapy: a case series of corneal neurotrophic ulcers," *Cornea*, vol. 35, no. 4, pp. 451–455, 2016.

[20] *Evaluation of Safety and Efficacy of rhNGF in Patients with Stage 2 and 3 Neurotrophic Keratitis (REPARO)*, ClinicalTrials.gov, https://www.clinical-trials.gov/ct2/show/NCT01756456.

[21] A. Lambiase, P. Rama, S. Bonini, G. Caprioglio, and L. Aloe, "Topical treatment with nerve growth factor for corneal neurotrophic ulcers," *New England Journal of Medicine*, vol. 338, no. 17, pp. 1174–1180, 1998.

[22] S. López-Plandolit, M. C. Morales, V. Freire, J. Etxebarría, and J. A. Durán, "Plasma rich in growth factors as a therapeutic agent for persistent corneal epithelial defects," *Cornea*, vol. 29, no. 8, pp. 843–848, 2010.

[23] T. Castillo, M. Pouliot, H. Kim, and J. Dragoo, "Comparison of growth factor and platelet concentration from commercial platelet-rich plasma separation systems," *American Journal of Sports Medicine*, vol. 39, no. 2, pp. 266–271, 2010.

[24] A. Nurden, "Platelets, inflammation and tissue regeneration," *Thrombosis and Haemostasis*, vol. 105, no. 1, pp. S13–S33, 2011.

[25] R. E. Marx, "Platelet-rich plasma (PRP): what is PRP and what is not PRP?," *Implant Dentistry*, vol. 10, no. 4, pp. 225–228, 2001.

[26] L. Senzel, D. Gnatenko, and W. Bahou, "The platelet proteome," *Current Opinion in Hematology*, vol. 16, no. 5, pp. 329–333, 2009.

[27] L. Drago, M. Bortolin, C. Vassena, S. Taschieri, and M. del Fabbro, "Antimicrobial activity of pure platelet-rich plasma against microorganisms isolated from oral cavity," *BMC Microbiology*, vol. 13, no. 1, pp. 47–51, 2013.

[28] J. Lee, M. Kim, S. Ha, and H. Kim, "Autologous platelet-rich plasma eye drops in the treatment of recurrent corneal erosions," *Korean Journal of Ophthalmolog*, vol. 30, no. 2, pp. 101–107, 2016.

[29] M. Figueroa, A. Govetto, and P. Arriba-Palomero, "Short-term results of platelet-rich plasma as adjuvant to 23-G vitrectomy in the treatment of high myopic macular holes," *European Journal of Ophthalmology*, vol. 26, no. 5, pp. 491–496, 2016.

[30] H. Cakmak, C. Dereli, M. Can, and N. Cagil, "A novel graft option after pterygium excision: platelet-rich fibrin for conjunctivoplasty," *Eye*, vol. 31, no. 11, pp. 1606–1612, 2017.

[31] A. Panda, M. Jain, M. Vanathi, T. Velpandian, S. Khokhar, and T. Dada, "Topical autologous platelet-rich plasma eye drops for acute corneal chemical injury," *Cornea*, vol. 31, no. 9, pp. 989–993, 2012.

11

Internal Astigmatism and Its Role in the Growth of Axial Length in School-Age Children

Liangcheng Wu,[1] **Chenghai Weng**,[1] **Fei Xia**,[1] **Xiaoying Wang**,[1,2] **and Xingtao Zhou**[2]

[1]*Department of Ophthalmology, Jing'an District Centre Hospital of Shanghai, Fudan University, Shanghai, China*
[2]*Department of Ophthalmology and Vision Science, Eye and ENT Hospital, Shanghai Medical College, Fudan University, Shanghai, China*

Correspondence should be addressed to Xingtao Zhou; xingtaozhou@163.com

Academic Editor: Ewa Mrukwa-Kominek

Objectives. To explore the role of internal astigmatism (IA) in the growth of axial length (AL) in school-age children. *Methods.* Total astigmatism (TA), corneal astigmatism (CA), and AL of all children in Jing'an District 2nd Centre Primary School in Shanghai were measured. In IA, the difference between TA and CA was also calculated using vector analysis. The association of axial length with IA, genders, and age was analyzed using linear regression. The difference of IA between both eyes was also calculated. The AL between both eyes was compared using paired samples t-test when DIA = 0 D, <0.5 D, and ≥0.5 D. *Results.* Six hundred and twelve cases (98.23%) in 623 children aged 7–12 yrs older entered into the study. Genders, age, and IA all affected AL. This could be represented by a linear regression line in the form $AL = 21.46 - 0.43 * \text{gender} + 0.22 * \text{age} + 0.46 * IA$ (male = 1, female = 2, $t = 7.01$, $P < 0.01$ for sex; $t = 11.6$, $P < 0.01$ for age; and $t = 6.6$, $P < 0.01$ for IA; $R^2 = 0.16$). The AL in the eye with larger IA was also longer when DIA was larger than 0.5 D ($t = 2.65$, $P < 0.01$). *Conclusions.* IA was observed to be associated with AL and might be a risk factor of the onset and progress of myopia in school-age children.

1. Introduction

Myopia is becoming a common public health problem worldwide especially in eastern Asian countries [1]. The myopia-related complications are major causes of visual impairments and blindness [1–3]. To explore the mechanism and risk factors of myopia is always the hot focus of myopia study. It is well known but still under debate that astigmatism takes an important role in the creation and progress of myopia in the growth and development stage of humans and some animals. Many studies supported that astigmatism was a risk factor for myopia progress or creation [4–6]. But not all studies have shown an association between the presence of astigmatism and the progression of myopic refractive errors. Czepita and Filipiak reported that a negative correlation was found between cornea astigmatism (CA) and myopia progress, and a positive correlation was observed between TA and myopia [7]. Astigmatism or total astigmatism (TA) consists of CA and internal astigmatism (IA). TA and CA can be independently measured. The difference between the two, internal astigmatism (IA), is thought to arise from the internal optics of the eye, including asymmetries related to the crystalline lens [8]. We speculate that IA may play a more important role in the progress or creation of myopia. In the present study, we examined TA, CA, and axial length (AL) for all children in Jing'an District 2nd Centre Primary School in Shanghai, and the purpose was to explore the role of IA in the growth of eye axial length.

2. Methods

The study was based on a school survey and was approved by the Jing'an District Hospital Ethics Committee and conducted in accordance with the principles of the Declaration of Helsinki. The study was a part of routine school refraction screening program and was performed in Jing'an District 2nd

Centre Primary School. Jing'an District 2nd Central Primary School was a school with 5 grades, 20 classes, and 623 children including 335 male and 288 females in 2016. All children were asked to test for uncorrected visual acuity, presenting visual acuity, refraction, and axial length. The eyeball axial length was measured by a commercial instrument (IOLMaster; Carl Zeiss Meditec AG, Jena, Germany). Noncycloplegic autorefraction was performed using an Auto Ref-Keratometer (HRK-7000A; HUVITZ Co. Ltd., Korea). In fully automated mode, the Auto Ref-Keratometer performed at least five autorefractions in each eye and gave a standardized value as its output.

TA, CA, and IA were expressed in negative correcting cylinder form and were described at the corneal vertex surface. So the vertex distance was set as zero during autorefractor examination and TA was given in the autorefractor output. CA axis was set along the K_{min} meridian. We calculated CA based on the autokeratometry reading using a corneal refractive index of 1.3375. This takes into account the negative refractive power of the posterior corneal surface [8]. CA was calculated as $K_{min} - K_{max}$, where K_{min} represents the meridian with the least refractive power and K_{max} the meridian with the greatest refractive power. IA was calculated as the vector difference between TA and CA and was detailed described in other studies [8, 9].

The difference of IA between both eyes (DIA) was also calculated; these children were divided into 3 groups according to the DIA including DIA = 0 D, DIA <0.5 D, and DIA ≥ 0.5 D.

2.1. Statistical Analysis. Statistical analysis was performed using SPSS software version 13 (SPSS Inc., Chicago, IL). IA and DIA were expressed as absolute value (positive value) in statistical process. The age, AL, and IA in between both genders were compared using independent-samples t-test. Paired-samples t-test was used to compare AL between both eyes when DIA = 0 D, DIA < 0.5 D, and DIA ≥ 0.5 D. Linear regression was used to analyze relationship between AL and age, relationship between IA and age, relationship between AL and IA, and relationship between AL and some factors including age and genders along with IA. The sex ratio between boys and girls in various ages was compared using a chi-square test. $P < 0.05$ was considered as statistically significant.

3. Results

Six hundred and twelve cases (98.23%) in 623 children aged 7–12 yrs older were enrolled into the study, including 330 boys and 282 girls. Four children were excluded from the study because of being absent from school and 7 because of obtaining unreliable data. The distribution of age in both genders was showed in Figure 1; the average age between genders was not significantly different (independent-samples t-test: 9.51 ± 1.59 yrs for boys versus 9.41 ± 1.56 yrs for girls, $t = 0.79$, and $P > 0.05$), and there was no significant difference in sex ratio between boys and girls in all ages (chi-square test: $\chi^2 = 6.81$, $P > 0.05$). The refractive errors including sphere and TA, CA, and AL along with DIA were showed in Table 1.

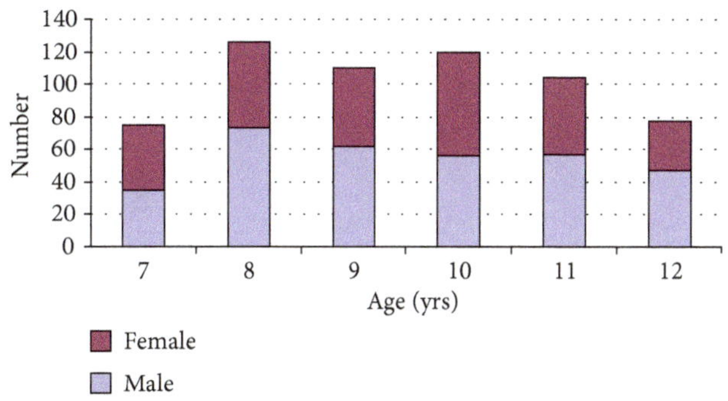

FIGURE 1: The distribution of gender at various age in 623 children.

3.1. Association of AL with IA, Age, and Gender. The AL of boys was 23.46 ± 0.92 mm, and that of girls was 23.01 ± 0.99 mm. The AL of boys was longer significantly than that of girls (independent-samples t-test: $t = 6.57$, $P < 0.001$). There was a linear relationship between AL and age in both genders (linear regression analysis: $t = 10.56$, $P < 0.001$ in male; $t = 9.14$, $P < 0.001$ in female; Figure 2).

The IA was 0.61 ± 0.46(−D) in boys and 0.66 ± 0.41(−D) in girls; there was no significant difference between genders (independent-samples t-test: $t = 1.88$, $P > 0.05$). IA maintained stable with age in both genders (linear regression analysis: $t = 0.56$, $P > 0.05$ in male; $t = 0.053$, $P > 0.05$ in female). But a linear relationship was found between AL and IA (linear regression analysis: $t = 6.27$, $P < 0.001$ in male; $t = 3.68$, $P < 0.001$ in female; Figure 2).

Linear regression analysis showed that genders, age, and IA all affected AL. This could be represented by a linear regression line in the form $AL = 21.46 - 0.43 * gender + 0.22 * age + 0.46 * IA$ (male = 1, female = 2; $t = 7.01$, $P < 0.01$ for sex; $t = 11.6$, $P < 0.01$ for age; and $t = 6.6$, $P < 0.01$ for IA; $R^2 = 0.16$).

3.2. Association of AL with DIA. The DIA was −0.38 ± 0.42(D) in male and −0.33 ± 0.33(D) in female; the difference was not significant between genders (independent-samples t-test: $t = 1.62$, $P > 0.05$) and also did not vary with age (one-way ANOVA: $F = 0.66$, $P > 0.05$ in male; $F = 0.18$, $P > 0.05$ in female), but when DIA was larger than 0.5 D, the axial length with larger IA was also longer (pared-samples t-test: $t = 2.65$, $P < 0.01$) and was showed in Table 2.

4. Discussion

Cycloplegic refraction was a need in school-age children due to high accommodation. However, cycloplegic refraction was difficult to perform in school. AL is the primary determinant of nonsyndromic myopia. It is a parameter representing the combination of anterior chamber depth, lens thickness, and vitreous chamber depth of the eye. The AL elongation in children can be related to the normal growth of the eyeball and, thus, affect the refractive status of the eye. Considering the

Table 1: Axial length, IA, and DIA in school children in Jing'an District 2nd Primary School 2016.

Age (yrs)	Axial length (mm)		Sphere (−D)		TA (−D)		CA (−D)		IA (−D)		DIA (−D)	
	Male	Female	Male	Female	Male	Female	Male	Female	Male	Female	Male	Female
7	22.93 ± 0.56	22.56 ± 0.58	0.16 ± 0.36	0.29 ± 1.13	0.91 ± 0.93	0.6 ± 0.44	0.92 ± 0.89	0.6 ± 0.52	0.60 ± 0.37	0.61 ± 0.36	0.34 ± 0.24	0.31 ± 0.30
8	23.15 ± 0.72	22.60 ± 0.78	0.31 ± 0.77	0.41 ± 0.97	0.89 ± 0.75	0.85 ± 0.56	0.84 ± 0.70	0.85 ± 0.62	0.63 ± 0.57	0.64 ± 0.37	0.43 ± 0.62	0.35 ± 0.30
9	23.41 ± 0.84	22.94 ± 0.93	0.37 ± 0.65	0.64 ± 1.29	0.79 ± 0.62	0.84 ± 0.75	0.83 ± 0.67	0.84 ± 0.74	0.58 ± 0.37	0.72 ± 0.42	0.36 ± 0.26	0.35 ± 0.34
10	23.37 ± 0.77	23.08 ± 0.93	0.51 ± 0.97	0.78 ± 1.30	0.85 ± 0.63	0.76 ± 0.58	0.88 ± 0.65	0.75 ± 0.60	0.63 ± 0.45	0.61 ± 0.43	0.41 ± 0.40	0.31 ± 0.39
11	23.71 ± 1.02	23.26 ± 1.19	0.97 ± 1.31	1.11 ± 1.40	0.89 ± 0.72	1.04 ± 0.85	0.88 ± 0.74	1.02 ± 0.83	0.57 ± 0.42	0.69 ± 0.48	0.31 ± 0.36	0.32 ± 0.39
12	24.16 ± 1.06	23.78 ± 1.06	1.22 ± 1.37	1.67 ± 1.65	1.05 ± 0.79	0.90 ± 0.49	1.10 ± 0.84	0.84 ± 0.51	0.68 ± 0.49	0.71 ± 0.35	0.40 ± 0.40	0.32 ± 0.34
Average	23.45 ± 0.92	23.01 ± 0.99	0.58 ± 1.04	0.76 ± 1.34	0.89 ± 0.73	0.83 ± 0.64	0.90 ± 0.74	0.82 ± 0.66	0.61 ± 0.46	0.66 ± 0.41	0.38 ± 0.42	0.33 ± 0.33

TA: total astigmatism; CA: corneal astigmatism; IA: internal astigmatism; DIA: difference of internal astigmatism between both eyes. The axial length of boys was longer significantly than that of girls ($t = 8.14$, $P < 0.001$). A linear relationship between axial length and age was found in both genders ($t = 10.56$, $P < 0.001$ in male; $t = 9.14$, $P < 0.001$ in female). And there was no significant difference in IA and DIA between genders ($t = 1.88$, $P > 0.05$ for IA; $t = 1.63$, $P > 0.05$). IA and DIA did not grow significantly with age in both genders ($t = 0.56$, $P > 0.05$ in male, and $t = 0.053$, $P > 0.05$ in female, resp.).

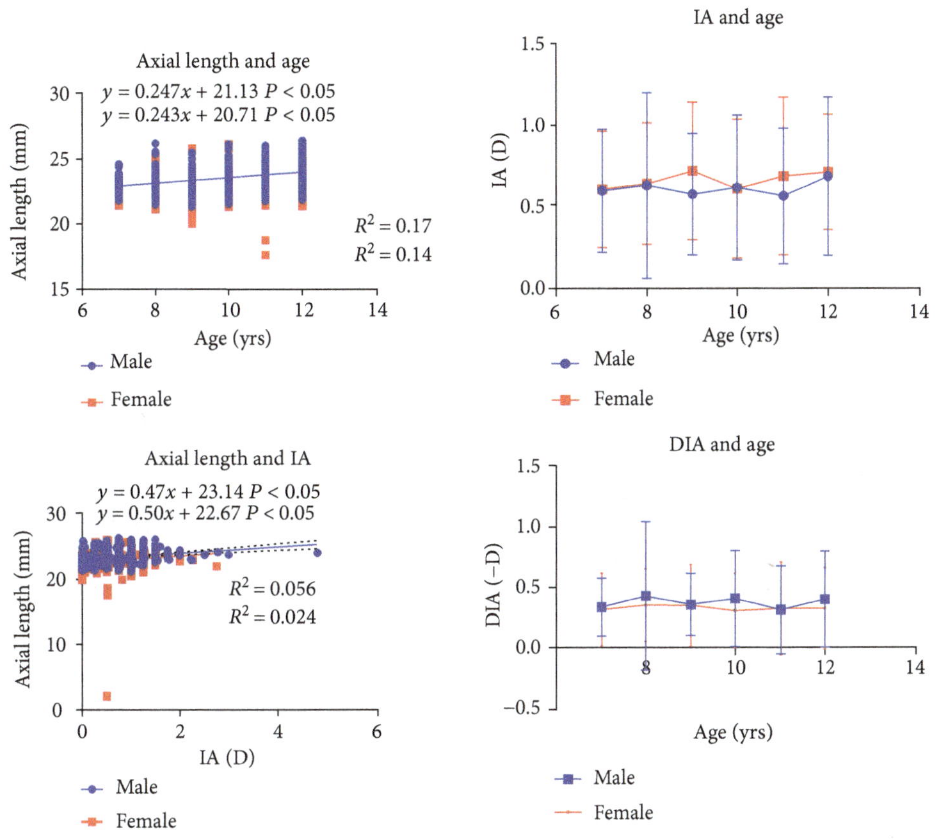

Figure 2: The relationship between axial length and age as well as the relationship between internal astigmatism age.

Table 2: The axial length in different DIA.

Group	Cases	Axial length in the eye with less IA (mm)	Axial length in the eye with larger IA (mm)	t	P
DIA = 0 D	128	23.27 ± 0.99 (right eye)	23.29 ± 0.96 (left eye)	0.89	>0.05
0 < DIA< 0.5 D	292	23.22 ± 0.92	23.24 ± 0.95	0.44	>0.05
DIA ≥ 0.5 D	192	23.17 ± 0.95	23.28 ± 0.97	2.65	<0.05

DIA: difference of internal astigmatism between both eyes; IA: internal astigmatism.

contribution of AL, lens power, and corneal power together using multiple linear regression analyses, AL can explain up to 96% of the variation of refraction in populations [10]. The AL is a valid parameter for monitoring myopic progression [10, 11]. In our study, the AL was used to evaluate the refractive status and the growth of the eyeball in school-age children.

Our study showed that genders, age, and IA all affected the AL. A linear relationship was found between AL and IA. In fact, many factors including age, genders, outdoor activities, ethics, refraction correction pattern, and so on all affect the AL growth. In order to exclude these disturbing factors, we compared the AL difference between both eyes when DIA = 0 D, 0–0.5 D, and ≥0.5 D. The eye with larger IA had also a longer AL ($P < 0.05$) when the DIA was more than 0.5 D, which suggested that IA might be a stimulus factor of myopia progress or occurrence.

One study showed that it was possible that astigmatism was a passive byproduct of abnormal posterior axial eye growth [12]. They pointed out that axial eye growth might alter anterior ocular structures through stretching and the fact that changes in axial length correlated significantly with changes in corneal power or lens power during early infancy. Although these results seem to be contradictory, we still speculate that IA was a stimulus factor of AL growth rather than the outcome of AL elongation. Firstly, IA was independent from age, which meant that AL growth with age did not increase IA. Secondly, the AL growth mainly led to increase of CA [12]. Thirdly, the conclusion from the animal experiment was based on eyeball abnormal growth [12], and in the present study, most patients were less than 26 mm.

Blurred image focusing on the retina was considered the mechanism of myopia occurrence or progress. Deprivation of a focused retinal image can cause high myopia in primates and chicks, and peripheral retinal hyperopic defocus imposing peripheral hyperopic defocus produces axial myopia [13, 14]. Even with spectacle corrections, IA can create a blurred retinal image especially in the peripheral retina because there is an axial distance between the corrected spectacle and the intraocular lens (the internal astigmatism location). The study confirmed the linear relationship between AL growth and IA. It is this line of reasoning, along with reports of an association between astigmatism and the onset of myopia in animal experiment [4].

We acknowledge certain limitations in our study. Firstly, the present study had a cross-sectional design based on a single elementary school. The conclusion should be applied with caution and need to be further studied in the future. Secondly, AL was used as the only parameter for monitoring myopia progress in the study. In fact, other ocular structures such as the cornea, aqueous humor, lens, and the vitreous humor also contribute to the refractive status of a given human eye. The ratio between the AL and corneal radius may be a better indicator of myopia [15]. Thirdly, our study does not analyze the relationship between AL and TA (CA) and the relationship between high myopia and high astigmatism. Finally, in the corneal refractive astigmatism calculated from autoref, the results were rather coarse; it is better to use some advanced machine to measure corneal astigmatism, such as IOL master [16].

In conclusion, IA was observed to be associated with axial length and might be a risk factor of the onset and progress of myopia in school-age children.

Conflicts of Interest

No author has conflicts of interest to report.

Acknowledgments

This work was supported by the Clinical Multicenter Cooperation Project of Shanghai Science and Technology Commission (no.: 17411950200 and no.: 17411950208), the Eye Disease Prevention Personnel Training Plan of Shanghai, China (no.:15GWZK0601-QJGG02), the Shanghai Shenkang Hospital Development Center (Grant no. SHDC12016207), and the Health and Family Planning Committee of Pudong New District of Shanghai (Grant no. PW2014D-1).

References

[1] P. C. Wu, H. M. Huang, H. J. Yu, P. C. Fang, and C. T. Chen, "Epidemiology of myopia," *Asia-Pacific Journal of Ophthalmology*, vol. 5, no. 6, pp. 386–393, 2016.

[2] F. Xia, L. Wu, C. Weng, and X. Zhou, "Causes and three-year incidence of irreversible visual impairment in Jing-an District, Shanghai, China from 2010–2015," *BMC Ophthalmology*, vol. 17, no. 1, p. 216, 2017.

[3] L. C. Wu, X. H. Sun, X. T. Zhou, and C. H. Wen, "Unrecognized and unregistered blindness in people 70 or older in Jing'an District, Shanghai, China," *International Journal of Ophthalmology*, vol. 6, no. 3, pp. 321–326, 2013.

[4] C. CHG and C. S. Kee, "Effects of optically imposed astigmatism on early eye growth in chicks," *PLoS One*, vol. 10, no. 2, article e0117729, 2015.

[5] J. D. Twelker, J. M. Miller, D. L. Sherrill, and E. M. Harvey, "Astigmatism and myopia in Tohono O'odham Native American children," *Optometry & Vision Science*, vol. 90, no. 11, pp. 1267–1273, 2013.

[6] F. Rezvan, A. Yekta, H. Hashemi et al., "The association between astigmatism and spherical refractive error in a clinical population," *Iranian Journal of Ophthalmology*, vol. 23, no. 4, pp. 37–42, 2011.

[7] D. Czepita and D. Filipiak, "Role of astigmatism in the creation of myopia," *Klinika Oczna*, vol. 105, no. 6, pp. 385-386, 2003.

[8] Y. C. Liu, P. Chou, R. Wojciechowski et al., "Power vector analysis of refractive, corneal, and internal astigmatism in an elderly Chinese population: the Shihpai Eye Study," *Investigative Ophthalmology & Visual Science*, vol. 52, no. 13, pp. 9651–9657, 2011.

[9] S. Marasini, "Pattern of astigmatism in a clinical setting in Maldives," *Journal of Optometry*, vol. 9, no. 1, pp. 47–53, 2015.

[10] W. Meng, J. Butterworth, F. Malecaze, and P. Calvas, "Axial length of myopia: a review of current research," *Ophthalmologica*, vol. 225, no. 3, pp. 127–134, 2011.

[11] S. W. Cheung and P. Cho, "Validity of axial length measurements for monitoring myopic progression in orthokeratology," *Investigative Ophthalmology & Visual Science*, vol. 54, no. 3, pp. 1613–1615, 2013.

[12] C. Kee and L. Deng, "Astigmatism associated with experimentally induced myopia or hyperopia in chickens," *Investigative Ophthalmology & Visual Science*, vol. 49, no. 3, pp. 858–867, 2008.

[13] J. Yang, P. S. Reinach, S. Zhang et al., "Changes in retinal metabolic profiles associated with form deprivation myopia development in guinea pigs," *Scientific Reports*, vol. 7, no. 1, article 2777, 2017.

[14] A. Benaventepérez, A. Nour, and D. Troilo, "Axial eye growth and refractive error development can be modified by exposing the peripheral retina to relative myopic or hyperopic defocus," *Investigative Ophthalmology & Visual Science*, vol. 55, no. 10, pp. 6765–6773, 2014.

[15] X. He, H. Zou, L. Lu et al., "Axial length/corneal radius ratio: association with refractive state and role on myopia detection combined with visual acuity in Chinese schoolchildren," *PLoS One*, vol. 10, no. 2, article e0111766, 2015.

[16] M. Shajari, C. Cremonese, K. Petermann, P. Singh, M. Müller, and T. Kohnen, "Comparison of axial length, corneal curvature, and anterior chamber depth measurements of 2 recently introduced devices to a known biometer," *American Journal of Ophthalmology*, vol. 178, pp. 58–64, 2017.

12

Mutation Spectrum of the *ABCA4* Gene in a Greek Cohort with Stargardt Disease: Identification of Novel Mutations and Evidence of Three Prevalent Mutated Alleles

Kamakari Smaragda,[1] **Kokkinou Vassiliki**,[1] **Koutsodontis George**,[1] **Stamatiou Polixeni**,[1] **Giatzakis Christoforos**,[2] **Anastasakis Anastasios**,[3] **Aslanides Ioannis Minas**,[4] **Koukoula Stavrenia**,[5] **Panagiotoglou Theoni**,[6] **Datseris Ioannis**,[7] **and Tsilimbaris K. Miltiadis**[6]

[1]*Ophthalmic Genetics Unit, OMMA Ophthalmological Institute of Athens, Athens, Greece*
[2]*DNAbiolab, Cretan Center for Research and Development of Applications on Genetics and Molecular Biology, Heraklion, Crete, Greece*
[3]*Department of Clinical Electrophysiology of Vision, Athens Eye Hospital, Glyfada, Athens, Greece*
[4]*Department of Ophthalmology, Emmetropia Mediterranean Eye Institute, Heraklion, Crete, Greece*
[5]*Ophthalmica Institute of Ophthalmology and Microsurgery, Thessaloniki, Greece*
[6]*Department of Ophthalmology, University of Crete School of Medicine, Heraklion, Greece*
[7]*Department of Retinal Disorders, OMMA Ophthalmological Institute of Athens, Athens, Greece*

Correspondence should be addressed to Kamakari Smaragda; kamakari@hotmail.gr

Academic Editor: Robert B. Hufnagel

Aim. To evaluate the frequency and pattern of disease-associated mutations of *ABCA4* gene among Greek patients with presumed Stargardt disease (STGD1). *Materials and Methods.* A total of 59 patients were analyzed for *ABCA4* mutations using the ABCR400 microarray and PCR-based sequencing of all coding exons and flanking intronic regions. MLPA analysis as well as sequencing of two regions in introns 30 and 36 reported earlier to harbor deep intronic disease-associated variants was used in 4 selected cases. *Results.* An overall detection rate of at least one mutant allele was achieved in 52 of the 59 patients (88.1%). Direct sequencing improved significantly the complete characterization rate, that is, identification of two mutations compared to the microarray analysis (93.1% versus 50%). In total, 40 distinct potentially disease-causing variants of the *ABCA4* gene were detected, including six previously unreported potentially pathogenic variants. Among the disease-causing variants, in this cohort, the most frequent was c.5714+5G>A representing 16.1%, while p.Gly1961Glu and p.Leu541Pro represented 15.2% and 8.5%, respectively. *Conclusions.* By using a combination of methods, we completely molecularly diagnosed 48 of the 59 patients studied. In addition, we identified six previously unreported, potentially pathogenic *ABCA4* mutations.

1. Introduction

Stargardt disease (STGD1, OMIM 248200) is a juvenile-onset form of macular dystrophy (MD) [1]. It is inherited mainly in an autosomal recessive manner and is one of the most frequent causes of MD in childhood [2]. The disease is characterized by loss of photoreceptor cells in the macula and affects 1 in 10,000 individuals [3]. STGD1 is associated with the appearance of orange-yellow flecks around the macula and accumulation of lipofuscin—a combination of fluorescent by-products of the visual cycle—in the choroid. This accumulation appears to have toxic effects on the retinal pigment epithelium [4].

Mutations in the *ABCA4* (gene ID: 24; OMIM: 601691) gene have been described in *ABCA4*-associated retinopathies, including STGD1, cone-rod dystrophy (CRD), retinitis pigmentosa (RP), and retinal dystrophy [1, 5]. *ABCA4* is a large gene that consists of 50 exons located in chromosome 1p13. It is a member of the subfamily A of the ATP-binding cassette (ABC) transporters that is expressed in the retinal photoreceptors. This gene is involved in the transport and clearance of all-transretinal aldehyde, a by-product of the retinoid cycle of vision, and other essential molecules across the disc membrane into the cytoplasm [6–8]. It is the only gene whose mutations are known to be associated with autosomal recessive STGD1 [3]. Over 800 disease-causing mutations have been identified to date in *ABCA4*-associated phenotypes. The *ABCA4* mutation spectrum ranges from single base substitutions to deletions of several exons, although the majority of reported changes are missense mutations [9–11]. Numerous genetic studies on STGD1 patients have revealed that the disease-associated *ABCA4* alleles are extraordinarily heterogeneous. While some founder mutations accounting for a significant proportion of disease alleles have been identified in specific ethnic groups, hundreds of extremely rare or private variants have also been identified [12–14].

In this study, we used a combination of the ABCR400 microarray analysis and direct sequencing of the entire coding sequence of *ABCA4* gene to investigate the frequency and pattern of disease-associated mutations and polymorphisms in a large cohort of Greek patients with presumed STGD1. Our data extend the mutational spectrum of the *ABCA4* gene and, in addition, facilitate the screening of *ABCA4* mutations in Greek patients by identifying a set of three prevalent alleles.

2. Methods

This study adhered to the tenets of the Declaration of Helsinki and the ARVO statement of human subjects and was approved by the Human Subjects Review Committee at the University Hospital of Heraklion, Crete. Informed written consent was obtained for all study participants.

All patients were referred for genotyping after a clinical diagnosis of presumed Stargardt disease was put from treating ophthalmologists. A complete medical and familial history (including consanguineous marriages) was obtained from each patient. Age of symptom onset was documented. Familial STGD1 cases had to be compatible with autosomal recessive inheritance.

2.1. Mutation Screening of the ABCA4 Gene. Total genomic DNA was extracted from whole blood samples on an iPrep purification instrument using the iPrep PureLink gDNA Blood Kit (Invitrogen, Life Technologies, Carlsbad, CA) according to the manufacturer's instructions. A group of 30 Greek STGD1 patients were analyzed for variants on the ABCR400 microarray version 11.0 including 513–558 alterations (http://www.asperbio.com), as described elsewhere [15]. A second independent group of 29 patients and 8 patients from the microarray group were analyzed by direct sequencing of all 50 exons and intron-exon junctions of the *ABCA4* gene following PCR amplification with PCR primers designed using the Web Primer program. To test for deep intronic sequence variants [16] in 4 patients, primer pairs *ABCA4*-Exon30.1 fwd (5′-CACCCGATCCC TGCTCTTTTTTAT-3′)/rev (5′-TTACATTTGTCCAGG GACCAAGG-3′) and *ABCA4*-Exon36.1 fwd (5′-ACAGGG ATCATTATGACATCAACCCC-3′)/rev (5′-AGCTACATC TCTCTCCATAGGCTCAGA-3′) were used to amplify and sequence a 406- and 596-bp fragment within *ABCA4* intervening sequences 30 and 36, respectively. All primer sequences are shown in Supplementary Table 1. We followed the methods of Kamakari et al. [17] for PCR and Sanger sequencing conditions. Specifically, PCR reactions were performed in a 25 μl total reaction volume, containing 50–100 ng genomic DNA, 2.5 μl of 10x PCR buffer (w/o $MgCl_2$), 3 μl of 10 mM dNTPs mix, 0.75 μl of 50 mM $MgCl_2$, 1.75 μl of 10 μM forward primer, 1.75 μl of 10 μM reverse primer, and 0.25 μl of 5 U/μl Platinum Taq DNA polymerase (Invitrogen, Life Technologies). Amplification was performed with the following cycling profile: incubation at 94°C for 5 min followed by 36 cycles of 45 sec denaturation at 94°C, 45 sec annealing at 58°C, and 45 sec elongation at 72°C. The last cycle was followed by a final extension of 3 min at 72°C. Excess primers and dNTPs were removed using exonuclease I and shrimp alkaline phosphatase, and PCR products were sequenced with the BigDye Terminator v3.1 Cycle Sequencing Kit (Applied Biosystems, Foster City, CA) according to the manufacturer's instructions. All sequences were analyzed in forward and reverse directions on an ABI3500 fluorescent sequencer (Applied Biosystems). Nucleotide sequences were compared with the published DNA sequence of *ABCA4* gene (GenBank accession number NG_011605.1 or NG_009073.1) and cDNA (GenBank accession number NM_000350.2). For the *ABCA4* gene, cDNA numbering +1 corresponds to A in the ATG translation initiation codon of ABCA4 transcript.

2.2. Multiplex Ligation-Dependent Probe Amplification. Multiplex ligation-dependent probe amplification (MLPA) reagents were obtained from MRC-Holland (SALSA MLPA kit P151-P152 ABCA4, Amsterdam), and the reactions were performed according to the manufacturer's instructions (MRC-Holland).

Whenever possible, segregation analysis was performed according to whether relatives were willing to offer clinical material.

3. Results

A total of 59 Greek patients with a presumed clinical diagnosis of STGD1 were screened for *ABCA4* mutations, including 25 males and 34 females. At least two cases reported consanguinity, and notably, two other cases had affected relatives across two successive generations which represent an atypical pattern of inheritance for the disease. The patients are presented in two groups. The first group of 30 patients was screened by an early version of the ABCR400 microarray chip (version 11.0) and the second group of 29 patients by direct sequencing. Direct sequencing was also performed as a complementary method in a subset of 8 patients of the microarray group with one identified mutation leading to the identification of the second mutant allele in 6 of them (Supplementary Table 2). Finally, additional sequencing of two regions in introns 30 and 36 as well as MLPA analysis in 4 patients with one single mutation from both subgroups did not identify the second mutant allele.

ABCR400 *Microarray Screening.* Of the 30 patients screened using the ABCR400 microarray, 15 (50%) were found to carry two disease-causing mutations whereas 8 were found to carry a single mutation in heterozygous state (26.7%) (Supplementary Table 2). No mutations were identified in 7 patients (23.3%).

Direct Sequencing and MLPA Analysis. Of the 29 patients screened by PCR-based Sanger sequencing, 27 (93.1%) were found to carry two disease-causing mutations whereas 2 carried a single mutation (6.9%) (Supplementary Table 2). In addition, direct sequencing was performed in the 8 patients of the microarray-analyzed group with one identified mutation leading to the identification of the second mutation in 6 of them. Conclusively, 4 patients from both subgroups remained with one identified mutation. These 4 patients were tested for the known pathogenic deep intronic mutations in introns 30 and 36 [16] and, in addition, screened for large deletions or duplications by MLPA analysis, but no second mutation was identified in them.

In addition, direct sequencing revealed several polymorphic variants in *ABCA4* gene summarized in Supplementary Table 3.

3.1. Frequency of Mutations. Altogether, 100 potentially disease-causing *ABCA4* alleles were identified in this cohort of 59 Greek patients presenting with presumed STGD1. Among these 100 mutant alleles, a total of 40 distinct mutations were identified (Table 1). However, three mutations (c.5714+5G>A, p.Gly1961Glu, and p.Leu541Pro (alone or as a complex allele with the p.Ala1038Val)) occurred at a significantly higher frequency, compared to other variants in this cohort (Supplementary Table 2, Table 1). The most frequent mutation c.5714+5G>A (intron 40) was detected in 19 alleles in 16 patients (13 heterozygous, 3 homozygous) accounting for 16.1% of the total number of alleles ($n = 118$). The second most frequent mutation p.Gly1961Glu was detected in 18 alleles in 18 patients (all heterozygous) accounting for 15.2% of the total number of alleles ($n = 118$). The third most frequent mutation p.Leu541Pro was detected in 15 alleles either as a single mutation (5 alleles) or as a complex allele with the p.Ala1038Val (10 alleles) in 14 patients (13 heterozygous, 1 homozygous) accounting for 12.7% ($n = 118$). p.Ala1038Val was not detected as a single allele (Supplementary Table 2, Table 1).

A few mutations were detected more than once, that is, p.Gly607Arg in 4 alleles in 4 patients (all heterozygous), accounting for 3.3% ($n = 118$), and p.Val1973* and the novel mutation c.5714+1G>C (intron 40) both found in 3 alleles in 2 patients each (1 heterozygous, 1 homozygous), each accounting for 2.45% ($n = 118$). In addition, mutations c.4352+1G>A (intron 29) first reported by us [18], p.Arg18Trp, p.Arg212Cys, and p.Arg1108Cys were detected each in 2 alleles in 4 patients (all heterozygous), each accounting for 1.6% ($n = 118$). In addition, the allelic variant p.Arg1108Leu of the latter mutation was found in 1 patient.

The remainder of 22 distinct mutations was detected once in heterozygosity each accounting for 0.8% ($n = 118$) (Supplementary Table 2, Table 1), including five of the six previously unreported potentially pathogenic mutations p.Trp12* (exon 1), p.Asn76Thr (exon 3), p.Ser673Argfs*6 (exon 14), p.Cys698Arg (exon 14), and c.4352+4A>C (intron 29). Mutations p.Asn76Thr and p.Cys698Arg and the previously reported p.Arg107*, p.Pro143Leu, p.Gly607Arg, and p.Trp1449* were detected in compound heterozygosity with the most frequent mutation c.5714+5G>A in intron 40. Mutations p.Arg290Trp, p.Gly607Arg, p.Ser673Argfs*6, c.4352+1G>A, p.Glu1087Lys, p.Arg1108Cys, p.Met1115Cysfs*33, p.Glu1271Gly, p.Gln1412*, p.Cys1488Arg, p.Ser1696Asn, c.5714+1G>C, p.Val1973*, and p.Arg2038Trp were detected in compound heterozygosity with the second most frequent mutation p.Gly1961Glu. Mutations p.Gly2146Asp and p.Arg1108Leu were detected in compound heterozygosity with c.4352+1G>A (intron 29) and p.Arg212Cys, respectively. Some of these once occurring mutations were detected in the same patient, namely, p.Arg18Trp and p.His1625Gln (patient ABCA4-20A), p.Glu1122Lys and p.Gly1591Arg (patient ABCA4-39A), and p.Arg220Cys and p.Gly607Arg (patient ABCA4-35A).

In 4 patients, only one mutant allele was identified even after the use of direct sequencing and MLPA, these mutant alleles being p.Asn380Lys, p.Arg1640Trp, and c.5714+5G>A (the latter in 2 patients).

The majority of the distinct mutations were evenly distributed along the exons of the *ABCA4* gene. Three different mutations were observed in exon 22 and two in each of exons 1, 4, 6, 13, 14, 23, 35, and 44 and introns 29 and 40; however, no accumulation in a specific exon was observed. No mutation was identified in exons 2, 5, 7, 10, 11, 15, 18–20, 24, 26, 27, 31, 32, 34, 37–41, 45, 46, and 48–50 which comprise 50% (25/50) of the exons of the *ABCA4* gene.

Twenty-six of the detected mutations were missense, 5 were splice defects, 6 were nonsense, and 3 were frameshift mutations (Table 1).

3.2. Novel Mutations. Six novel mutations, namely, p.Trp12* (exon 1), p.Asn76Thr (exon 3), p.Ser673Argfs*6 (exon 14), p.Cys698Arg (exon 14), c.4352+4A>C (intron 29) and c.5714+1G>C (intron 40), and c.4352+1G>A (intron 29) previously reported by us [18], were detected in this study. Two were missense, three were splicing mutations (two of which occur in intron 29), one nonsense, and one small deletion of 13 nucleotides leading to a frameshift mutation of the *ABCA4* gene. These seven distinct mutations were detected in 10 apparently unrelated patients, 9 in heterozygous, and 1 in homozygous state. p.Trp12* (exon 1), p.Asn76Thr (exon 3), p.Ser673Argfs*6 (exon 14), p.Cys698Arg (exon 14), and c.4352+4A>C (intron 29) were each detected once in heterozygosity in 5 respective patients, and c.5714+1G>C was detected twice in two patients (1 in homozygosity, 1 in heterozygosity) and c.4352+1G>A (in three patients in heterozygosity).

Of these, the mutations p.Asn76Thr and p.Cys698Arg were detected in compound heterozygosity with the most frequently detected mutation c.5714+5G>A (intron 40) in one male (ABCA4-47A, Supplementary Figures 1A and B) and

TABLE 1: Frequency of 40 distinct mutations detected in 59 Greek patients with presumed STGD1.

Mutation number	Amino acid change	Nucleotide change	Exon	Number of alleles detected	Frequency	References
1	p.Trp12*	c.36G>A	1	1	0.8%	This study
2	p.Arg18Trp	c.52C>T	1	2	1.6%	[33]
3	p.Asn76Thr	c.227A>C	3	1	0.8%	This study
4	p.Pro143Leu	c.428C>T	4	1	0.8%	[13]
5	p.Arg107*	c.319C>T	4	1	0.8%	[34]
6	NA	c.571-2A>T	Intron 5	1	0.8%	[35]
7	p.Arg212Cys	c.635C>T	6	2	1.6%	[33]
8	p.Arg220Cys	c.658C>T	6	1	0.8%	[11]
9	p.Arg290Trp	c.868C>T	8	1	0.8%	[36]
10	p.Asn380Lys	c.1140T>A	9	1	0.8%	[11]
11[a]	p.Leu541Pro	c.1622T>C	12	10	8.5%	[37]
12	p.Gly607Arg	c.1819G>A	13	4	3.3%	[10]
13	p.Asp645Asn	c.1933G>A	13	1	0.8%	[9]
14	p.Ser673Argfs*6	c.2019_2031del13	14	1	0.8%	This study
15	p.Cys698Arg	c.2092T>C	14	1	0.8%	This study
16	p.Ser795Argfs* 43	c.2385_2400delCTTACTGTCTCCGGTG	16	1	0.8%	[38]
17	p.Gln876*	c.2626C>T	17	1	0.8%	[39]
18	p.Ala1038Val	c.3113C>T	21	6	5.1%	[3]
19	p.Arg1108Cys	c.3322C>T	22	2	1.6%	[37]
20	p.Arg1108Leu	c.3323G>T	22	1	0.8%	[36]
21	p.Glu1087Lys	c.3259G>A	22	1	0.8%	[3]
22	p.Met1115Cysfs* 33	c.3342delC	23	1	0.8%	[36]
23	p.Glu1122Lys	c.3364G>A	23	1	0.8%	[9]
24	p.Glu1271Gly	c.3812A>G	25	1	0.8%	[40]
25	p.Gln1412*	c.4234C>T	28	1	0.8%	[12]
26	p.Trp1449*	c.4346G>A	29	1	0.8%	[9]
27	NA	c.4352+1G>A	Intron 29	3	2.5%	[18, 40, 41]
28	NA	c.4352+4A>C	Intron 29	1	0.8%	This study
29	p.Cys1488Arg	c.4462T>C	30	1	0.8%	[9]
30	p.Gly1591Arg	c.4771G>A	33	1	0.8%	[42]
31	p.Arg1640Trp	c.4918C>T	35	1	0.8%	[37]
32	p.His1625Gln	c.4875T>A	35	1	0.8%	[13]
33	p.Ser1696Asn	c.5087G>A	36	1	0.8%	[9]
34	NA	c.5714+5G>A	Intron 40	19	16.1%	[30]
35	NA	c.5714+1G>C	Intron 40	3	2.5%	This study
36	p.Gly1961Glu	c.5882G>A	42	18	15.2%	[43]
37	p.Val1973*	c.5917delG	43	3	2.5%	[10]
38	p.Leu2026Pro	c.6077T>C	44	1	0.8%	[44]
39	p.Arg2038Trp	c.6112C>T	44	1	0.8%	[3]
40	p.Gly2146Asp	c.6437G>A	47	1	0.8%	[36]

[a]4 times was detected as single and 6 times as complex with p.A1038V.

one female patient (ABCA4-27A, Supplementary Figures 2A and B), respectively. The age of onset for patient ABCA4-47A carrying the p.Asn76Thr was 52 years according to the patient who was initially erroneously diagnosed with age-related macular degeneration in 2012. He had a cataract surgery at the age of 42 and eventually diagnosed with presumed Stargardt disease of late onset.

The age of onset for patient ABCA4-27A carrying the novel potentially pathogenic missense mutation p.Cys698Arg was 13 years of age.

Mutation c.4352+4A>C (intron 29) was detected in 1 patient in compound heterozygosity with p.Arg18Trp (exon 1) (patient ABCA4-37A, Supplementary Figures 3A and 3B). The age at diagnosis for this patient was 15. Segregation analysis documented that the unaffected parents were heterozygous for each mutation with the c.4352+4A>C paternally inherited and the p. Arg18Trp maternally inherited whereas her affected sister carried both mutations (Supplementary Figure 3A).

c.4352+1G>A was detected in two unrelated patients in compound heterozygosity with p.Gly2146Asp (exon 47) in patient ABCA4-5A (Supplementary Figures 4A and 4B) and with the complex allele p.Leu541Pro/p.Ala1038Val (exons 12/21) in patient ATH44A, (Supplementary Figures 5A and B). For patient ATH44A, five additional family members including two affected siblings, their unaffected parents, and an unaffected maternal uncle were tested for the two mutations. Both affected siblings were compound heterozygous for the two mutations; the mother was a heterozygous carrier of the c.4352+1G>A and the father of the p.Leu541Pro/p.Ala1038Val (Supplementary Figure 5A) whereas the maternal uncle was free of mutation.

The c.5714+1G>C mutation was initially detected in homozygous state in one young female patient (ABCA4-31A, Supplementary Figures 6A–C). Five additional family members including her unaffected parents (ABCA4-31B, C), her two affected maternal third male cousins (ABCA4-33A, B), and their unaffected mother (ABCA4-33C) were tested for the novel mutation. All parents were found heterozygous carriers whereas the affected cousins were homozygous (Supplementary Figures 6A–6C). All three young patients were diagnosed with presumed Stargardt disease approximately at the age of 7. Furthermore, the same novel potentially pathogenic mutation was detected in a seemingly unrelated patient (ABCA4-14A, Supplementary Figures 7A and 7B) in compound heterozygosity with the p.Gly1961Glu mutation.

Genetic analysis of patient (ATH73A) revealed a novel nonsense mutation c.36G>A (p.Trp12*) and a previously reported mutation c.571-2A>T occurring in a compound heterozygous state in exon 1 and intron 5, respectively, in the ABCA4 gene (Supplementary Figures 8A and 8B). This mutation leads to premature truncation after just 12 amino acids, which is likely to render the protein to be nonfunctional or lead to nonsense-mediated mRNA decay. It is included in the SNP database (https://www.ncbi.nlm.nih.gov/snp/) (rs761209432); however, according to our knowledge, it has not been associated previously with disease.

The sixth mutation c.2019_2031delCATCGTCTTGGAG was detected in patient ATH-53A. It consists of a deletion of 13 nucleotides from c.2019 to c.2031 (Supplementary Figures 9A and 9B) which would cause a frameshift that changes codon Ser673 to Arg, leading to a premature stop codon at position 678 (p.Ser673Argfs*6). The predicted translation product from this allele would consist of 677 amino acid residues instead of the 2273 found in the mature protein. This mutation was detected in compound heterozygosity with the p.Gly1961Glu mutation. The disease onset for this patient was at the age of 17.

In silico analysis for missense variants using the predictive algorithms of "Sorting Intolerant From Tolerant" ((SIFT) in the public domain, http://sift.jcvi.org), Polymorphism Phenotyping v2 ((PolyPhen-2) in the public domain, http://genetics.bwh.harvard.edu/pph2), and Protein Variation Effect Analyzer ((PROVEAN) in the public domain, http://provean.jcvi.org/index.php) tools predicted novel changes p.Asn76Thr and p.Cys698Arg to have a deleterious effect, whereas novel changes c.4352+4A>C and c.5714+1G>C are predicted to affect normal splicing by the Human Splicing Finder ((HSF); in the public domain, http://www.umd.be/HSF3/ prediction tool (Supplementary Table 4)).

3.3. Results of Relatives. Allelic segregation analyses were performed in 11 families. A total of 37 relatives were tested (data not shown). The analysis of one family (F11) that showed atypical pattern of inheritance is presented in detail hereafter.

3.4. Family F11A: A Family with an Atypical Pattern of Inheritance. In this family, the male proband (F11A, Figure 1(a)) and one of his brothers (F11B, Figure 1(a)) were diagnosed with presumed STGD1 before school age. Their parents (F11M, F11L) were unaffected which supported an autosomal recessive pattern of inheritance. However, two paternal aunts (F11C and F11J) were also affected but the disease presented in their twenties. Genotyping using the ABCR400 microarray was performed initially in the proband (F11A) and in one of his two affected aunts (F11C). The analysis revealed the complex p.Leu541Pro/p.Ala1038Val mutation in both of them. The proband was homozygous for the detected mutation; however, his aunt was compound heterozygous with p.Gly1961Glu. Following the initial analysis, thirteen additional family members including the proband's six siblings, parents, paternal grandparents, paternal aunts, and paternal cousin were tested for the two aforementioned mutations. Their results shown in Figures 1(a)–1(f) confirmed that the proband's affected siblings presenting with an early onset severe form of the disease were homozygous for the p.Leu541Pro/p.Ala1038Val complex allele whereas his second affected aunt with the later onset milder phenotype was a compound heterozygote with the p.Gly1961Glu mutation. The proband's unaffected parents were found heterozygous carriers for the p.Leu541Pro/p.Ala1038Val mutation. In addition, the paternal grandmother was a heterozygous carrier of the p.Gly1961Glu mutation and his grandfather heterozygous for the p.Leu541Pro/p.Ala1038Val. The parents of the proband did not report consanguinity, but their

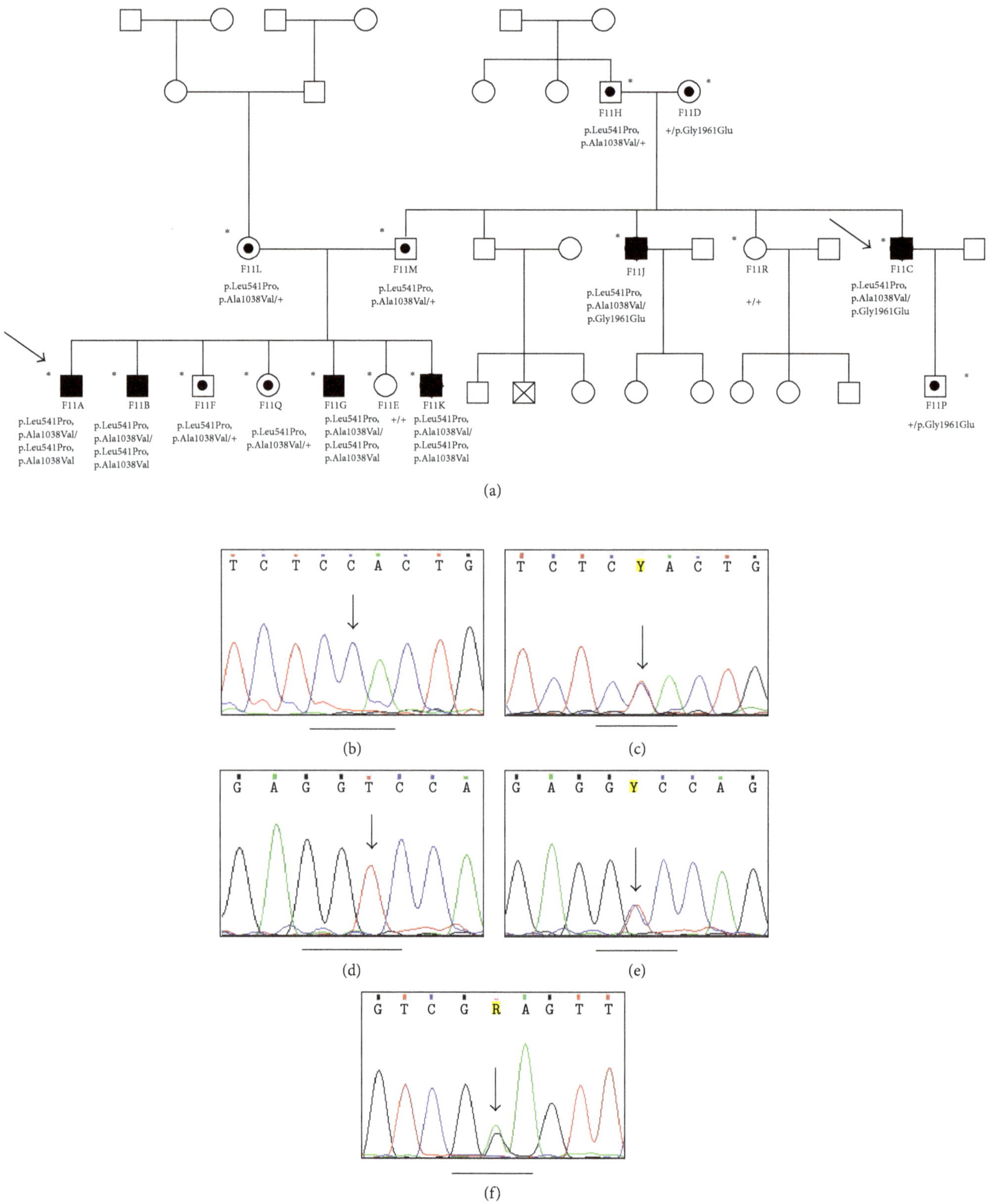

FIGURE 1: Family F11. (a) Pedigree of patients F11A and F11C (probands). Arrows indicate the probands. Affected and unaffected individuals are represented with black and open circles, respectively. Males are represented with a quadrant and females with a circle. The asterisk denotes the individuals genetically examined. A dot in a symbol denotes an unaffected carrier of the respective mutation. Pluses (+) denote the wild type alleles. (b, c, d, and e) Sequence chromatograms of the F11A and F11C showing the complex allele c.1622T>C/c.3113C>T (p.Leu541Pro/p.Ala1038Val) in homozygosity in proband F11A (b, d) and in heterozygosity in proband F11C (c, e). (f) Sequence chromatogram of the proband F11C showing the missense mutation c.5882G>A (p.Gly1961Glu) in heterozygosity on the second allele. The arrow indicates the position of the G to A substitution at the second nucleotide of codon 1961 encoded by GGA marked by a horizontal line.

ascendants originated from the same part of Northern Greece. Genotyping resolved the atypical pattern of inheritance of STGD1 disease in this family.

4. Discussion

Genetic analysis of 59 Greek patients with presumed STGD1 revealed 40 different mutations in the *ABCA4* gene and an overall detection rate of at least one mutant allele in 88.1% (52 patients) using a combination of the ABCR400 microarray, direct sequencing, and MLPA methods. Of these 52 patients, 48 were completely characterized (two mutant alleles detected) (81.3%) and 4 partially characterized (one mutant allele detected) (6.7%). This is well within the published range of biallelic mutation identification that ranges between 55% and 80% [19]. However, clinical heterogeneity and variable diagnostic criteria in our cohort of patients who were referred by a number of collaborating ophthalmologists may have led to uncertainties in clinical diagnosis in some of our patients.

Specifically, using the ABCR400 microarray screening method between the years 2006 and 2009 in 30 patients, two mutations were identified in 15 (50%), one mutation in 8 (26.7%), and no mutation in the remaining 7 (23.3%) cases. Valverde et al. [15] have reported similar mutation detection rates using the same microarray in a cohort of 76 patients, but Jaakson et al. [13] have reported somewhat lower detection rates (36.6% with two mutations and 24.4% with no mutations).

Using direct sequencing in 29 patients, both disease-causing mutations were identified in 27 (93.1%) whereas one mutation was identified in 2 patients (6.9%). Moreover, direct sequencing of *ABCA4*, used as a complementary method in 8 patients previously found to harbor one mutant allele using the microarray method of screening, led to the identification of a second mutant allele in 6 of them thus raising the complete characterization rate (identification of both mutant alleles) to 70% in this group. Overall, the use of direct sequencing as an initial screening method led to significantly higher complete characterization rate when compared to the microarray (93.1% versus 50%, resp.); therefore, it became the method of choice for *ABCA4* mutation screening by our group. These rates of detection parallel well with the recently published literature [20–22]. For example, in the study by Riveiro-Alvarez et al. [21], the mutation detection rate after complete *ABCA4* sequencing with Sanger sequencing or next generation sequencing (NGS) was 73.6% in arSTGD1 patients.

Most of the patients (42; $n = 59$) (71.1%) were compound heterozygotes. Only six patients were found to be homozygotes (Table 2). A single disease allele was found in 6.7% (4/59) of our cases. No disease allele was detected in 11.8% (7; $n = 59$) of our patients. Possible explanations for this may include erroneous clinical diagnosis, as well as the presence of disease-causing mutations in parts of the gene that were not screened, for example, deep into the introns or other regulatory regions and the presence of disease-causing mutations in other genes. The latter has proved to be the case in two of our ABCA4 negative patients which were found to harbor mutations in CRX and PROM1 genes (unpublished data).

Concurring with earlier studies [10, 23, 24], most *ABCA4* mutations are distributed throughout the entire coding sequence, and no mutational hotspots seem to exist. However, it is of note that 4 mutations lie in introns 29 and 40 (2 in each), 3 in exon 22 and 2 each in exons 1, 4, 6, 13, 14, 23, 35, and 44. In addition, mutations have been detected in half of the exons of the *ABCA4* gene in this cohort; therefore, perhaps initial *ABCA4* screening of Greek patients could include only this set of exons.

Most of the detected mutations were missense mutations (26), 5 were splice defects, 6 were nonsense, and 3 were frameshift mutations (Table 1).

A prevalent set of three mutant alleles composed of c.5714+5G>A representing 16.1% of all screened alleles (19/118), p.Gly1961Glu representing 15.2% (18/118), and p.Leu541Pro either as a single mutation or as a complex allele with the p.Ala1038Val representing 12.7% (15/118) was identified. Notably, of the 48 completely characterized subjects, 13 had two mutated alleles and 24 had one mutated allele from this high incidence set. Therefore, based on the mutation frequencies observed, one would expect that screening for these three mutations only would lead to complete genetic characterization of approximately 22% (13; $n = 59$) or partial genetic characterization of approximately 66.1% (39; $n = 59$) of Greek STGD1 patients providing strong indication of a true *ABCA4*-related retinopathy. Specifically, in our cohort, the most frequent mutation is the intronic splicing mutation IVS40+5G>A, accounting for 16.1% of all screened alleles (19/118). This is considerably higher than the frequency observed in other Europeans (3.9% in Spanish, 4.2% in Italian, and 8.6% in Hungarian patients) [15, 23, 24]. This mutation confers a milder phenotype, and this is especially true when the mutation is in homozygosity (3 patients in our cohort, H1, ATH35A, and ABCA4-44A) with an age of onset at the 4th decade; these patients consist half of the homozygotes in this cohort. The second most frequent mutation is p.Gly1961Glu with a frequency of 15.2% in our cohort of patients. This mutation is one of the most frequently mutated alleles in several populations analyzed. Its frequency ranges from 9% to 9.5% in some European countries or even lower in Spanish and Portuguese patients to 20-21% in Italian, Slovenian, and German patients. Its frequency of 15.2% in our cohort is comparable with the average frequency of 10% for the central European populations. The third most frequent mutation in Greek patients is p.Leu541Pro, alone or as a complex with p.Ala1038Val, with a frequency of 12.7% (15/118). This mutation is traditionally considered to be a German allele and is found in Germanic populations in general with a very low representation in other European populations, for example, 0.7% of the mutated alleles in an Italian cohort [25]. However, in our Greek cohort of patients, this is one of the three prevalent alleles. Although difficult to interpret, this high prevalence of the particular allele among Greek patients may be due to the fact that there has been a strong interaction and tight bonds between Greeks and Germans throughout the years with significant immigration from Greece to Germany starting around 1700. Moreover, it is known that in 1828, 31 Bavarian families came to Greece along with King Otto of Greece (http://www.greece-is.com/

little-bavaria-in-athens/) and were settled in Greece and their Hellenized offspring still living in Greece today. Moreover, it is estimated that between the 1960s and 1970s, 500,000 Greek young people migrated and approximately 30% of them returned to Greece. Considering these facts, a phenomenon of gene flow for this prevalent allele through intermarriage cannot be excluded. A similar hypothesis of gene flow has been used to explain the unusually high incidence of b-globin gene mutations in Germans. It has been hypothesized that mutations in two-thirds of the cases have been introduced from the Mediterranean [26, 27].

Six previously unreported potentially pathogenic mutations, namely, p.Trp12* (exon 1), p.Asn76Thr (exon 3), p.Cys698Arg (exon 14), p.Ser673Argfs*6 (exon 14), c.4352+4A>C (intron 29), and c.5714+1G>C (intron 40) were detected in this study. Their absence from the ExAC (Exome Aggregation Consortium) database and their in silico analysis for the investigation of their pathogenicity, as mentioned in Results, support their potential pathogenicity. In addition, segregating results in the cases of the c.4352+4A>C and c.5714+1G>C splice variants strengthen their potential pathogenicity. Interestingly, the novel splice mutation c.5714+1G>C in intron 40 was detected in two apparently unrelated patients, one male patient from the region of the western Greek islands in the Ionian sea and one female patient from the region of the Cyclades islands (Santorini) in the Aegean sea. It was detected in compound heterozygosity in the first patient and in homozygosity in the second patient. Parents of the second patient were found heterozygous for the mutation thus confirming the true homozygous state of the mutation in the patient. Furthermore, this second female patient who comes from the island of Santorini has two-thirds affected male cousins being siblings between them who were found to bear the same homozygous mutation. This family has other affected relatives across different generations once again proving the not so infrequent atypical pattern of inheritance in STGD1 families [28]. The family living in the same village of the island shared the information with us that there are many similarly affected patients in their village. We presume that they all bear the same homozygous mutation due to their common origin and endogamy, and we intend to offer a simple targeted testing to them per their request. It is of note that the paternal origin of the patient from the western Greek islands is from Santorini, and it would be interesting to verify that the c.5714+1G>C is his paternal allele, that is, the same which was detected in the patients from Santorini.

In addition, mutation c.4352+1G>A that was first described by our group in 2009 [18] was detected in two unrelated patients in our cohort in compound heterozygosity with p.Gly2146 (exon 47) (patient ABCA4-5A) or in conjunction with the complex allele p.Leu541Pro/p.Ala1038Val (exons 12/21) (patient ATH44A).

One family (F-F11) presented with an atypical pattern of inheritance of STGD1 with affected members of different age of onset in two successive generations. The male proband (F11A) and his brother (F11B) were diagnosed with presumed STGD1 before school age, whereas their parents were unaffected, and two paternal aunts (F11C and F11J) were diagnosed with the disease in their late twenties. Genotyping of the proband and one of his affected aunts revealed that the proband was homozygous for the p.Leu541Pro/p.Ala1038-Val, whereas his aunt was a compound heterozygote with the p.Gly1961Glu mutation. 13 additional family members were tested for these two mutations as described in Results. In summary, this family segregates two different pathogenic *ABCA4* variants. Based on the different age of onset of the disease in the proband and his other affected siblings and his affected aunts, we assume that the milder phenotype of the two affected aunts is likely due to the p.Gly1961Glu which has been previously associated with a late-onset, milder disease phenotype [28, 29]. Due to the high carrier frequency of disease-causing *ABCA4* alleles in the general population (1 : 20), pseudodominant inheritance in STGD1 has been described [9, 30–32].

All patients of this cohort were referred for genotyping from a network of collaborating ophthalmologists after a clinical diagnosis of presumed Stargardt was put. However, details of the phenotype were not always available thus precluding a systemic genotype-phenotype correlation. Future work towards this direction could provide additional helpful clinical data.

5. Conclusions

In summary, we report here the mutational spectrum of the *ABCA4* gene in a large Greek cohort, with successful identification of both disease-causing alleles at a rate of 81.3% (48/59). In addition, we report the identification of six novel potentially pathogenic mutations thus extending the spectrum of the *ABCA4* gene mutations and of three prevalent alleles which may facilitate the screening of Greek patients with *ABCA4*-related retinopathy. The complete genetic characterization of the patients will improve the accuracy of diagnosis and their counselling and also will assist in more effective patient selection of genetically confirmed participants for current and future clinical trials for *ABCA4*-associated retinal diseases.

Disclosure

This paper was previously presented as a poster in the following link: http://www.ashg.org/2009meeting/abstracts/fulltext/f10084.htm.

Conflicts of Interest

The authors declare that there is no conflict of interest regarding the publication of this paper.

Supplementary Materials

Supplementary Figure 1: family ABCA4-47. Supplementary Figure 2: family ABCA4-27. Supplementary Figure 3: family ABCA4-37. Supplementary Figure 4: family ABCA4-5. Supplementary Figure 5: F-ATH44. Supplementary Figure 6: F-ABCA4-31/33. Supplementary Figure 7: F-ABCA4-31/33. Supplementary Figure 8: F-ATH73. Supplementary Figure 9: F-ATH53. Supplementary Table 1: *ABCA4* PCR primer sequences. Supplementary Table 2: mutations detected in the

ABCA4 gene in a cohort of 59 Greek patients with presumed STGD1. Supplementary Table 3: polymorphic variants of the ABCA4 gene detected in Greek STGD patients. Supplementary Table 4: results of in silico analysis for 2 novel missense variants using the predictive algorithms SIFT, PolyPhen-2, and PROVEAN and for 2 novel splice variants using HSF prediction tool. *(Supplementary Materials)*

References

[1] V. North, R. Gelman, and S. H. Tsang, "Juvenile-onset macular degeneration and allied disorders," *Developments in Ophthalmology*, vol. 53, pp. 44–52, 2014.

[2] K. Zhang, M. Kniazeva, A. Hutchinson, M. Han, M. Dean, and R. Allikmets, "The *ABCR* gene in recessive and dominant Stargardt diseases: a genetic pathway in macular degeneration," *Genomics*, vol. 60, no. 2, pp. 234–237, 1999.

[3] R. Allikmets, "A photoreceptor cell-specific ATP-binding transporter gene (*ABCR*) is mutated in recessive Stargardt macular dystrophy," *Nature Genetics*, vol. 15, no. 3, pp. 236–246, 1997.

[4] L. J. Roberts, C. A. Nossek, L. J. Greenberg, and R. S. Ramesar, "Stargardt macular dystrophy: common *ABCA4* mutations in South Africa–establishment of a rapid genetic test and relating risk to patients," *Molecular Vision*, vol. 18, pp. 280–289, 2012.

[5] B. J. Klevering, A. F. Deutman, A. Maugeri, F. P. M. Cremers, and C. B. Hoyng, "The spectrum of retinal phenotypes caused by mutations in the *ABCA4* gene," *Graefe's Archive for Clinical and Experimental Ophthalmology*, vol. 243, no. 2, pp. 90–100, 2005.

[6] H. Sun, R. S. Molday, and J. Nathans, "Retinal stimulates ATP hydrolysis by purified and reconstituted ABCR, the photoreceptor-specific ATP-binding cassette transporter responsible for Stargardt disease," *The Journal of Biological Chemistry*, vol. 274, no. 12, pp. 8269–8281, 1999.

[7] A. V. Cideciyan, M. Swider, T. S. Aleman et al., "*ABCA4* disease progression and a proposed strategy for gene therapy," *Human Molecular Genetics*, vol. 18, no. 5, pp. 931–941, 2009.

[8] J. Weng, N. L. Mata, S. M. Azarian, R. T. Tzekov, D. G. Birch, and G. H. Travis, "Insights into the function of Rim protein in photoreceptors and etiology of Stargardt's disease from the phenotype in *abcr* knockout mice," *Cell*, vol. 98, no. 1, pp. 13–23, 1999.

[9] R. A. Lewis, N. F. Shroyer, N. Singh et al., "Genotype/phenotype analysis of a photoreceptor-specific ATP-binding cassette transporter gene, *ABCR*, in Stargardt disease," *American Journal of Human Genetics*, vol. 64, no. 2, pp. 422–434, 1999.

[10] A. Rivera, K. White, H. Stöhr et al., "A comprehensive survey of sequence variation in the *ABCA4* (*ABCR*) gene in Stargardt disease and age-related macular degeneration," *American Journal of Human Genetics*, vol. 67, no. 4, pp. 800–813, 2000.

[11] A. R. Webster, E. Héon, A. J. Lotery et al., "An analysis of allelic variation in the *ABCA4* gene," *Investigative Ophthalmology & Visual Science*, vol. 42, no. 6, pp. 1179–1189, 2001.

[12] A. Maugeri, M. A. van Driel, D. J. van de Pol et al., "The 2588G->C mutation in the *ABCR* gene is a mild frequent founder mutation in the Western European population and allows the classification of *ABCR* mutations in patients with Stargardt disease," *American Journal of Human Genetics*, vol. 64, no. 4, pp. 1024–1035, 1999.

[13] K. Jaakson, J. Zernant, M. Külm et al., "Genotyping microarray (gene chip) for the *ABCR* (*ABCA4*) gene," *Human Mutation*, vol. 22, no. 5, pp. 395–403, 2003.

[14] F. Simonelli, F. Testa, J. Zernant et al., "Genotype-phenotype correlation in Italian families with Stargardt disease," *Ophthalmic Research*, vol. 37, no. 3, pp. 159–167, 2005.

[15] D. Valverde, R. Riveiro-Alvarez, S. Bernal et al., "Microarray-based mutation analysis of the *ABCA4* gene in Spanish patients with Stargardt disease: evidence of a prevalent mutated allele," *Molecular Vision*, vol. 12, pp. 902–908, 2006.

[16] T. A. Braun, R. F. Mullins, A. H. Wagner et al., "Non-exomic and synonymous variants in *ABCA4* are an important cause of Stargardt disease," *Human Molecular Genetics*, vol. 22, no. 25, pp. 5136–5145, 2013.

[17] S. Kamakari, G. Koutsodontis, M. Tsilimbaris, A. Fitsios, and G. Chrousos, "First report of *OPA1* screening in Greek patients with autosomal dominant optic atrophy and identification of a previously undescribed OPA1 mutation," *Molecular Vision*, vol. 20, pp. 691–703, 2014.

[18] S. Kamakari, P. Stamatiou, T. Panagiotoglou, C. Tsika, and M. Tsilimbaris, "Microarray-based mutation analysis of the ABCA4 gene in Greek patients with Stargardt disease: evidence of three mutated alleles," *Investigative Ophthalmology & Visual Science*, vol. 50, no. 13, p. 4118, 2009.

[19] F. Jiang, Z. Pan, K. Xu et al., "Screening of *ABCA4* gene in a Chinese cohort with Stargardt disease or cone-rod dystrophy with a report on 85 novel mutations," *Investigative Ophthalmology & Visual Science*, vol. 57, no. 1, pp. 145–152, 2016.

[20] J. Aguirre-Lamban, R. Riveiro-Alvarez, S. Maia-Lopes et al., "Molecular analysis of the *ABCA4* gene for reliable detection of allelic variations in Spanish patients: identification of 21 novel variants," *The British Journal of Ophthalmology*, vol. 93, no. 5, pp. 614–621, 2009.

[21] R. Riveiro-Alvarez, M. A. Lopez-Martinez, J. Zernant et al., "Outcome of *ABCA4* disease-associated alleles in autosomal recessive retinal dystrophies: retrospective analysis in 420 Spanish families," *Ophthalmology*, vol. 120, no. 11, pp. 2332–2337, 2013.

[22] J. Zernant, Y. A. Xie, C. Ayuso et al., "Analysis of the *ABCA4* genomic locus in Stargardt disease," *Human Molecular Genetics*, vol. 23, no. 25, pp. 6797–6806, 2014.

[23] A. Fumagalli, M. Ferrari, N. Soriani et al., "Mutational scanning of the ABCR gene with double-gradient denaturing-gradient gel electrophoresis (DG-DGGE) in Italian Stargardt disease patients," *Human Genetics*, vol. 109, no. 3, pp. 326–338, 2001.

[24] J. Hargitai, J. Zernant, G. M. Somfai et al., "Correlation of clinical and genetic findings in Hungarian patients with Stargardt disease," *Investigative Ophthalmology & Visual Science*, vol. 46, no. 12, pp. 4402–4408, 2005.

[25] I. Passerini, A. Sodi, B. Giambene, A. Mariottini, U. Menchini, and F. Torricelli, "Novel mutations in of the *ABCR* gene in Italian patients with Stargardt disease," *Eye*, vol. 24, no. 1, pp. 158–164, 2010.

[26] B. Vetter, C. Schwarz, E. Kohne, and A. E. Kulozik, "Beta-thalassaemia in the immigrant and non-immigrant German

populations," *British Journal of Haematology*, vol. 97, no. 2, pp. 266–272, 1997.

[27] E. Kohne and E. Kleihauer, "Hemoglobinopathies: a longitudinal study over four decades," *Deutsches Ärzteblatt International*, vol. 107, no. 5, pp. 65–71, 2010.

[28] T. R. Burke, G. A. Fishman, J. Zernant et al., "Retinal phenotypes in patients homozygous for the G1961E mutation in the *ABCA4* gene," *Investigative Ophthalmology & Visual Science*, vol. 53, no. 8, pp. 4458–4467, 2012.

[29] W. Cella, V. C. Greenstein, J. Zernant-Rajang et al., "G1961E mutant allele in the Stargardt disease gene *ABCA4* causes bull's eye maculopathy," *Experimental Eye Research*, vol. 89, no. 1, pp. 16–24, 2009.

[30] F. P. Cremers, D. J. van de Pol, M. van Driel et al., "Autosomal recessive retinitis pigmentosa and cone-rod dystrophy caused by splice site mutations in the Stargardt's disease gene *ABCR*," *Human Molecular Genetics*, vol. 7, no. 3, pp. 355–362, 1998.

[31] A. N. Yatsenko, N. F. Shroyer, R. A. Lewis, J. R. Lupski et al., "Late-onset Stargardt disease is associated with missense mutations that map outside known functional regions of *ABCR* (*ABCA4*)," *Human Genetics*, vol. 108, no. 4, pp. 346–355, 2001.

[32] W. Lee, Y. Xie, J. Zernant et al., "Complex inheritance of *ABCA4* disease: four mutations in a family with multiple macular phenotypes," *Human Genetics*, vol. 135, no. 1, pp. 9–19, 2016.

[33] S. Gerber, J. M. Rozet, T. J. van de Pol et al., "Complete exon-intron structure of the retina-specific ATP binding transporter gene (*ABCR*) allows the identification of novel mutations underlying Stargardt disease," *Genomics*, vol. 48, no. 1, pp. 139–142, 1998.

[34] T. R. Burke, R. Allikmets, R. T. Smith, P. Gouras, and S. H. Tsang, "Loss of peripapillary sparing in non-group I Stargardt disease," *Experimental Eye Research*, vol. 91, no. 5, pp. 592–600, 2010.

[35] S. Rossi, F. Testa, M. Attanasio et al., "Subretinal fibrosis in Stargardt's disease with fundus flavimaculatus and *ABCA4* gene mutation," *Case Reports in Ophthalmology*, vol. 3, no. 3, pp. 410–417, 2012.

[36] C. E. Briggs, D. Rucinski, P. J. Rosenfeld, T. Hirose, E. L. Berson, and T. P. Dryja, "Mutations in *ABCR* (*ABCA4*) in patients with Stargardt macular degeneration or cone-rod degeneration," *Investigative Ophthalmology & Visual Science*, vol. 42, no. 10, pp. 2229–2236, 2001.

[37] J. M. Rozet, S. Gerber, E. Souied et al., "Spectrum of ABCR gene mutations in autosomal recessive macular dystrophies," *European Journal of Human Genetics*, vol. 6, no. 3, pp. 291–295, 1998.

[38] https://www.ncbi.nlm.nih.gov/clinvar/variation/99132/.

[39] S. Stenirri, I. Fermo, S. Battistella et al., "Denaturing HPLC profiling of the *ABCA4* gene for reliable detection of allelic variations," *Clinical Chemistry*, vol. 50, no. 8, pp. 1336–1343, 2004.

[40] J. Zernant, C. Schubert, K. M. Im et al., "Analysis of the *ABCA4* gene by next-generation sequencing," *Investigative Ophthalmology & Visual Science*, vol. 52, no. 11, pp. 8479–8487, 2011.

[41] P. J. Ernest, C. J. Boon, B. J. Klevering, L. H. Hoefsloot, and C. B. Hoyng, "Outcome of *ABCA4* microarray screening in routine clinical practice," *Molecular Vision*, vol. 15, pp. 841–847, 2009.

[42] T. Eisenberger, C. Neuhaus, A. O. Khan et al., "Increasing the yield in targeted next-generation sequencing by implicating CNV analysis, non-coding exons and the overall variant load: the example of retinal dystrophies," *PLoS One*, vol. 8, no. 11, p. e78496, 2013.

[43] R. Allikmets, N. F. Shroyer, N. Singh et al., "Mutation of the Stargardt disease gene (*ABCR*) in age-related macular degeneration," *Science*, vol. 277, no. 5333, pp. 1805–1807, 1997.

[44] H. L. Schulz, F. Grassmann, U. Kellner et al., "Mutation spectrum of the *?* gene in 335 Stargardt disease patients from a multicenter German cohort-impact of selected deep intronic variants and common SNPs," *Investigative Ophthalmology & Visual Science*, vol. 58, no. 1, pp. 394–403, 2017.

13

HLA-C Alleles and Cytomegalovirus Retinitis in Brazilian Patients with AIDS

Tânia Gisela Biberg-Salum,[1] Maria de Lourdes Veronese Rodrigues,[2] Ana Paula Morais Fernandes,[3] Neifi Hassan Salum Deghaide,[4] Jayter Silva de Paula,[2] Erick C. Castelli,[5] Celso Teixeira Mendes-Junior,[6] and Eduardo Antonio Donadi[4,7]

[1]*Ribeirao Preto Medical School, University of São Paulo, University for Development of Pantanal Region (UNIDERP), São Paulo, SP, Brazil*
[2]*Department of Ophthalmology, Otorhinolaryngology and Head and Neck Surgery, Ribeirao Preto Medical School, University of São Paulo, São Paulo, SP, Brazil*
[3]*Department of General and Specialized Nursing, Nursing School of Ribeirao Preto, University of São Paulo, São Paulo, SP, Brazil*
[4]*Molecular Immunology Laboratory and HLA Hemocentro, Ribeirão Preto Medical School University Hospital, Ribeirão Preto, Brazil*
[5]*School of Medicine, Department of Pathology and Molecular Genetics and Bioinformatics Laboratory, São Paulo State University, Botucatu, SP, Brazil*
[6]*Departamento de Química, Laboratório de Pesquisas Forenses e Genômicas, Faculdade de Filosofia, Ciências e Letras de Ribeirão Preto, Universidade de São Paulo, 14040-901 Ribeirão Preto, SP, Brazil*
[7]*Division of Immunology, Department of Internal Medicine, Ribeirao Preto Medical School, University of São Paulo, São Paulo, SP, Brazil*

Correspondence should be addressed to Ana Paula Morais Fernandes; anapaula@eerp.usp.br

Academic Editor: Anna Nowinska

Purpose. Since cytomegalovirus retinitis (CR) is an important cause of visual impairment among AIDS patients and *HLA-C* alleles have been associated with AIDS disease outcome, we typed *HLA-C* locus in patients with AIDS exhibiting or not CR. *Methods.* Three groups of individuals were studied: (i) 49 patients with AIDS and CR (Group I), (ii) 161 patients with AIDS without CR (Group II), and (iii) 202 healthy HIV-negative individuals (Group III). *HLA-C* typing was performed using commercial kits. *Results.* The *HLA-C*∗07 allele group was underrepresented in AIDS patients with CR ($P = 0.005$) when compared to controls or when compared to AIDS patients without CR ($P = 0.006$). The *HLA-C*∗05 allele group was overrepresented in Group II in comparison to Group III ($P = 0.017$). The frequency of the *HLA-C*∗16 allele group was increased in Group III in comparison to Group II ($P = 0.004$). *Conclusion.* The *HLA-C*∗07 allele group conferred protection against the development of CR in Brazilian AIDS patients, whereas the *HLA-C*∗05 and *HLA-C*∗16 allele groups were associated with AIDS susceptibility or protection, respectively.

1. Introduction

Cytomegalovirus retinitis (CR) is the most common ocular opportunistic infection in patients with AIDS, often leading to blindness [1]; however, among patients who experience immune recovery after antiretroviral treatment (ART), an important reduction in the incidence of CR has been reported [2]. Despite recent advances in treatment, CR continues to rise challenging diagnostic and therapeutic questions since not all patients respond to ART [3].

Progression to AIDS has been strongly associated with the human leukocyte antigen B (*HLA-B*) alleles, particularly

HLA-B∗57 and *HLA-B*∗27 allele groups (protection), and *HLA-B*∗35 (susceptibility), due to the restricted recognition of HIV epitopes by cytotoxic immune system cells [4]. An increasing body of evidence has pointed out the role of HLA-C on HIV-1 disease progression. *HLA-C* gene diversity has an impact on HIV infection, particularly a polymorphism located at the promoter region of the *HLA-C* gene (-35C/T), for which the -35C variant has been associated with low viral load and high *HLA-C* mRNA [5].

We have previously reported that susceptibility to CR was associated with *HLA* alleles associated with rapid progression to AIDS, especially *HLA-B35* [6]. To further understand the impact of *HLA-C* polymorphism on CR development among Brazilian patients with AIDS, we evaluated the *HLA-C* allele polymorphism in patients presenting or not CR.

2. Materials and Methods

2.1. Subjects. An observational case-control study was carried out, using DNA samples obtained from patients with AIDS and from healthy individuals, stored in a DNA Sample Bank (Banco de Amostras do Núcleo de Pesquisa em Imunogenética (BANPI)), approved by the local Ethics Committee #7581/2007). All the 210 patients with AIDS were regularly registered at the Brazilian Ministry of Health and were followed up at the University Hospital of the Ribeirão Preto Medical School, the officially recognized hospital to follow-up these patients.

Group I consisted of DNA samples from 49 patients with AIDS presenting CR (38 men aged 21–77 years, median = 35 years), collected regardless of the evolutionary phase or the antiviral treatment of retinochorioiditis. CR was diagnosed by at least two experienced observers, and concordance between them was considered to be a *sine qua non* condition for patient inclusion. Clinical evaluation was performed by indirect binocular ophthalmoscopy, using a Heine Omega 100® ophthalmoscope (Herrsching, Germany), and a 20 diopter Nikon® lens (Melville, USA) under mydriasis produced by the local use of 1% tropicamide (Mydriacyl®, Alcon, São Paulo, Brazil). The $CD4^+$ cell count ranged from 1 to 368 cells/mm^3 (median = 31), and the viral load ranged from 400 to 8,500,000 copies/mL (median = 85,000). Only 19 (43.2%) of these patients were on antiretroviral therapy. The time since the diagnosis of AIDS ranged from 1–105 months (median = 22 months), and the number of systemic opportunistic infections preceding CR ranged from 0–6 (median = 3). The most frequent infections included candidiasis, neurotoxoplasmosis, pneumocystosis, and neurocryptococcosis.

Group II consisted of DNA samples obtained from 161 patients with AIDS (102 men aged 21–62 years, median = 37 years), randomly selected after performing the ophthalmologic examination excluding the presence of CR and exhibiting no changes of the choroid and retina or any other doubtful retinal diagnosis. The $CD4^+$ cell count ranged from 4 to 1164 cells/mm^3 (median = 588), and the viral load ranged from 80 to 2,000,000 copies/mL (median = 85,000). Time since the diagnosis of AIDS ranged from 1–108 months (median = 20 months), and these patients experienced 0–8 systemic previous opportunistic infections (median = 2), the most frequent being candidiasis, neurotoxoplasmosis, tuberculosis, and neurocryptococcosis.

Group III consisted of DNA samples from 202 healthy individuals (146 men aged 18–59 years, median = 33 years), exhibiting negative serology for HIV-1.

2.2. HLA-C Typing. Patient DNA was obtained from peripheral venous blood collected during the patient follow-up at Unit for the Treatment of Infectious Diseases (UETDI), and healthy control DNA was obtained from bone marrow donors.

HLA-C typing was carried at the Laboratory of Molecular Immunology of HCFMRP-USP, using a commercial kit (Micro SSP DNA Typing Tray, One Lambda, Canoga Park, CA).

2.3. Statistical Analyses. Intergroup differences were determined by the two-tailed Fisher exact test, with calculation of the odds ratio (OR) and 95% confidence interval (95% CI). The level of significance was set at $P \leq 0.05$ in all analyses. In addition, the etiologic fraction (EF) was calculated to determine how much each allele, genotype, or haplotype contributed to susceptibility to CR. The preventive fraction (PF), which estimates how much these same three factors contribute to protection against CR, was also calculated.

3. Results

The *HLA-C*∗07 allele group was underrepresented in Group I compared to Group II (OR: 0.4233, 95% CI: 0.2246–0.9782, $P = 0.006$), yielding a PF of 0.1531 (Table 1).

When the *HLA-C* allele frequencies were compared between Groups I and III, an underrepresentation of the *HLA-C*∗07 allele group was also observed for Group I (OR: 0.4192, 95% CI: 0.2246–0.7822, $P = 0.005$), conferring a PF of 0.1553 (Table 2).

The *HLA-C*∗05 allele group was overrepresented in Group II in comparison to Group III (OR: 2.2045, 95% CI: 1.1665–4.1665, $P = 0.017$), conferring an EF of 0.0455. The frequency of the *HLA-C*∗16 allele group was increased in Group III in comparison to Group II (OR: 0.3580, 95% CI: 0.1737–0.7380, $P = 0.004$), exhibiting a PF of 0.0524 (Table 3).

4. Discussion

It has been recognized that CR is a condition leading to reduced visual acuity and blindness in patients with AIDS patients; however, with the advent of the more effective antiretroviral therapy, a reduction in the frequency and in the severity of CR has been observed. Notwithstanding, in less favored regions, due to the lack of treatment or incorrect use of medications, or even in more privileged regions due to immunosuppression for organ transplantation, CR continues to deserve special attention.

Table 1: *HLA-C* allele frequencies compared between Groups I (patients with AIDS and CR) and II (patients with AIDS without CR).

Allele	Group I (%)	*N*	Group II (%)	*N*	OR	Preventive fraction	*P* value
*HLA-C**01	5.10	5	1.55	5			
*HLA-C**02	5.10	5	3.10	10			
*HLA-C**03	9.18	9	10.24	33			
*HLA-C**04	18.36	18	16.45	53			
*HLA-C**05	6.12	6	8.07	26			
*HLA-C**06	8.16	8	6.52	21			
*HLA-C**07	13.30	13	22.67	73	0.4233	0.1531	0.0063
*HLA-C**08	2.04	2	3.10	10			
*HLA-C**10	0	0	0.31	1			
*HLA-C**12	6.12	6	5.27	17			
*HLA-C**13	0	0	0.31	1			
*HLA-C**14	0	0	1.86	6			
*HLA-C**15	5.1	5	3.41	11			
*HLA-C**16	7.14	77	3.10	10			
*HLA-C**17	5.1	5	3.41	11			
*HLA-C**18	0.0	0	1.55	5			

HLA-C = major histocompatibility complex, class I, C; OR = odds ratio.

Table 2: *HLA-C* allele frequencies compared between Groups I (patients with AIDS and CR) and III (healthy HIV-negative individuals).

Allele	Group I (%)	Group III (%)	*N*	OR	Preventive fraction	*P* value
*HLA-C**01	5.1	1.73	7			
*HLA-C**02	5.1	5.70	23			
*HLA-C**03	11.2	6.93	28			
*HLA-C**04	22.4	15.33	62			
*HLA-C**05	7.1	3.96	16			
*HLA-C**06	9.2	9.90	40			
*HLA-C**07	13.3	26.73	106	0.4192	0.1553	0.0054
*HLA-C**08	2.0	5.70	23			
*HLA-C**10	0.0	0.0	0			
*HLA-C**12	6.1	6.43	26			
*HLA-C**13	0.0	0.0	0			
*HLA-C**14	0.0	2.22	9			
*HLA-C**15	6.1	3.48	14			
*HLA-C**16	7.1	8.17	33			
*HLA-C**17	5.1	2.97	13			
*HLA-C**18	0.0	0.74	4			

HLA-C = major histocompatibility complex, class I, C; OR = odds ratio.

Table 3: *HLA-C* allele frequencies compared between Groups II (patients with AIDS without CR) and III (healthy HIV-negative individuals).

Allele	Group II (%)	Group III (%)	Etiologic fraction	OR	Preventive fraction	*P* value
*HLA-C**01	1.5	1.7				
*HLA-C**02	3.4	5.7				
*HLA-C**03	10.8	6.9				
*HLA-C**04	17.6	15.3				
*HLA-C**05	8.3	4.0	0.0455	2.2045		0.0169
*HLA-C**06	7.7	9.9				
*HLA-C**07	26.5	26.7				
*HLA-C**08	3.4	5.7				
*HLA-C**10	0.3	0.0				
*HLA-C**12	5.9	6.4				
*HLA-C**13	0.3	0.0				
*HLA-C**14	1.9	2.2				
*HLA-C**15	3.7	3.5				
*HLA-C**16	3.1	8.2		0.3580	0.0524	0.0041
*HLA-C**17	4.0	3.0				
*HLA-C**18	1.5	0.7				

HLA-C = major histocompatibility complex, class I, C; OR = odds ratio.

In the present study, the *HLA-C*∗07* allele group was underrepresented in AIDS patients with CR, when compared to patients with AIDS without CR and when compared to healthy controls, indicating that the allele group is a protective factor against CR development. Considering that CD4 cell counts observed for patients with AIDS exhibiting CR (1 to 368 cells/mm^3, median = 31) were very different from patients with AIDS without CR (4–1164 cells/mm^3, median = 588), one may argue that CD4 cell count could be a confounding variable. To circumvent this problem, we compared patients with CR with those without CR, stratified according to the CD4 cell counts, that is, (i) patients with AIDS without CR (exhibiting CD4 ≤ 800 cells/mm^3; 4 to 778 cells/mm^3, median = 215) versus patients with AIDS and CR (exhibiting CD4 ≤ 368 cells/mm^3; 1 to 368 cells/mm^3, median = 31) and (ii) patients with AIDS without CR (exhibiting CD4 ≤ 100 cells/mm^3; 4 to 99 cells/mm^3, median = 49) versus patients with AIDS and CR (exhibiting CD4 ≤ 100 cells/mm^3; 1 to 90 cells/mm^3, median = 29). The first comparison revealed that the *HLA-C*∗07* allele group was overrepresented in patients with AIDS without CR ($P = 0.0163$), and the second comparison showed that the HLA-C∗07 allele group was also overrepresented in patients with AIDS without CR ($P = 0.0298$), indicating that the number of CD4 cells counts did not bias the results, and the *HLA-C*∗07* allele group did protect against CR development in patients with AIDS.

HLA-C alleles have been associated with protection against AIDS development, particularly for patients exhibiting the -35C allele upstream of the *HLA-C* gene, which has been reported to be associated with high cellular expression of HLA-C molecules and protection against HIV [7, 8]. Notably, many alleles of the *HLA-C*∗07* group have been associated with the -35T allele that contributes to low HLA-C expression and relatively high risk of disease progression [9]. Then, according to the -35CT dimorphism hypothesis, one should expect that an increased frequency of *HLA-C*∗07* alleles is associated with the -35T upstream allele, a fact that was not observed in the present study. Although the -35CT hypothesis is very attractive to explain AIDS outcome due to the immune modulatory role of the *HLA-C* molecule, the complete structure of the *HLA-C* gene (regulatory and coding regions) has not been completely studied. Further studies encompassing larger groups of patients with AIDS exhibiting CR as well as the study of the complete *HLA-C* gene could unravel the role of the gene in the susceptibility to CR. Besides the association with CR, the frequency of the *HLA-C*∗05* allele group was increased in patients with AIDS, irrespective of the presence or not of CR, indicating that this allele group is associated with AIDS susceptibility. On the contrary, patients with AIDS exhibited a reduced frequency of the *HLA-C*∗16* allele group, indicating a protective factor against the AIDS development.

HLA molecules have a relevant role on the control of HIV infection. Classic examples are the association of *HLA-B*∗57* and *HLA-B*∗35* with a slower or faster progression of the disease, respectively [10]. Regarding the HLA-C molecules, Silva et al. [11] reported that the *HLA-B*∗04*, -*B*∗57*, and -*C*∗18* alleles were associated with a low viral load in HIV-infected Brazilian patients. The present results expand the knowledge about the impact of *HLA-C* alleles on CR susceptibility; however, the major limitation of this cross-sectional study is the number of patients with AIDS exhibiting CR, a condition that has been drastically decreased due to the availability of ART.

5. Conclusion

The *HLA-C*∗07* allele conferred protection against the development of CR in Brazilian patients with AIDS, whereas *HLA-C*∗05* and *HLA-C*∗16* allele groups were associated with susceptibility/protection against AIDS development. Considering that the etiologic and preventive fractions conferred by these alleles were low, one may assume that many other genes are implicated on disease development.

Conflicts of Interest

The authors declare that there are no conflicts of interest.

Acknowledgments

The authors would like to thank Maria Cecilia Onofre for the collaboration in the organization of the manuscript. They would also like to thank Foundation for Support of Teaching, Research and Assistance (FAEPA) for article processing charges.

References

[1] G. Huang, Q. Jiang, M. Li, Y. Lu, and Z. Wang, "Retrospective study of cytomegalovirus retinitis complicated with acquired immunodeficiency syndrome," *International Journal of Clinical and Experimental Medicine*, vol. 8, no. 6, pp. 9537–9542, 2015.

[2] D. A. Jabs, A. Ahuja, M. L. Van Natta, A. T. Lyon, S. Yeh, and R. Danis, "Long-term outcomes of cytomegalovirus retinitis in the era of modern antiretroviral therapy: results from a United States Cohort," *Ophthalmology*, vol. 122, no. 7, pp. 1452–1463, 2015.

[3] A. Timperley, H. Taha, and S. Das, "Management of cytomegalovirus retinitis in HIV infection in the era of highly active antiretroviral therapy," *International Journal of STD & AIDS*, vol. 26, no. 10, pp. 757-758, 2015.

[4] M. Carrington and S. J. O'Brien, "The influence of *HLA* Genotype on AIDS," *Annual Review of Medicine*, vol. 54, no. 1, pp. 535–551, 2003.

[5] M. Carrington, A. A. Bashirova, and P. J. McLaren, "On stand by: host genetics of HIV control," *AIDS*, vol. 27, no. 18, pp. 2831–2839, 2013.

[6] A. P. Fernandes, M. A. G. Gonçalves, R. B. Zavanella, J. F. C. Figueiredo, E. A. Donadi, and M. L. V. Rodrigues, "HLA markers associated with progression to AIDS are also associated with susceptibility to cytomegalovirus retinitis," *AIDS*, vol. 17, no. 14, pp. 2133–2136, 2003.

[7] E. Raymond, V. Tricottet, D. Samuel, M. Reynès, H. Bismuth, and J. L. Misset, "Epstein-Barr virus-related localized hepatic lymphoproliferative disorders after liver transplantation," *Cancer*, vol. 76, no. 8, pp. 1344–1351, 1995.
[8] R. Thomas, R. Apps, Y. Qi et al., "HLA-C cell surface expression and control of HIV/AIDS correlate with a variant upstream of HLA-C," *Nature Genetics*, vol. 41, no. 12, pp. 1290–1294, 2009.
[9] T. W. Corrah, N. Goonetilleke, J. Kopycinski et al., "Reappraisal of the relationship between the HIV-1-protective single-nucleotide polymorphism 35 kilobases upstream of the HLA-C gene and surface HLA-C expression," *Journal of Virology*, vol. 85, no. 7, pp. 3367–3374, 2011.
[10] K. D. Squires, M. Monajemi, C. F. Woodworth, M. D. Grant, and M. Larijani, "Impact of APOBEC mutations on CD8+ T cell recognition of HIV epitopes varies depending on the restricting HLA," *Journal of Acquired Immune Deficiency Syndromes*, vol. 70, no. 2, pp. 172–178, 2015.
[11] E. M. Silva, A. X. Acosta, E. J. Santos et al., "HLA-Bw4-B*57 and Cw*18 alleles are associated with plasma viral load modulation in HIV-1 infected individuals in Salvador, Brazil," *Brazilian Journal of Infectious Diseases*, vol. 14, no. 5, pp. 468–475, 2010.

Functional and Structural Outcomes of Temporal Zone II-Sparing Laser Photocoagulation Combined with Intravitreal Bevacizumab in Retinopathy of Prematurity

Eoi Jong Seo and Joo Yong Lee

Department of Ophthalmology, Asan Medical Center, University of Ulsan College of Medicine, Seoul, Republic of Korea

Correspondence should be addressed to Joo Yong Lee; ophthalmo@amc.seoul.kr

Academic Editor: Enrico Peiretti

Background/Aim. The aim of the study was to investigate the outcomes of temporal Zone II-sparing laser photocoagulation combined with intravitreal bevacizumab (IVB) in patients with Type 1 retinopathy of prematurity (ROP) in Zone I. *Methods.* Medical records of 74 eyes of 37 infants were analysed. Only infants with Type 1 ROP in Zone I were included. Thirty-two eyes were treated with temporal-sparing laser + IVB. Both Zone I and temporal Zone II were spared to minimise potential visual field loss. Forty-two eyes were treated with laser alone conventionally. Early treatment outcomes, late complications, and refractive errors were analysed. *Results.* The mean gestational age and birth weight of the enrolled patients were 25.7 ± 2.5 weeks and 798.8 ± 440.2 g, respectively. In the combined treatment group, plus sign regression was achieved faster (12.1 ± 6.2 days vs. 25.6 ± 21.3 days, $p = 0.011$) and retreatment was required less (0% vs. 23.8%, $p = 0.004$) than in the laser-alone group. Retinal/preretinal haemorrhages occurred more often in the laser-alone group (42.9% vs. 9.4%, $p = 0.002$). Normal development of temporal retinal vessels was also observed in twelve eyes in the combined treatment group. No differences in late complications or refractive errors were observed between the groups. *Conclusion.* Temporal Zone II-sparing laser treatment combined with IVB showed good early treatment outcome and temporal retinal vessels development.

1. Introduction

Retinopathy of prematurity (ROP), a vasoproliferative disease associated with underdevelopment of the retina, is a leading cause of severe impairment of visual function in childhood [1]. Mild cases show spontaneous regression. However, some cases progress to a severe form of the disease and show retinal haemorrhage and tractional retinal detachment, which require surgical interventions such as vitrectomy [2, 3]. The Early Treatment for Retinopathy of Prematurity Cooperative Group (ETROP) trial established laser photocoagulation as an effective approach to stop disease progression in Type 1 ROP [4].

However, confluent laser scars on the retinal periphery may cause visual field restriction after the treatment. The area where laser photocoagulation was performed becomes atrophic, eventually restricting the patient's peripheral visual field. Several efforts have been made to reduce the area of laser photocoagulation using the recently highlighted intravitreal bevacizumab (IVB) treatment [5–8]. But IVB monotreatment showed delayed reactivation and caused devastating retinal sequelae in some cases [9]. Recent studies reported that posterior pole-sparing laser photocoagulation combined with IVB produced favourable outcomes [6, 7, 10, 11].

To minimise the visual field restriction caused by laser treatment, we saved a larger area in Type 1 ROP, including temporal Zone II, to maximise the combination effect compared with that in previously reported studies, which spared Zone I or the posterior pole. The functional and long-term structural outcomes were analysed.

2. Materials and Methods

This study, performed retrospectively, followed the tenets of the Helsinki declaration and was approved by the Institutional Review Board of Asan Medical Center. Informed consent was obtained from all parents after providing an explanation of laser photocoagulation and off-label use of bevacizumab, if indicated. Potential risks and side effects of IVB were explained. After thorough consideration, all parents agreed to the treatment involving laser photocoagulation with/without IVB.

The medical records of preterm infants who received laser photocoagulation alone or combined with IVB, and had been followed for at least 6 months in the period from Mar 2013 to Sep 2016 at Asan Medical Center, Seoul, Korea, were collected. Peripheral retinal laser photocoagulation was indicated when the fundus examination revealed Type 1 ROP in Zone I. Only infants with ROP in Zone I were included in the current study. Infants who received laser treatment due to Zone II ROP were excluded.

Two distinctive patterns of treatment were performed (Figure 1). In one group, eyes were treated with laser photocoagulation only. Laser photocoagulation was done using an 810 nm laser indirect ophthalmoscope (LIO). In these cases, LIO treatment was performed conventionally in the entire avascular area from the retinal ridge to the ora serrata. These patients were defined as the LIO-alone group. In the other group, patients were treated with both LIO and IVB (0.5 mg/0.02 mL). When combined with IVB, LIO treatment spared Zone I and temporal Zone II to minimise potential visual field loss. These patients were classified as the temporal-sparing LIO + IVB group. The treatment choice was determined by a retinal specialist (JYL) depending on the severity of ROP. In cases of aggressive posterior ROP (AP-ROP), poor pupillary dilation, or media opacity, combined laser treatment with IVB was performed instead of laser-only treatment.

Before treatment and during follow-ups, the fundus was examined by indirect ophthalmoscopy and wide-field photography, if indicated. A RetCam (Clarity Medical Systems, Pleasanton, CA, USA) was employed to record the severity of ROP, extent of the laser scar, regression of new vessels, and development of peripheral retinal vessels after treatment. Patient baseline characteristics such as gestational age at birth, birth weight, multiplicity, APGAR score, ventilator care, and O_2 therapy period were collected. A series of comorbid systemic diseases associated with ROP, such as necrotising enterocolitis, respiratory distress syndrome, ligated patent ductus arteriosus, bronchopulmonary dysplasia, sepsis, intrauterine growth restriction, poor weight gain, hydrocephalus, and intraventricular haemorrhage, were also documented.

Early treatment outcomes/complications as well as late structural/functional complications were analysed based on fundus photographs and medical records. At 6–12 months after treatment, all treated infants underwent measurement of refractive errors by manual cycloplegic refraction performed by a skilled paediatric ophthalmologist. The results were recorded as measurements of spherical and cylinder astigmatism, and the spherical equivalent. These were also divided into the categories of emmetropia, mild (0–3 D), moderate (3–6 D), or high (>6 D) myopia, and hyperopia.

Statistical analysis was performed using SPSS for Windows (version 21.0, SPSS, Inc., Chicago, IL). The independent *t*-, Fisher's exact, and Pearson's Chi-square tests were used. p values < 0.05 were considered to be statistically significant.

3. Results

A total of 74 eyes of 37 infants were analysed. Thirty-two eyes of 16 infants were treated with temporal-sparing LIO + IVB, and 42 eyes of 21 infants were treated with LIO alone. The mean follow-up period was 19.7 ± 9.0 months. Out of the 32 eyes treated with temporal-sparing LIO + IVB, 10 (31.3%) showed AP-ROP. With the exception of the follow-up period being shorter in the temporal-sparing LIO + IVB group, there were no statistically significant differences in baseline characteristics and comorbid conditions between the two groups (Table 1).

Treatment outcomes and complications are shown in Table 2. After both treatments, all eyes showed complete regression of plus sign. However, plus sign regression was faster in the group combining LIO treatment with IVB compared with the LIO-only group (12.1 ± 6.2 vs. 25.6 ± 21.3 days, $p = 0.011$). Ten eyes in the LIO-alone group required retreatment after a mean 25 days from the initial treatment, while all eyes in the temporal-sparing LIO + IVB group were stabilised after the first treatment ($p = 0.004$). Among the eyes requiring retreatment, 6 eyes were treated with LIO + IVB and 4 eyes were treated with additional LIO only. Retinal/preretinal haemorrhages were found more frequently in the LIO-alone group (9.4% vs. 42.9%, $p = 0.002$). No reports of endophthalmitis or adverse systemic safety issues related to IVB were found. Among late complications, structural complications like macular dragging or optic disc atrophy tended to occur frequently in patients treated with LIO alone. Functional complications such as strabismus or nystagmus showed no tendency between the groups. Refractive error measurements were performed 10.4 ± 5.0 months after treatment. No statistically significant differences were found between the two groups in the spherical equivalent ($p = 0.293$) and refractive error ($p = 0.130$) distributions.

Among the 32 eyes treated with temporal-sparing LIO + IVB, 24 eyes of 12 infants were able to analyse the retinal periphery with wide-field fundus photography after 1 month of treatment. The others were not able to do so because of poor peripheral visualisation. Normal development of temporal retinal vessels was observed in the 12 eyes (50%) of 6 infants. Vessel development progressed close to the laser scar, and the avascular area was barely visible (Figure 2). In the other 12 eyes, no or little vessel development was observed, and most of the avascular area remained. Among these, 5 eyes (both eyes of 2 infants, the left eye of 1 infant) showed a persistent avascular area even 3 months after treatment (Figure 3). No significant correlation between the presence of a persistent avascular area and any other patient characteristic was found.

4. Discussion

In the present study, the functional and structural outcomes in patients with Type 1 ROP were compared between those who underwent temporal Zone II-sparing laser photocoagulation combined with IVB and conventional laser

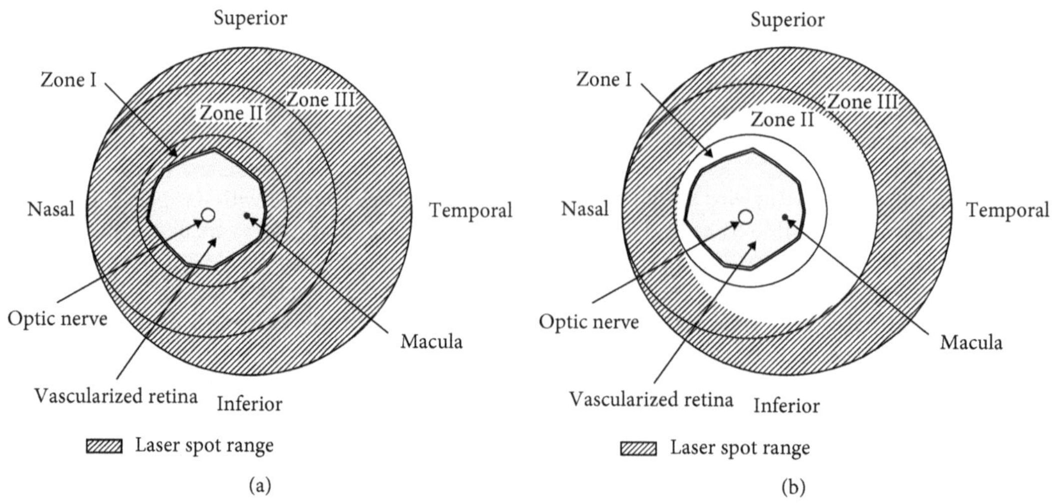

FIGURE 1: Diagrammatic images of the two different treatment methods. In conventional laser photocoagulation, laser spots covered the entire avascular area, including Zones I, II, and III (a). When both Zone I and temporal Zone II areas were spared, intravitreal bevacizumab was added (b). Slash lines indicate the laser spot range.

TABLE 1: Baseline characteristics of the subjects.

	Temporal-sparing LIO + IVB	LIO alone	p value
Number of infants (eyes)	16 (32)	21 (42)	
Gestational age at birth (weeks)	25.1 ± 1.3	26.2 ± 3.0	0.169‡
Birth weight (g)	673.1 ± 145.8	594.5 ± 557.3	0.132‡
Follow-up period (weeks)	84.4 ± 36.9	117.4 ± 43.6	0.020‡
Eyes with aggressive posterior ROP (%)	10 (31.3)	0 (0)	<0.001*
Multiplicity (%)			0.502*
Single	9 (56.3)	12 (57.1)	
Twins	6 (37.5)	9 (42.9)	
Triplets	1 (6.2)	0 (0.0)	
APGAR score			
1 minute	3.1 ± 2.2	4.0 ± 1.6	0.186‡
5 minutes	5.2 ± 2.7	6.1 ± 1.1	0.155‡
Ventilator care period (days)	75.6 ± 29.0	67.1 ± 35.0	0.427‡
O2 therapy period (days)	96.9 ± 30.3	88.4 ± 42.9	0.485‡
Comorbid conditions			
NEC operation (%)	5 (31.3)	2 (9.5)	0.095*
PDA ligation (%)	12 (75.0)	20 (95.2)	0.144†
RDS (%)	15 (93.8)	21 (100)	0.432†
BPD ≥ moderate (%)	5 (31.3)	12 (57.1)	0.117†
Sepsis (%)	11 (68.8)	12 (57.1)	0.471*
IUGR (%)	2 (12.5)	7 (33.3)	0.248†
Poor weight gain (%)	15 (93.8)	16 (76.2)	0.206†
Hydrocephalus (%)	2 (12.5)	7 (33.3)	0.248†
IVH (%)			0.448*
None	4	2	
Grade I-II	9	14	
Grade III-IV	3	5	

Continuous variables are shown as mean ± SD; *chi-square analysis; †Fisher's exact test; ‡Student's t-test; NEC, necrotising enterocolitis; PDA, patent ductus arteriosus; RDS, respiratory distress syndrome; BPD, bronchopulmonary dysplasia; IUGR, intrauterine growth restriction; IVH, intraventricular haemorrhage.

photocoagulation alone. Wider preservation of the retina after regression of ROP was observed in eyes treated with temporal-sparing laser therapy combined with IVB compared with those treated with laser photocoagulation alone. Eyes undergoing the combined treatment required retreatment less frequently and showed faster regression of plus sign compared with eyes treated with LIO alone. Refractive changes and the incidence of long-term complications showed no differences between the two treatments. In 50% of eyes treated with the combined therapy, normal development of the peripheral retina was observed after complete regression of ROP.

TABLE 2: Comparison of treatment outcomes, ocular complications, and refractive errors.

	Temporal-sparing LIO + IVB	LIO alone	p value
Early treatment outcome			
Plus sign disappeared (%)	32 (100)	42 (100)	
Time to plus sign regression (days)	12.1 ± 6.2	25.6 ± 21.3	0.011‡
Retreatment (%)	0 (0)	10 (23.8)	0.004†
Time to retreatment (days)		25.0 ± 14.4	
Retinal/preretinal hmr (%)	3 (9.4)	18 (42.9)	0.002*
Vitreous hmr (%)	0 (0)	4 (9.5)	0.129†
Ocular inflammation (%)	0 (0)	0 (0)	
Endophthalmitis (%)	0 (0)	0 (0)	
Adverse systemic safety issues (%)	0 (0)	0 (0)	
Late complications			
Macular dragging (%)	0 (0)	5 (11.9%)	0.065†
Optic disc atrophy (%)	4 (12.5)	8 (19.0%)	0.449*
Strabismus (%)	10 (31.3)	14 (33.3)	0.850*
Nystagmus (%)	6 (18.8)	6 (14.3)	0.606*
Amblyopia (%)	8 (25.0)	10 (23.8)	0.906*
Cataract (%)	0 (0)	0 (0)	
Microcornea (%)	0 (0)	0 (0)	
Angle closure glaucoma (%)	0 (0)	0 (0)	
Refractive errors			
Measurement period (months)	9.7 ± 4.2	11.0 ± 5.6	0.464‡
Spherical equivalent (D)	−0.43 ± 0.58	−0.94 ± 2.69	0.293‡
Emmetropia (%)	7 (21.9)	16 (38.0)	0.130*
Mild myopia (0–3 D) (%)	20 (62.5)	22 (52.4)	
Moderate myopia (3–6 D) (%)	0 (0)	0 (0)	
High myopia (>6 D) (%)	0 (0)	2 (4.8)	
Hyperopia (%)	5 (15.6)	2 (4.8)	

Continuous variables are shown as mean ± SD; *chi-square analysis; †Fisher's exact test; ‡Student's t-test; hmr, haemorrhage.

Temporal Zone II area was chosen to be spared in the current study. Saving the nasal area would be more beneficial in saving the temporal visual field in binocular vision. However, as shown in Figure 1, the temporal area is larger, and it is mainly responsible for the retinal avascularity and has spatial closeness with the macula. Saving the maximum amount of retina adjacent to the macula could enhance the central visual field, which is crucial for the functional vision.

Because retinal atrophy and photoreceptor damage are inherent sequelae of laser photocoagulation, IVB monotherapy might be a good option to achieve ROP regression with a good anatomical outcome. However, several findings of delayed reactivation were reported in IVB monotherapy, sometimes as late as 3 years posttreatment [9, 12–14]. Moreover, when recurrences occur, their locations and patterns may be altered compared with the original pathology [9, 13, 15]. Several efforts have been made to combine laser photocoagulation and IVB to minimise retinal damage and maximise treatment efficacy, including studies combining IVB therapy with Zone I or posterior pole-sparing laser treatment [10, 16, 17]. We performed eccentric laser photocoagulation on the avascular area sparing the temporal Zone II area and injected bevacizumab simultaneously. While maximising the effect of combined IVB and laser therapy, we were able to save a larger area of the retina compared with the previously published reports, in which only Zone I or the posterior pole was saved. The long-term outcomes of our treatment were not different from those of conventional laser therapy alone, while better visual function, such as wider visual field acquisition, can be expected.

As in previous reports [5, 7, 8], combining IVB and laser therapy in one treatment produced better structural outcomes than did laser treatment alone. In the present study, plus sign regression was faster and retreatment was required less frequently in the combined therapy group compared with the laser-only group (Table 2). Based on the pathogenesis of ROP, a surge of VEGF excreted from the wide avascular retina plays a key role in neovascularisation [18, 19]. The rapid VEGF-lowering effect of injected bevacizumab is beneficial for stabilisation of the retinal vasculature. The diminished laser ablation of the retina in combination therapy resulted in fewer retinal/preretinal haemorrhages (Table 2). Given that the ocular environment is proangiogenic and proinflammatory, fibrin-rich preretinal haemorrhage can be a possible risk for fibrovascular membrane formation [20]. The rapid stabilisation of ROP achieved with IVB may underlie the decrease in structural complications in long-term follow-up. In the present study, macular dragging was more frequently observed in the LIO-alone group with a marginal significance ($p = 0.065$).

In spite of the advantages of IVB use in ROP treatment, delayed reactivation is a major concern. However, there was no reactivation in both groups followed up for 103.1 ± 43.6 weeks PMA in the current study. The follow-up period was shorter in the combined treatment group (84.4 ± 36.9 vs.

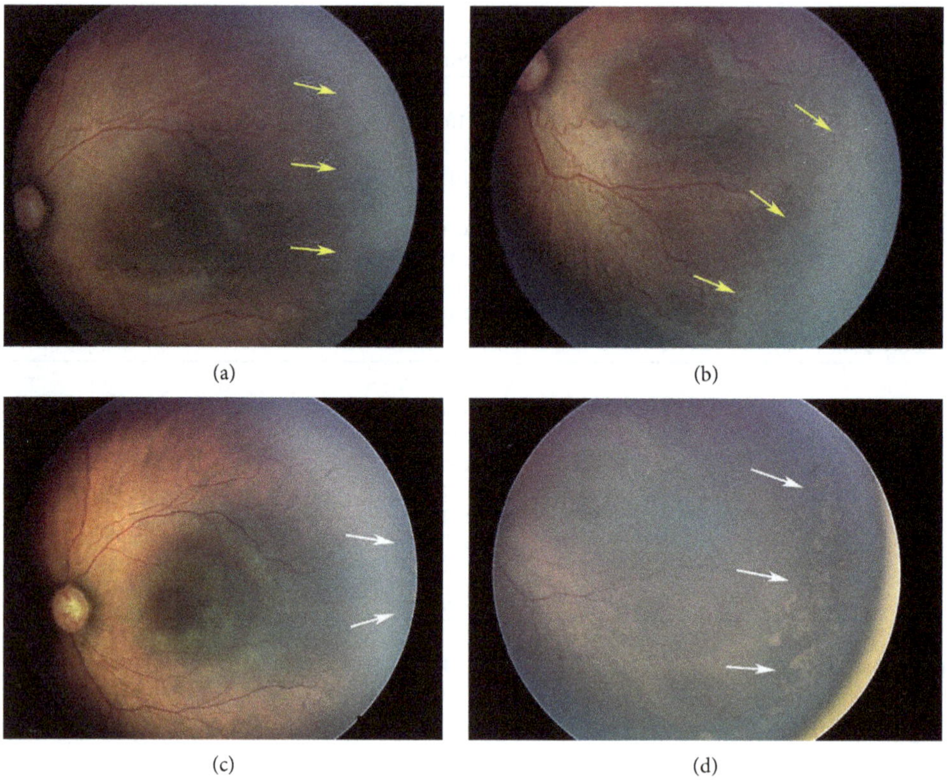

FIGURE 2: A male infant born at a gestational age of 27 weeks showed Type 1 ROP at 32 weeks PMA. (a, b) An avascular area was observed and is indicated with yellow arrows. Temporal-sparing LIO combined with IVB was performed. Two weeks after treatment, temporal retinal vessels had reached the laser-treated Zone II area. (c, d) The edge of the vascularized retina is indicated with white arrows. Reactivation of ROP was not observed through 137 weeks of follow-up.

117.4 ± 43.6 weeks). Nonetheless, given that the mean time to recurrence was 19.2 ± 8.6 weeks after bevacizumab treatment in the BEAT-ROP study, our follow-up period was long enough to analyse long-term efficacy [8]. Another case series [9] reported reactivation of ROP after IVB monotherapy as late as at 69 weeks PMA. When IVB was combined with Zone I-sparing laser treatment, neither reactivation nor retinal detachment was reported for 83.6 weeks PMA [21]. Treatment of ROP with bevacizumab followed by prophylactic laser therapy also showed no reactivation for 125 weeks PMA [17]. Taken together with our findings, these results demonstrate that combining laser therapy with IVB treatment is a safe way to prevent delayed reactivation of ROP.

After treatment, there was no difference in mean spherical equivalent between the two groups at 6 months. Over 80% of the infants showed emmetropia or mild myopia. In a meta-analysis of 11 studies of a total of 378 eyes with intravitreal anti-VEGF treatment in ROP, the average spherical equivalent refractive error reported after anti-VEGF monotherapy ranged from +0.75 D to −3.75 D [22]. In the BEAT-ROP study, ROP-severity-matched eyes receiving anti-VEGF therapy were found to have significantly lower myopia than those receiving peripheral laser ablation at average of 2.5 years [23]. Further observation of refractive errors should be required to obtain refractive error differences.

As demonstrated in Figure 2, 12 out of 24 eyes treated with IVB showed normal development of the peripheral retina in this study. Peripheral retinal development after IVB treatment was reported in multiple previous studies [5, 6, 17, 24, 25]. Lepore et al. reported various abnormalities such as abnormal branching or shunts at the retinal periphery of bevacizumab-treated eyes [25]. It is unclear whether these peripheral vessels act as normal vasculature, leading to normal peripheral retinal development. However, because ablation with laser certainly destroys the retinal structure, preservation of as much viable retina as possible should be good for the patient's potential visual field. Five eyes (20.8%) in the current study showed persistent avascular areas 3 months after temporal-sparing laser treatment combined with IVB. If it persists further, the avascular area can be worrisome because it can be a source of VEGF that can potentially lead to the late reactivation of ROP. Although there were no infants with late reactivation of ROP in the present study, a longer study is needed to identify the possibility of using additional laser treatment for the persistent avascular areas.

There have been reports that performing laser treatment in combination with bevacizumab injection increases the systemic levels of the drug, which decreases the levels of systemic VEGF and could possibly be associated with decreased neurodevelopmental outcomes [26, 27]. The use of laser can alter the blood retinal barrier, potentially increasing

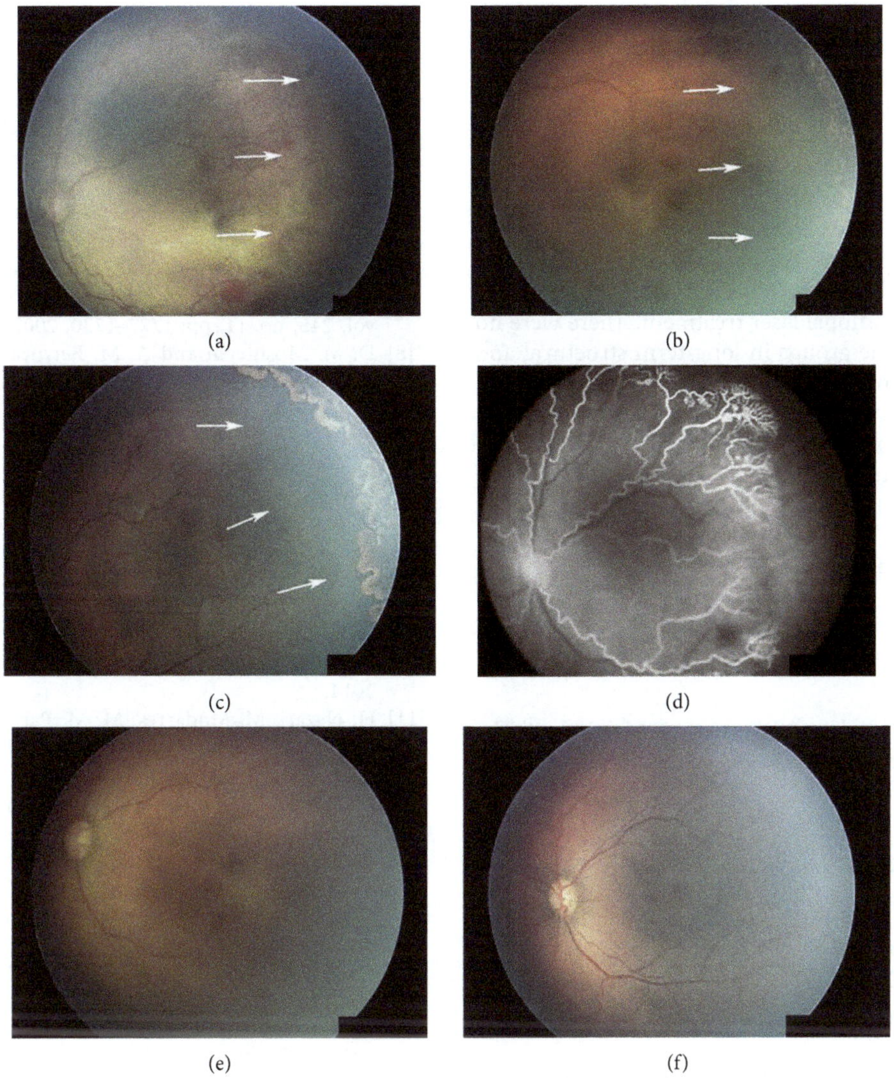

FIGURE 3: Examples of eyes with persistent avascular areas after temporal-sparing LIO + IVB. Avascular areas are indicated with white arrows. (a, d) Pretreatment fundus image and fluorescein angiograph. (b, e) Two weeks after treatment, the plus sign had disappeared but the temporal avascular area persisted. (c, f) Three months after treatment, plus sign was absent but the temporal avascular area had not decreased compared with the previous exam.

the anti-VEGF absorption into the systemic flow. Within the follow-up period of our study, no neurodevelopmental delay related to IVB was observed. Further studies would be helpful in revealing the influence of IVB on the systemic VEGF.

Our study has several limitations. Besides the retrospective nature of the study design and small sample size, the major limitation is that multiple systemic and environmental factors influencing the treatment outcome, such as oxygen supply, nutrient concentration, intrauterine environment, and perinatal issues, may have been different between the treatment groups. We confirmed that major systemic risks were not significantly different between the two groups in Table 1, but other factors could still play confounding roles. Another limitation is the possibility of a selection bias due to the treatment method being chosen by a single ophthalmologist. However, as mentioned above and shown in Table 1, the more severely affected eyes tended to be treated with temporal-sparing LIO + IVB. Finally, we could not measure peripheral visual function as a treatment outcome. Because subjects were infants, the conventional visual field test could not be performed. Retinal microperimetry could be used instead to clarify the functional outcome of the peripheral retina. When the infants are grown enough to undergo the visual field test, a quantitative comparison can be performed.

Despite its limitations, the present study is valuable in that we demonstrated good structural and functional outcomes in minimally threatened visual fields and visualised them with wide-field fundus photography and fluorescein angiography. The previous studies had limitations in treatment standardisation or diagnosis because of a lack of images. We adopted a wide-field fundus-imaging system to determine the ROP stage, plus sign regression, retinal haemorrhages, extent of the avascular area, laser ablated area, and peripheral vessel advancement. This visualisation allowed us to standardise treatment and perform an appropriate comparison.

5. Conclusions

Temporal-sparing laser treatment combined with intravitreal bevacizumab showed better early treatment outcomes compared with conventional laser treatment. There were no differences between the groups in long-term structural and functional complications, including delayed reactivation. Because of the preservation of the viable retina with peripheral vessel development and the low reactivation rate, temporal Zone II-sparing laser photocoagulation combined with intravitreal bevacizumab could be a good choice for Type 1 ROP patients to achieve complete regression while minimising peripheral field defects.

Disclosure

The topic was presented at 2017 Annual Meeting of The Korean Retina Society, Seoul, Korea, December 1-2, 2017.

Conflicts of Interest

The authors declare that there are no conflicts of interest regarding the publication of this paper.

Acknowledgments

This work was funded by grants from Asan Institute for Life Sciences (2014-7206), Asan Medical Center, Seoul, Republic of Korea.

References

[1] C. Gilbert, "Retinopathy of prematurity: a global perspective of the epidemics, population of babies at risk and implications for control," *Early Human Development*, vol. 84, no. 2, pp. 77–82, 2008.

[2] P. Bhende, L. Gopal, T. Sharma, A. Verma, and R. K. Biswas, "Functional and anatomical outcomes after primary lens-sparing pars plana vitrectomy for Stage 4 retinopathy of prematurity," *Indian Journal of Ophthalmology*, vol. 57, no. 4, pp. 267–271, 2009.

[3] P. K. Shah, V. Narendran, N. Kalpana, and K. A. Tawansy, "Anatomical and visual outcome of stages 4 and 5 retinopathy of prematurity," *Eye*, vol. 23, no. 1, pp. 176–180, 2009.

[4] Early Treatment For Retinopathy of Prematurity Cooperative Group, "Revised indications for the treatment of retinopathy of prematurity: results of the early treatment for retinopathy of prematurity randomized trial," *Archives of Ophthalmology*, vol. 121, no. 12, pp. 1684–1694, 2003.

[5] H. A. Mintz-Hittner, K. A. Kennedy, and A. Z. Chuang, "Efficacy of intravitreal bevacizumab for stage 3+ retinopathy of prematurity," *New England Journal of Medicine*, vol. 364, no. 7, pp. 603–615, 2011.

[6] J. Y. Lee, J. B. Chae, S. J. Yang, Y. H. Yoon, and J. G. Kim, "Effects of intravitreal bevacizumab and laser in retinopathy of prematurity therapy on the development of peripheral retinal vessels," *Graefe's Archive for Clinical Experimental Ophthalmology*, vol. 248, no. 9, pp. 1257–1262, 2010.

[7] E. J. Chung, J. H. Kim, H. S. Ahn, and H. J. Koh, "Combination of laser photocoagulation and intravitreal bevacizumab (Avastin) for aggressive zone I retinopathy of prematurity," *Graefe's Archive for Clinical Experimental Ophthalmology*, vol. 245, no. 11, pp. 1727–1730, 2007.

[8] D. M. Moshfeghi and A. M. Berrocal, "Retinopathy of prematurity in the time of bevacizumab: incorporating the BEAT-ROP results into clinical practice," *Ophthalmology*, vol. 118, no. 7, pp. 1227-1228, 2011.

[9] J. Hu, M. P. Blair, M. J. Shapiro, S. J. Lichtenstein, J. M. Galasso, and R. Kapur, "Reactivation of retinopathy of prematurity after bevacizumab injection," *Archives of Ophthalmology*, vol. 130, no. 8, pp. 1000–1006, 2012.

[10] R. Kim and Y. C. Kim, "Posterior pole sparing laser photocoagulation combined with intravitreal bevacizumab injection in posterior retinopathy of prematurity," *Journal of Ophthalmology*, vol. 2014, Article ID 257286, 5 pages, 2014.

[11] H. Nazari, M. Modarres, M. M. Parvaresh, and K. Ghasemi Falavarjani, "Intravitreal bevacizumab in combination with laser therapy for the treatment of severe retinopathy of prematurity (ROP) associated with vitreous or retinal hemorrhage," *Graefe's Archive for Clinical Experimental Ophthalmology*, vol. 248, no. 12, pp. 1713–1718, 2010.

[12] S. Ittiara, M. P. Blair, M. J. Shapiro, and S. J. Lichtenstein, "Exudative retinopathy and detachment: a late reactivation of retinopathy of prematurity after intravitreal bevacizumab," *Journal of American Association for Pediatric Ophthalmology and Strabismus*, vol. 17, no. 3, pp. 323–325, 2013.

[13] J. J. Chan, C. P. Lam, M. K. Kwok et al., "Risk of recurrence of retinopathy of prematurity after initial intravitreal ranibizumab therapy," *Scientific Reports*, vol. 6, no. 1, article 27082, 2016.

[14] A. R. Hajrasouliha, J. M. Garcia-Gonzales, M. J. Shapiro, H. Yoon, and M. P. Blair, "Reactivation of retinopathy of prematurity three years after treatment with bevacizumab," *Ophthalmic Surgery, Lasers and Imaging Retina*, vol. 48, no. 3, pp. 255–259, 2017.

[15] R. D. Patel, M. P. Blair, M. J. Shapiro, and S. J. Lichtenstein, "Significant treatment failure with intravitreous bevacizumab for retinopathy of prematurity," *Archives of Ophthalmology*, vol. 130, no. 6, pp. 801-802, 2012.

[16] J. M. Yoon, D. H. Shin, S. J. Kim et al., "Outcomes after laser versus combined laser and bevacizumab treatment for type 1 retinopathy of prematurity in zone I," *Retina*, vol. 37, no. 1, pp. 88–96, 2017.

[17] J. M. Garcia Gonzalez, L. Snyder, M. Blair, A. Rohr, M. Shapiro, and M. Greenwald, "Prophylactic peripheral laser and fluorescein angiography after bevacizumab for retinopathy of prematurity," *Retina*, vol. 38, no. 4, pp. 764–772, 2017.

[18] G. Cavallaro, L. Filippi, P. Bagnoli et al., "The pathophysiology of retinopathy of prematurity: an update of previous and recent knowledge," *Acta Ophthalmologica*, vol. 92, no. 1, pp. 2–20, 2014.

[19] M. E. Hartnett, "Pathophysiology and mechanisms of severe retinopathy of prematurity," *Ophthalmology*, vol. 122, no. 1, pp. 200–210, 2015.

[20] J. Ma, M. Mehta, G. Lam et al., "Influence of subretinal fluid in advanced stage retinopathy of prematurity on proangiogenic response and cell proliferation," *Molecular Vision*, vol. 20, pp. 881–893, 2014.

[21] J. Kim, S. J. Kim, Y. S. Chang, and W. S. Park, "Combined intravitreal bevacizumab injection and zone I sparing laser photocoagulation in patients with zone I retinopathy of prematurity," *Retina*, vol. 34, no. 1, pp. 77–82, 2014.

[22] H. A. Mintz-Hittner and M. M. Geloneck, "Review of effects of anti-VEGF treatment on refractive error," *Eye and Brain*, vol. 8, pp. 135–140, 2016.

[23] M. M. Geloneck, A. Z. Chuang, W. L. Clark et al., "Refractive outcomes following bevacizumab monotherapy compared with conventional laser treatment: a randomized clinical trial," *JAMA Ophthalmology*, vol. 132, no. 11, pp. 1327–1333, 2014.

[24] H. A. Mintz-Hittner, M. M. Geloneck, and A. Z. Chuang, "Clinical management of recurrent retinopathy of prematurity after intravitreal bevacizumab monotherapy," *Ophthalmology*, vol. 123, no. 9, pp. 1845–1855, 2016.

[25] D. Lepore, G. E. Quinn, F. Molle et al., "Intravitreal bevacizumab versus laser treatment in type 1 retinopathy of prematurity: report on fluorescein angiographic findings," *Ophthalmology*, vol. 121, no. 11, pp. 2212–2219, 2014.

[26] T. Sato, K. Wada, H. Arahori et al., "Serum concentration of bevacizumab (avastin) and vascular endothelial growth factor in infants with retinopathy of prematurity," *American Journal of Ophthalmology*, vol. 153, no. 2, pp. 327.e1–333.e1, 2012.

[27] W. C. Wu, C. P. Shih, R. Lien et al., "Serum vascular endothelial growth factor after bevacizumab or ranibizumab treatment for retinopathy of prematurity," *Retina*, vol. 37, no. 4, pp. 694–701, 2017.

15

Effect of Hyaluronic Acid/Trehalose in Two Different Formulations on Signs and Symptoms in Patients with Moderate to Severe Dry Eye Disease

Klemens Fondi,[1] **Piotr A. Wozniak**,[1,2] **Doreen Schmidl**,[1] **Ahmed M. Bata**,[1] **Katarzyna J. Witkowska**,[1] **Alina Popa-Cherecheanu**,[3,4] **Leopold Schmetterer**,[1,5,6,7,8] **and Gerhard Garhöfer**[1]

[1]*Department of Clinical Pharmacology, Medical University of Vienna, Vienna, Austria*
[2]*Department of Ophthalmology, Medical University of Warsaw, Warsaw, Poland*
[3]*Carol Davila University of Medicine and Pharmacy, Bucharest, Romania*
[4]*Department of Ophthalmology, Emergency University Hospital, Bucharest, Romania*
[5]*Center for Medical Physics and Biomedical Engineering, Medical University of Vienna, Vienna, Austria*
[6]*Singapore Eye Research Institute, Singapore National Eye Centre, Singapore*
[7]*Lee Kong Chian School of Medicine, Nanyang Technological University, 59 Nanyang Drive, Singapore 637459*
[8]*Visual Science Academic Clinical Programme, Duke-NUS, Singapore*

Correspondence should be addressed to Gerhard Garhöfer; gerhard.garhoefer@meduniwien.ac.at

Academic Editor: Maurizio Uva

Purpose. This randomized, observer-masked, crossover study investigated the effect of two hyaluronic acid/trehalose-based containing formulations, with different physical properties, on the signs and symptoms in patients with moderate to severe dry eye disease (DED). *Methods.* In one group, patients received a mixture of sodium hyaluronate and trehalose (HT, Thealoz Duo®) for use during the day. In the other group, patients received a more viscous formulation consisting of hyaluronic acid, trehalose, and carbomer (HTC-gel, Thealoz Duo Gel) to use pro re nata. Both groups used HTC-gel before going to bed. Clinical standard tests for DED were performed at the beginning and end of each one-week period. Further, patient satisfaction including quality of sleep was assessed using a visual analogue scale. *Results.* Corneal fluorescein and conjunctival lissamine green staining scores decreased, and tear breakup time (BUT) increased for both groups ($p < 0.001$ each). Mean instillation frequency was 3.1 ± 2.6 drops/day when using HT and 1.9 ± 2.2 drops/day when using HTC-gel ($p = 0.02$). A significant improvement in the quality of sleep was observed with both treatments ($p = 0.01$). *Conclusions.* Our results show improvement in signs and symptoms of DED in both groups. While instillation of HTC-gel resulted in a lower instillation frequency, both formulations of trehalose showed good clinical efficacy. This trial is registered with NCT02980913.

1. Introduction

Dry eye disease (DED) is a frequent ocular disorder occurring especially in the elderly [1]. DED affects both the tears and the ocular surface and may produce symptoms that range from slight ocular discomfort up to a considerable reduction of quality of life caused by corneal damage, decreased vision, and pain [2, 3]. Although in recent years important progress has been made in the understanding of DED and its pathogenesis, tear supplementation is still a mainstay of therapy for DED.

Most tear supplements function as topical lubricants and are therefore designed to moisten the ocular surface. This is achieved by complex formulations, including a large variety of surfactants, emulsifiers, and electrolytes, which differ considerably between products [4–6]. Recently, trehalose, a potent osmo- and bioprotectant [6, 7], and castor oil [8, 9] have been introduced to tear supplements to exert biological effects beyond lubrication.

One major determinant of clinical efficacy, along with patient compliance, is the residency time of the topical lubricant therapy on the ocular surface. A short ocular residency time requires frequent instillation of the product [7, 10], which in turn limits patient compliance and quality of life. In principle, this can be overcome by increasing the viscosity of the lubricant formulation. This has been confirmed by a variety of studies showing that higher viscosity of the formulation is related to a longer ocular residence time [11–13]. Although this may lead to a better lubrication of the ocular surface, administration of gel-based topical lubricants is not well tolerated by all patients, because it may impact quality of vision. Thus, some treatment regimens use gels mainly as an evening therapy. Evidence from clinical studies regarding the effect of different administration schemes for high-viscous eye drops is, however, sparse.

Although a large number of different topical lubricants are currently approved and used in clinical routine, not much information is available on the clinical effect of different treatment schemes according to the formulation. The current study was designed to investigate the clinical effect of a new topical treatment with a lachrymal substitute gel, containing trehalose, hyaluronic acid, and carbomer (Thealoz Duo Gel, HTC-gel), compared to the use of artificial tears containing trehalose and hyaluronic acid (Thealoz Duo, HT) during the day. Both groups used the gel formulation before going to sleep. As a secondary aim, the effect of therapy on sleep-related parameters, daily work, and impact on daily activities was assessed. Further, the voluntary instillation frequency of the two different treatment schemes was also recorded.

2. Materials and Methods

2.1. Subjects. The study was performed in accordance with the Declaration of Helsinki and the Good Clinical Practice (GCP) guidelines of the European Union. The study protocol was approved by the Ethics Committee of the Medical University of Vienna. Forty male and female patients with moderate to severe DED were included according to the inclusion/exclusion criteria outlined below. All subjects gave written informed consent after detailed personal explanation.

Participating subjects underwent a prestudy screening, which was carried out within the 2 weeks before the first study day. The screening examination included a medical history for general and ocular conditions (including duration of DED), pregnancy test in women with childbearing potential, subjective assessment of symptoms of DED using the Ocular Surface Disease Index (OSDI) questionnaire, ophthalmic examination including visual acuity using the ETDRS acuity charts, slit-lamp biomicroscopy and indirect funduscopy, measurement of breakup time (BUT), Schirmer I test, and measurement of intraocular pressure (IOP).

Patients with moderate to severe dry eye disease were included based on the following criteria: OSDI $\geq$ 22 and BUT $\leq$ 10 s or Schirmer I test between 2 mm and 5 mm. Further inclusion criteria were age of at least 18 years, normal ophthalmic findings except DED, ametropia <6 diopters, and a history of DED for at least 3 months. The eye with the lower BUT was chosen as the study eye. If BUT was identical for both eyes, the eye with the lower Schirmer I test was chosen. If Schirmer I test results were also identical for both eyes, the right eye was used for study purposes.

The following exclusion criteria were defined for the present study: treatment with any ophthalmic drug except topical lubricants, intake of systemic NSAIDS, immunosuppressants, corticosteroids, or any medication which could affect lachrymal function (e.g., antidepressants, anxiolytics, neuroleptics, antihistamines, cholinergics, antimuscarines, phenothiazin, and beta-blockers). Further exclusion criteria were ocular surgery in the month preceding the study, known hypersensitivity to one of the administered products, pregnancy, planned pregnancy or lactating, participation in a clinical trial in the four weeks preceding the study, symptoms of a clinically relevant illness in the two weeks before the first study day, presence or a history of a severe medical condition as judged by the clinical investigator, and wearing of contact lenses.

2.2. Treatment Regimen. The following treatments were compared: one group received sodium hyaluronate/trehalose-based eye drops (HT, Thealoz Duo Eye Drops; Laboratoires Thea, France) instilled pro re nata (PRN) during the day for one week. The second treatment group received a sodium hyaluronate/trehalose/carbomer gel (HTC-gel, Thealoz Duo Gel, Laboratoires Thea, France) again instilled PRN for one week. Both treatment groups were asked to instill the HTC-gel at night time before going to sleep. After the first treatment period, the patients crossed over to the alternative treatment.

2.3. Study Design and Experimental Paradigm. The present study was performed in a randomized, observer-masked two-way crossover design. Forty patients with moderate to severe DED who matched the in/exclusion criteria described above were included in the study. A schematic drawing explaining the study design is given in Figure 1.

Before the first randomization period, a 7-day washout period was scheduled. During this period, patients were handed out eye drops containing hyaluronic acid (Hyabak®, Laboratoires Thea, France) to use until three days before the start of the study. Thereafter, patients used saline eye drops (Hydrabak, Laboratoires Thea, France) until the first study day. Patients were asked to stop all topical lubricants 12 hours before the first study day. In addition, patients were handed out a diary to document instillation frequencies and times.

After the 7-day washout period, patients were randomized to receive either HT or HTC-gel for one week. Both groups used HTC-gel before going to sleep. After another washout period for 1 week, patients crossed over to the alternative treatment for one week.

During the study, patients were instructed to record instillation frequencies in a diary. In addition, clinical standard tests for DED, such as measurement of breakup time (BUT), corneal fluorescein, and conjunctival lissamine green staining, Schirmer I test, and completion of the Ocular Surface Disease Index (OSDI) questionnaire were performed at the beginning and end of each crossover period.

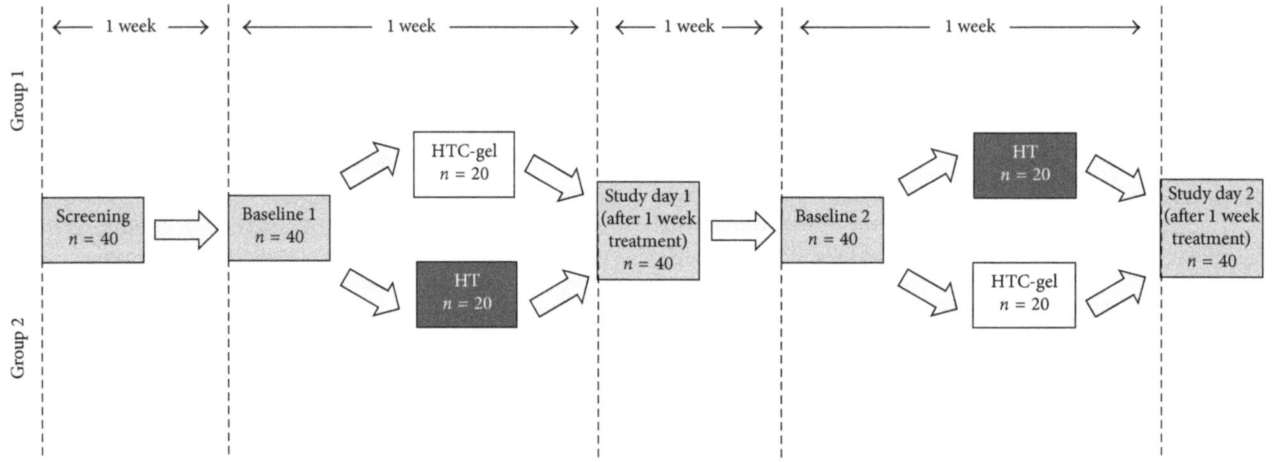

FIGURE 1: Randomization process and study design.

3. Methods

3.1. Breakup Time. Tear breakup time was measured following the guidelines described in the report of the TFOS International Dry Eye Workshop [14]. Five microliters of Minims-Fluorescein Sodium 2.0% eye drops was applied in the conjunctival sac of the eye, and the patients were instructed to blink naturally to distribute the fluorescein. The patients were asked to stare straight ahead without blinking, until told otherwise. By means of a stopwatch, the time between last complete blink and first appearance of a dry spot was recorded. The slit-lamp magnification was set at 10x, the background illumination intensity was kept constant (cobalt blue light), and a yellow filter was used to enhance observation of the tear film over the entire cornea. The mean value of three consecutive measurements was used for analysis.

3.2. Corneal Fluorescein Staining. Minims-Fluorescein Sodium 2.0% eye drops were used to detect corneal epithelial defects using cobalt blue light and a yellow filter. As a grading scale for corneal damage, the NEI/Industry Workshop guidelines were used [15]. The cornea was divided into five sectors (central, superior, inferior, nasal, and temporal), each of which was scored on a scale of 0–3, with 0 meaning no staining and 3 meaning maximum staining, with a maximal overall score of 15 (Figure 2).

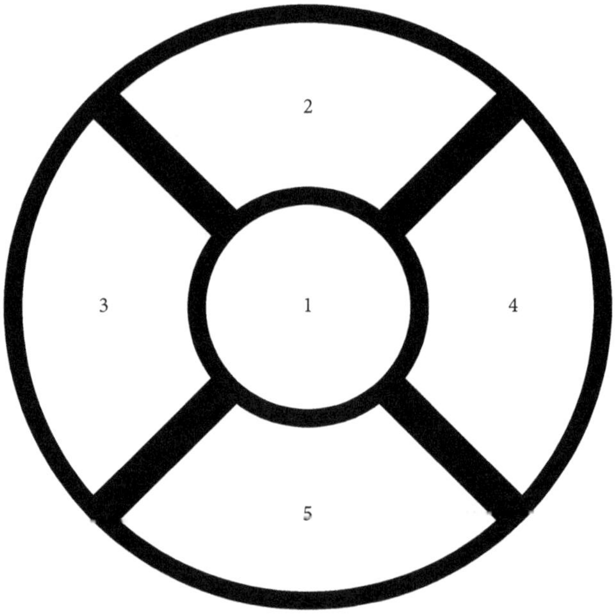

FIGURE 2: Divisions of the cornea according to the NEI/Industry Workshop guidelines [15].

3.3. Conjunctival Staining with Lissamine Green. Lissamine green (LG, EasyOpht, Italy) was used to detect conjunctival defects. Before placing the strip in the lower fornix of the eye, a drop of sterile saline was added to the strip. As grading scale for conjunctival damage, the NEI/Industry Workshop guidelines were used [15]. Both nasally and temporally, the conjunctiva was divided into a superior paralimbal area, an inferior paralimbal area, and a peripheral area with a grading scale of 0–3, with 0 meaning no staining and 3 meaning maximum staining, with a maximal score of 9 for the nasal and temporal conjunctiva, respectively.

3.4. Schirmer I Test. Schirmer I test without anesthesia was performed following the guidelines published in the report of the TFOS International Dry Eye Workshop [14]. Schirmer paper strips were inserted in the eye over the lower lid margin, midway between the middle and outer third. The patient was asked to close the eye, and after 5 minutes, the wetting of the Schirmer paper was measured.

3.5. Intraocular Pressure. Intraocular pressure (IOP) was measured with a slit-lamp mounted Goldmann applanation tonometer. Before each measurement, one drop of oxybuprocaine hydrochloride (4.0 mg/mL) combined with sodium fluorescein (0.8 mg/mL) was used for local anesthesia.

3.6. Ocular Surface Disease Index (OSDI). Symptoms of dry eye were assessed using the OSDI. The questionnaire underlying the OSDI is specifically designed for patients with DED and asks patients about the frequency of specific

Table 1: Changes in clinical signs and symptoms after 1 week treatment with either a gel containing hyaluronic acid, trehalose, and carbomer (HTC-gel) or eye drops containing hyaluronic acid (HT) PRN.

	HTC-gel		HT		
	Baseline	After 1-week treatment	Baseline	After 1-week treatment	p value (time effect, ANOVA)
Breakup time (s)	3.5 ± 1.7	4.2 ± 1.7	3.4 ± 1.4	4.3 ± 1.9	<0.001
Corneal fluorescein staining (0–15)	3.5 ± 2.3	2.7 ± 2.1	3.1 ± 1.7	2.2 ± 1.4	<0.001
Conjunctival lissamine green staining (0–18)	4.5 ± 2.8	3.5 ± 2.6	4.4 ± 2.5	2.8 ± 2.3	<0.001
Schirmer test I (mm)	11.6 ± 9.6	11.0 ± 9.2	12.2 ± 10.6	13.0 ± 10.4	0.88
Ocular surface disease index (OSDI, 0–100)	37.3 ± 21.4	36.1 ± 21.5	37.3 ± 19.9	33.4 ± 20.2	0.06

symptoms and their impact on vision-related functioning. Results are reported on a scale from 0 to 100, whereas "0" means no symptoms of DED.

3.7. Patient's Satisfaction and Questionnaires. Patient satisfaction scores were determined using a 100 mm VAS on which 0 means no symptoms and 100 means the worst possible discomfort. Patients were asked to mark the 100 mm line at the corresponding value on the VAS. The following parameters were assessed using VAS: patient satisfaction when awakening, feeling of swollen eyelid when awakening, ocular comfort during the night, and quality of sleep.

The effect of therapy on daily work and impact on daily activities was assessed using a 4-grade scale (0 = absent, 1 = present but not disturbing, 2 = disturbing but not interfering with daily life, and 3 = very distressing and interfering with daily activities).

3.8. Data Analysis. Statistical analysis was done "per protocol." To detect differences between the two treatment groups, a repeated measures ANOVA model was applied. Planned comparisons within the ANOVA model were performed to assess differences in clinical signs, subjective parameters, and instillation frequency between time points and groups. A p level of 0.05 or less was considered significant. Baseline values were reported using descriptive results (frequencies and percentages or mean and standard deviation). To detect differences in variables that were based on a 4-point scale, Kruskal–Wallis ANOVA was used. All statistical analyses were carried out using CSS Statistica (Version 6.0, Tulsa, Oklahoma, US).

4. Results

A total of 45 patients with dry eye disease aged between 20 and 72 years were included, of which 40 completed the study according to the protocol (age: 43.7 ± 12.3 years, mean ± SD). Of those participants, 12 patients were male and 28 patients were female. Two patients had to be excluded because they took prohibited medication, 1 patient withdrew consent and 2 patients were lost to follow up. The mean duration of DED in the whole study group was 6.9 ± 6.1 years. Mean OSDI score at screening was 51.8 ± 15.5.

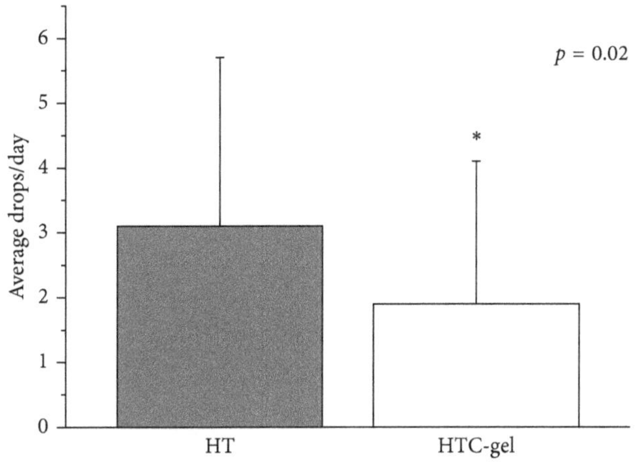

Figure 3: Difference in the frequency of use when using a gel containing hyaluronic acid, trehalose, and carbomer (HTC-gel) PRN compared to using eye drops containing hyaluronic acid and trehalose (HT) PRN.

After one week of treatment, BUT significantly increased and corneal fluorescein staining score significantly decreased ($p < 0.001$ each) in both study groups. In addition, a significant decrease in lissamine green staining scores was observed in both groups after one week of treatment ($p < 0.001$). In both groups, OSDI tended to decrease after one week of treatment ($p = 0.06$). No significant changes in Schirmer I test scores were observed ($p = 0.88$). Absolute values for these parameters are shown in Table 1.

During HT treatment, the frequency of instillation was 3.2 ± 2.6 times per day. When treated with HTC-gel, the frequency of instillation was significantly lower (1.9 ± 2.2 times per day, $p = 0.02$) compared to the HT treatment (Figure 3).

When looking at the VAS scores, a significant improvement in the quality of sleep was observed with both treatment regimens ($p = 0.01$, Table 2, Figure 4). For the other parameters evaluated, no significant changes occurred, although a tendency towards improvement in mean VAS scores for all parameters taken together was observed (Table 2).

The Kruskal–Wallis ANOVA revealed no differences in terms of changes of the impact on work and daily activities between the two study groups. This was also true after one week of treatment in either of the two groups (data not

Table 2: Changes in the visual analogue scale (VAS) for each question after 1 week treatment with either a gel containing hyaluronic acid, trehalose, and carbomer (HTC-gel) or eye drops containing hyaluronic acid (HT) PRN.

	Baseline	Study day	p value (time effect, ANOVA)	p value (between groups)
	"What is your global satisfaction concerning your eyes when awakening in the morning?"			
HT	26.9 ± 22.5	25.0 ± 22.8	0.48	0.59
HTC-gel	27.1 ± 26.0	26.8 ± 25.1		
	Feeling of swollen eyelid when awakening			
HT	23.9 ± 23.8	21.9 ± 24.5	0.68	0.38
HTC-gel	24.9 ± 25.5	25.6 ± 25.2		
	Subjective evaluation of ocular comfort during the night			
HT	25.7 ± 23.1	26.2 ± 24.2	0.56	0.36
HTC-gel	27.0 ± 25.0	24.9 ± 23.3		
	Quality of sleep			
HT	29.8 ± 30.6	23.9 ± 26.4	**0.01**	0.87
HTC-gel	30.7 ± 29.8	25.5 ± 29.1		
	Mean VAS score			
HT	26.7 ± 21.3	23.7 ± 20.7	0.08	0.67
HTC-gel	27.5 ± 23.6	25.7 ± 22.5		

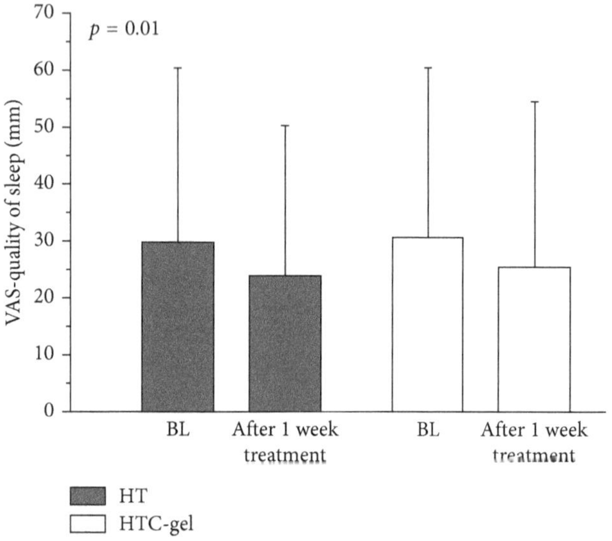

Figure 4: Patients' quality of sleep on the VAS at baseline and after one-week treatment with a gel containing hyaluronic acid, trehalose, and carbomer (HTC-gel) PRN compared to using eye drops containing hyaluronic acid and trehalose (HT) PRN.

shown). No changes in IOP or visual acuity were observed during the course of the study (data not shown).

5. Discussion

The data of the current study indicate that treatment with Thealoz Duo Gel alone or with Thealoz Duo eye drops combined with the gel before going to bed, led to a comparable improvement in BUT, corneal fluorescein, and conjunctival lissamine green staining scores. Both treatment regimens also significantly improved patients' quality of sleep. Further, the use of eye drops with higher viscosity during daytime was associated with a lower instillation frequency compared to the combination of the less viscous formulation during the day and the lubricant gel at night.

Modern tear replacement therapies are usually based on complex formulations consisting of different chemical components such as cellulose derivates, polyacrylic acid, or hyaluronic acid. Although the latter components exert good lubricant effects, new topical DED therapies also include agents that exert effects beyond wetting of the ocular surface, in particular, small organic molecules such as trehalose, L-carnitine, or some polyols such as erythritol [6, 16]. There is increasing evidence now that these osmoprotectants directly protect cells against hyperosmolarity, which is one of the main causes of cell death and inflammation in DED [6].

However, despite many efforts, there is currently no gold standard for the topical therapy for DED. A common problem and an important limitation in the treatment with topical lubricants is that the association between clinical effects and different treatment schemes is only insufficiently described [7, 10]. In particular, data from clinical trials regarding the influence of viscosity on instillation frequency and clinical efficacy are sparse.

The data of the current study indicate that both treatment regimens led to a comparable improvement in clinical signs of DED. It is worth noting that this improvement in clinical variables was observed even after a short-time treatment of one week. In particular, BUT, corneal fluorescein, and conjunctival lissamine green staining scores were significantly improved in both groups to a similar degree. This indicates that a strong beneficial effect on clinical signs is present with both treatment regimens, and that the treatment scheme may be adapted to the patients' preference.

A significant improvement in patient's quality of sleep was observed with both treatment regimens. This is of special importance since several studies have reported that poor sleep quality is associated with DED and the severity of symptoms [17, 18]. Further, patients' symptoms, as measured in this study using the OSDI score, showed a tendency towards improvements in both groups, but this effect did not reach the level of significance. Again, no significant difference was observed between the two treatment groups, indicating that although the HTC-gel treatment requires less frequent instillation, the patient-related benefit seems to be comparable.

Furthermore, our results show that the instillation frequency is significantly lower when patients were using HTC-gel during the day in comparison to the less viscous HT formulation. It is reasonable to suggest that the reason for this finding is related to the physical properties of the two formulations under the study. The HTC-gel used in the current trial contains a carbomer component in addition to hyaluronic acid/trehalose, which are the main components of the HT formulation. It has been hypothesized that carbomer comprising gels significantly extend the contact time of solutes or suspended solids with the corneal surface [19]. Therefore, it can be expected that using a HTC-gel formulation will lead to a less frequent instillation frequency, which is also reflected in the data of the current study.

The physical properties of the HT combination may well explain the lack of clinical difference between the two formulations, although the treatment frequency was higher in the HT group. Although the HT formulation does not contain a high-viscous component, it shows a long residency time on the ocular surface. In particular, it has been shown in a previous study that eye drops containing trehalose and hyaluronic acid, that were also used in the present study, increase tear film thickness as measured with a ultrahigh resolution optical coherence tomography system for as long as 240 minutes, indicating long corneal residence time [20].

In the current study, we have used a two-way crossover design, which is usually considered the gold standard in clinical trials. However, one prerequisite for this study design is that patients start on the same severity level at the beginning of both treatment periods and that no overhang effect of the treatment is present. This was achieved by a 7-day washout period, which was scheduled before start of each treatment period. Furthermore, the washout allows the study to detect effects largely independent from the previous treatments, which is also been previously described as a beneficial way to improve the clinical trial design in DED [21]. It has, however, to be noted that a washout period with saline may, in principle, influence tear film stability and impact the ocular surface. To minimize this effect, only in the last 3 of 7 days, saline solution was used whereas patients received hyaluronic acid for the other days.

Further, no active control or placebo group was included in the study. However, one of the strengths of a crossover design is that each subject receives all treatments and therefore acts as its own control, which considerably reduces confounding covariates. Given that the main aim of this study was to compare the two different treatment regimens, we do not assume that it limits the conclusions of the study.

Finally, our study indicates that the safety profile of both treatment regimens was excellent. No change in any of the safety parameters was observed, and adverse events that occurred during the course of the study were mild. This is also reflected in the VAS scores of patients' satisfaction that showed a trend towards improvement.

Some limitations need to be considered when interpreting the results of our study. First, for feasibility reasons, the treatment time was limited to one week before patients crossed over to the alternative treatment. Thus, it cannot be fully excluded that the limited observation period was not sufficient to detect differences in clinical parameters between the two treatment regimens. This is also reflected in the clinical parameters, such as staining and BUT. Although both variables show a statistical significant improvement, longer studies are needed to assess the full clinical effect of the treatments.

Furthermore, the sample size of the current study was limited to 40 patients. Although the crossover design used in the current study is considered to be the gold standard for clinical studies because every patient acts as his/her own control, which provides additional power in comparison to parallel group studies, a larger sample size with longer observation periods may be necessary to detect subtle differences in signs and symptoms.

6. Conclusions

In conclusion, the data of the current study showed that both formulations containing trehalose and hyaluronic acid induced a significant improvement in BUT, corneal fluorescein, and conjunctival lissamine green staining scores and patient's quality of sleep after 1 week of use. Further, although the instillation frequency was lower when using the HTC-gel formulation compared to the more liquid HT eye drops, no statistical difference was found between the two treatment regimens regarding the improvement of clinical measures and symptoms of DED. Therefore, both trehalose-based treatment schemes are effective in patients with DED and can be adapted according to patient's preferences regarding the formulation.

Conflicts of Interest

The authors declare that there are no conflicts of interest regarding the publication of this paper.

Acknowledgments

The present study was sponsored by Laboratoires Thea, Clermont Ferrand, France.

References

[1] F. Stapleton, M. Alves, V. Y. Bunya et al., "TFOS DEWS II epidemiology report," *Ocular Surface*, vol. 15, no. 3, pp. 334–365, 2017.

[2] Q. Le, X. Zhou, L. Ge, L. Wu, J. Hong, and J. Xu, "Impact of dry eye syndrome on vision-related quality of life in a non-clinic-based general population," *BMC Ophthalmology*, vol. 12, no. 1, p. 22, 2012.

[3] Y. Mizuno, M. Yamada, Y. Miyake, and Dry Eye Survey Group of the National Hospital Organization of Japan,

"Association between clinical diagnostic tests and health-related quality of life surveys in patients with dry eye syndrome," *Japanese Journal of Ophthalmology*, vol. 54, no. 4, pp. 259–265, 2010.

[4] E. M. Messmer, "Osmoprotection as a new therapeutic principle," *Ophthalmologe*, vol. 104, no. 11, pp. 987–990, 2007.

[5] G. N. Foulks, "Pharmacological management of dry eye in the elderly patient," *Drugs and Aging*, vol. 25, no. 2, pp. 105–118, 2008.

[6] C. Baudouin, P. Aragona, E. M. Messmer et al., "Role of hyperosmolarity in the pathogenesis and management of dry eye disease: proceedings of the OCEAN group meeting," *Ocular Surface*, vol. 11, no. 4, pp. 246–258, 2013.

[7] L. Jones, L. E. Downie, D. Korb et al., "TFOS DEWS II management and therapy report," *Ocular Surface*, vol. 15, no. 3, pp. 575–628, 2017.

[8] T. Hasegawa, H. Amako, T. Yamamoto, M. Tazawa, and Y. Sakamoto, "Corneal-protective effects of an artificial tear containing sodium hyaluronate and castor oil on a porcine short-term dry eye model," *Journal of Veterinary Medical Science*, vol. 76, no. 9, pp. 1219–1224, 2014.

[9] C. Maissa, M. Guillon, P. Simmons, and J. Vehige, "Effect of castor oil emulsion eyedrops on tear film composition and stability," *Contact Lens and Anterior Eye*, vol. 33, no. 2, pp. 76–82, 2010.

[10] M. E. Johnson, P. J. Murphy, and M. Boulton, "Carbomer and sodium hyaluronate eyedrops for moderate dry eye treatment," *Optometry and Vision Science*, vol. 85, no. 8, pp. 750–757, 2008.

[11] J. R. Paugh, A. L. Nguyen, H. A. Ketelson, M. T. Christensen, and D. L. Meadows, "Precorneal residence time of artificial tears measured in dry eye subjects," *Optometry and Vision Science*, vol. 85, no. 8, pp. 725–731, 2008.

[12] H. Zhu and A. Chauhan, "Effect of viscosity on tear drainage and ocular residence time," *Optometry and Vision Science*, vol. 85, no. 8, pp. E715–E725, 2008.

[13] S. Bandlitz, C. Purslow, P. J. Murphy, and H. Pult, "Time course of changes in tear meniscus radius and blink rate after instillation of artificial tears," *Investigative Ophthalmology and Visual Science*, vol. 55, no. 9, pp. 5842–5847, 2014.

[14] DEWS, "Methodologies to diagnose and monitor dry eye disease: report of the Diagnostic Methodology Subcommittee of the International Dry Eye Workshop (2007)," *Ocular Surface*, vol. 5, no. 2, pp. 108–152, 2007.

[15] M. A. Lemp, "Report of the National Eye Institute/Industry Workshop on clinical trials in dry eyes," *CLAO Journal*, vol. 21, no. 4, pp. 221–232, 1995.

[16] G. R. Snibson, J. L. Greaves, N. D. Soper, J. M. Tiffany, C. G. Wilson, and A. J. Bron, "Ocular surface residence times of artificial tear solutions," *Cornea*, vol. 11, no. 4, pp. 288–293, 1992.

[17] M. Ayaki, M. Kawashima, K. Negishi, T. Kishimoto, M. Mimura, and K. Tsubota, "Sleep and mood disorders in dry eye disease and allied irritating ocular diseases," *Scientific Reports*, vol. 6, no. 1, article 22480, 2016.

[18] M. Kawashima, M. Uchino, N. Yokoi et al., "The association of sleep quality with dry eye disease: the Osaka study," *Clinical Ophthalmology*, vol. 10, pp. 1015–1021, 2016.

[19] C. G. Wilson, Y. P. Zhu, M. Frier, L. S. Rao, P. Gilchrist, and A. C. Perkins, "Ocular contact time of a carbomer gel (GelTears) in humans," *British Journal of Ophthalmology*, vol. 82, no. 10, pp. 1131–1134, 1998.

[20] D. Schmidl, L. Schmetterer, K. J. Witkowska et al., "Tear film thickness after treatment with artificial tears in patients with moderate dry eye disease," *Cornea*, vol. 34, no. 4, pp. 421–426, 2015.

[21] G. D. Novack, P. Asbell, S. Barabino et al., "TFOS DEWS II clinical trial design report," *Ocular Surface*, vol. 15, no. 3, pp. 629–649, 2017.

16

A Comparative Study of Characteristics and Outcomes of Patients with Proved and Suggested Sarcoid Uveitis Occurring after Ophthalmic Procedure

Yvan Jamilloux[1] **Aude Taleb,**[1,2] **Audrey De Parisot,**[1] **Laurent Pérard,**[3] **Carole Burillon,**[4] **Christiane Broussolle,**[1] **Laurent Kodjikian**[2] **and Pascal Sève**[1]

[1]*Department of Internal Medicine, Hôpital de la Croix Rousse, Hospices Civils de Lyon, Université Claude Bernard Lyon 1, Lyon, France*
[2]*Department of Ophthalmology, Hôpital de la Croix Rousse, Hospices Civils de Lyon, Université Claude Bernard Lyon 1, Lyon, France*
[3]*Department of Internal Medicine, Hôpital Edouard Herriot, Hospices Civils de Lyon, Université Claude Bernard Lyon 1, Lyon, France*
[4]*Department of Ophthalmology, Hôpital Edouard Herriot, Hospices Civils de Lyon, Université Claude Bernard Lyon 1, Lyon, France*

Correspondence should be addressed to Yvan Jamilloux; yvanjamilloux@hotmail.com

Academic Editor: Hamid Ahmadieh

Purpose. To describe patients with new onset sarcoid uveitis occurring after an ophthalmic procedure and compare them with patients with sarcoid uveitis without ocular procedure. *Methods.* Retrospective analysis of case records from patients with post-ophthalmic procedure sarcoid uveitis seen at our institution between April 2004 and October 2016. Patients with a previous history of uveitis were not included. Each patient was randomly matched with four controls from our incident cohort of new onset sarcoid uveitis without ophthalmic procedure. *Results.* We identified 11 patients (8.5%) from our incident cohort of sarcoid uveitis (n = 130), who were all women, with a postophthalmic procedure uveitis (mostly after cataract surgery (36%)). These patients were older (69.7 vs 52.7 years) and presented more synechiae than controls. After a mean follow-up of 30 (3–60) months, there was no significant difference between the postprocedure and the control group with regard to demography, clinical presentation, disease course, treatment, and outcome. *Conclusions.* Sarcoid uveitis has similar characteristics in patients with new onset sarcoid uveitis after or without ophthalmic procedure. As a consequence, ophthalmic intervention should be seen as a potential trigger of latent sarcoidosis.

1. Introduction

Ocular surgery may be responsible for new onset uveitis as a part of postcataract surgical inflammation [1]. Other types of chronic inflammation (defined by a duration >6 weeks) can occur after an ocular surgery: endophthalmitis [2] (the most severe), or Irvine–Gass syndrome (the most frequent) [3] or sympathetic ophthalmia [4]. Other acute inflammatory reactions (duration <6 weeks) can occur after ophthalmic procedure, such as phacoantigenic uveitis, toxic anterior segment [5] syndrome, or toxic endothelial cell destruction [6].

Sarcoidosis is a systemic inflammatory disorder of unknown etiology, characterized by noncaseating epithelioid-cell granulomas, which primarily affects the lungs and the lymphatics. The spectrum of ocular manifestations is wide and highly variable; almost any part of the eye and other orbital structures can be affected [7, 8]. Ocular involvement may coexist with symptomatic or asymptomatic systemic disease manifestations, but may precede systemic involvement by several years [7, 8]. In retrospective series of biopsy-proven sarcoidosis, symptomatic uveitis affects 20–50% of patients [8], with 80% of these cases being diagnosed within the first year, of which 30% have uveitis as a presenting manifestation [7]. Uveitis is the most frequent ocular manifestation and may affect up to 20–30% of sarcoidosis patients [1].

Because patients can present with new onset sarcoid uveitis occurring after an ophthalmic procedure, we aimed at describing such cases and comparing them with patients with sarcoid uveitis without ocular procedure.

2. Patients and Methods

2.1. Patients. Case records of patients who were seen at one of the two departments of Internal Medicine and at one of the two departments of Ophthalmology of the Lyon University Hospitals between April 2004 and October 2016 were analyzed retrospectively.

Patients were included if

(i) uveitis occurred no more than one year after ophthalmic procedure;

(ii) a biopsy analysis showed noncaseating granuloma or if patient met the Abad's modified criteria [9, 10]. According to these criteria, patients had *presumed* sarcoidosis if they had at least two of the following four criteria: typical changes on a chest radiograph or chest computed tomography (CT), predominantly CD4 lymphocytosis on bronchoalveolar lavage (BAL) fluid analysis, elevated serum angiotensin converting enzyme (ACE) levels, or a high gallium or 18F-labelled deoxyglucose positron emission tomography (^{18}FDG-PET) uptake. If only one criterion was fulfilled, it was considered as a *possible* sarcoidosis.

Patients with a previous history of uveitis, those who had uveitis before ocular procedure, and those with other possible causes of uveitis (including endophthalmitis [2] and Irvine–Gass syndrome [11] with isolated macular edema on OCT and/or on fluorescein angiogram without any other inflammatory signs such as vitritis and vasculitis) were not included.

2.2. Control Group. Patients with postophthalmic procedure uveitis were compared with control subjects presenting sarcoid uveitis but no history of ophthalmic procedure. Patients in the control group were randomly selected using a computerized algorithm among the 130 incident cases of sarcoid uveitis recorded in the Lyon University Hospitals. Each patient with postophthalmic procedure sarcoid uveitis was matched with 4 controls.

2.3. Ethical Statement. The institutional review board of the *Hospices Civils de Lyon* gave its approval to retrospectively review the records. According to the French law (no. 2004-806, August 9, 2004) and because the data were collected retrospectively and patient management was not modified, this study did not require further research ethics committee approval.

2.4. Data Collection. Clinical and laboratory data were collected and analyzed using a standardized form: medical history, presenting symptoms, ophthalmic and systemic manifestations, sites of tissue biopsies, C-reactive protein (CRP), blood lymphocytes count, liver tests, calcemia, and serum ACE at diagnosis. Chest X-rays were rated according to the Scadding criteria. Results of other imaging findings (including chest CT), pulmonary function tests, bronchoscopies with BAL, cardiac investigations, detailed medical treatments, and disease outcome were also recorded when available.

2.5. Ophthalmic Examination. Ophthalmologic data, which included assessment of the best-corrected visual acuity (BCVA), intraocular pressure, complete biomicroscopic examination and optical coherence tomography (OCT), and fluorescein and indocyanine green angiographies, were collected at diagnosis and during follow-up by ophthalmologists. Uveitis was classified according to the Standardization of Uveitis Nomenclature (SUN) [12].

2.6. Statistical Analysis. Continuous variables were expressed as means (±standard deviation) and compared between groups using a Mann–Whitney test. Categorical variables were expressed as percentages and compared between groups with a Chi-square test or Fisher's exact test as appropriate. *P* values were considered significant when they were <0.05. Statistical analysis was performed with the R software (version 3.4.5, the R company).

3. Results

3.1. Case Reports. Detailed case reports are supplied in the Supplementary Materials (available here).

3.2. Global Characteristics of Patients. Among the 130 incident cases of sarcoid uveitis seen at our institution, we identified 11 patients (8.5%) who were diagnosed after an ophthalmic procedure. The patients' general characteristics are summarized in Table 1. All patients were women, with a mean age of 69 (27–88) years. Ocular procedures included cataract surgery ($n = 4$), YAG capsulotomy ($n = 2$), vitreoretinal surgery ($n = 2$), trabeculectomy ($n = 1$), vitreous injection ($n = 1$), and laser therapy ($n = 1$). No sign or sequelae of intraocular inflammation existed before ophthalmic procedure. The mean delay between the ophthalmic procedure and uveitis was 3.6 months (1–12 months).

Sarcoidosis was histologically proven in seven patients (minor salivary glands biopsy, $n = 2$; fine-needle aspiration of mediastinal nodes, $n = 2$; conjunctival nodule biopsy, $n = 2$; and gastric biopsy, $n = 1$).

Ophthalmologic findings consisted of chronic ($n = 10$), bilateral ($n = 6$), granulomatous ($n = 8$) uveitis involving the anterior segment ($n = 3$), the vitreous ($n = 1$), and the retina or choroid ($n = 1$), or a panuveitis ($n = 7$). One patient had elevated intraocular pressure. Five patients had unilateral uveitis, but only three had an ophthalmic procedure performed on the symptomatic eye. In our tertiary center, preoperative chest X-ray is not performed routinely for patients undergoing cataract surgery. Thoracic imaging

TABLE 1: Clinical, ophthalmic, radiologic, and histopathologic features of patients with postophthalmic procedure sarcoid uveitis.

Patient#	Sex	Age	Ophthalmic procedure	Timeline	Unilateral/OU	Anatomical form	Uveitis					
							Granulomatous	Vasculitis	Choroiditis	Edema	Systemic involvement	Sarcoidosis diagnosis
1	F	69	Cataract	1	OU	Pan	+	–	–	Macular		MSG, bronchial, gastric biopsies
2	F	76	Cataract	3 + 10	OU	Pan	–	–	–	Macular		*Negative*
3	F	82	Cataract	12	OU	Pan	+				Conjunctival nodule	Conjunctival nodule biopsy
4	F	31	Preretinal haemorrhage + macular hole	2	OU	Pan	+	+/+	–	ERM + papilledema		MSG biopsy
5	F	67	Glaucoma	5	OU	Pan	+EIOP	–	+	Macular	Sicca syndrome + conjunctival nodule weight loss	Gastric biopsy
6	F	81	Cataract	1	OU	A/I	+	–	–	Macular	Dyspnea	Positive ^{18}FDG-PET
7	F	69	Retinal detachment	8	Unilateral	Pan	+	Venous	+			Abad's criteria
8	F	88	Cataract + YAG capsulotomy	1	Unilateral	I/P	+	–	–	Macular	Cough	Bronchial biopsy
9	F	83	Intravitreal aflibercept	1	Unilateral	A	+	–	–			*Negative*
10	F	70	Membrane peeling	5	Unilateral	A					Cough	Lymph node fine needle aspiration
11	F	58	YAG capsulotomy	4	Unilateral	I/P	–	–	–	Macular papilledema	Conjunctival nodule	Conjunctival nodule biopsy

F = female, age in years, OU = both eyes, A = anterior, I = intermediate, P = posterior, Pan = panuveitis, EIOP = elevated intraocular pressure, ERM = epiretinal membrane, ADP = adenopathy, MSG = minor salivary glands, and ^{18}FDG-PET = ^{18}F-labelled deoxyglucose positron emission tomography.

performed at the time of diagnostic workup showed abnormalities suggestive of sarcoidosis in nine cases: chest X-ray ($n = 1/11$), chest CT scan ($n = 9/11$), and nuclear imaging ($n = 8/11$).

All patients had postoperative inflammation. Eight patients received topical steroids and six required a systemic treatment by steroids for a mean duration of 14 (0–30.4) months. Other therapies were needed in two patients (methotrexate and hydroxychloroquine). Among the five patients who still had a treatment at last visit, four were not symptomatic anymore. Treatments and visual prognoses are shown in Table 2.

3.3. Comparison of Postophthalmic Procedure Patients with Controls. Both groups were statistically similar in terms of gender, ethnicity, chest CT imaging results, and the other organs involvement. As a consequence of random matching, patients were older in the study group than in the control group. The prevalence of ophthalmic signs varied according to the group considered, with more synechiae and a trend for more granulomatous uveitis in the postprocedure group. Otherwise, there were no significant differences between groups with regard to the presence of an ocular hypertony, multifocal choroiditis, CSME, vasculitis, and papilledema. The groups were no different in terms of follow-up and in terms of recovery or treatment at the last visit (Table 3).

4. Discussion

To our knowledge, the present study is the first series of patients with postophthalmic procedure sarcoid uveitis and the first case-control series comparing these patients with patients without ocular intervention. In our tertiary center, postoperative sarcoid uveitis represents 8.5% of our sarcoid uveitis cohort.

New onset uveitis is one of the potential causes of postoperative inflammation occurring after a cataract surgery. This diagnosis is considered in patients with chronic postoperative inflammation, in which etiologies include chronic endophthalmitis and lens-related inflammation [7, 8]. Postoperative recurrence of uveitis in uveitic patients is a well-known complication [3, 13, 14]. Anterior chamber inflammation is also a potential side effect after a trabeculoplasty [15]. Anterior chamber inflammation may also be seen in 0.4–33.5% of patients after capsulotomy, but persistent vitritis is rare and no complication has been reported [16]. To avoid such bias, we excluded all patients with a previous history of uveitis and all patients had a fundus examination before eye procedures.

Sarcoidosis etiology remains unknown but several infectious agents have been postulated as triggering factors [17]. However, there is no definite evidence that sarcoidosis is an infectious disease; rather, sarcoidosis is considered as an exaggerated immune response to pathogen-associated molecular patterns of killed and/or partly degraded (myco) bacteria which persist within immune cells and resist degradation [17, 18]. For example, some patients have been reported as developing sarcoidosis after cardiac [19] or bone marrow transplantations [20, 21], suggesting the transmission of a potential activator of the disease. Therefore, we hypothesize that ophthalmic procedures may act as a trigger of (latent) sarcoidosis. The fact that systematic fundus examination was performed before eye procedures and did not detect signs of sarcoidosis, along with the occurrence of bilateral and contralateral sarcoid uveitis, reinforces such an hypothesis.

Our results show that ethnic distribution, laboratory features, treatment, and ophthalmologic outcome were similar in sarcoid uveitis patients after an ophthalmologic procedure or spontaneously. Nevertheless, postophthalmic procedure sarcoid uveitis seemed to affect more frequently women than men. This sex ratio in sarcoid uveitis has already been reported in other larger studies, yet not so predominantly [8, 22–24]. We also noticed an older age at onset in the postprocedure group. This can be due to the random matching of patients or because the number of patients who need an ocular procedure tends to increase over age. The number of Caucasian patients in our series was also higher than that in other European studies [24–26]. Finally, patients with postophthalmic procedure sarcoid uveitis had significantly more synechiae. This result was in line with a previous series of 281 biopsy-proven sarcoidosis patients, in which 20–26% had posterior synechiae [13]. Although Evans et al. have reported that two-thirds of sarcoid uveitis was not granulomatous, we noted more granulomatous precipitates in the postprocedure group than in the control group [25]. This suggests that surgery/procedure increases the intraocular inflammation, as this is the case in the well-known postsurgical Irvine–Gass uveitis [27, 28]. Drancourt et al. also reported the case of a postcataract surgery uveitis that led to the diagnosis of Whipple disease [29]. Therefore, we can imagine that the ocular procedure may act as a trigger of inflammation in patients with latent sarcoidosis. Two patients were affected bilaterally. There is no evident explanation, but we can relate this situation with the physiopathology of sympathetic ophthalmia. Sympathetic ophthalmia is a rare bilateral granulomatous uveitis due to trauma or surgery in one eye [30]. The etiology is not well elucidated but might be secondary to the development of an autoimmune reaction to ocular antigens exposed during the traumatic or surgical event with T cells as primary mediators [31]. The main hypothesis is an immune dysregulation with an autoimmune inflammatory response against ocular self-antigens. A similar mechanism of autoimmune dysfunction in sarcoidosis might explain bilateral uveitis in our two patients.

Chest imaging was suggestive of sarcoidosis in 12.5% of chest X-rays and 82% of chest CTs with no statistical difference between groups. These data support the results of previous series and suggest that chest CT should be performed in patients with negative chest X-rays while sarcoidosis is highly suspected [32–34].

Finally, our study has some limitations. It is difficult to establish precisely the delay between the procedure and the onset of uveitis. We chose a maximum delay of 12 months between the ocular procedure and the onset of symptoms since chronic postoperative endophthalmitis may appear insidiously several months after an ophthalmic procedure. The design of the study, with single center and retrospective

TABLE 2: Treatment of patients with postophthalmic procedure sarcoid uveitis.

Patient	Initial treatment	Outcome of sarcoidosis after initial treatment	Adverse effects of treatment	Subsequent treatment	Final outcome		Final visual acuity		Treatment at the end of follow-up	Follow-up duration (months)
					Ophthalmic outcome	Other manifestations	OR	OS		
1	Topical CS	CSME OS	No	Systemic CS	Atrophic MFC	Pulmonary nodules progression on CT scan	20/20	20/25	Systemic CS 5 mg/day	52
2	DXM intravitreal implant		No	Systemic CS	CSME		20/50	20/25	Systemic CS 1 mg/day	36
3	DXM intravitreal implant	CSME OR with vitreomacular traction	No	Pars plana vitrectomy with membrane peel	No CSME		0	20/200	No	3
4	Systemic CS 70 mg/day	Retinal vasculitis OU CSME papilledema	No	No	ERM, and no inflammation		20/20	20/25	Systemic CS 4 mg/day	37
5	Topical + systemic CS 20 mg/day		Osteopenia, skin fragility cushing-like syndrome, and CS dependency	No	Persistent bilateral KP, and no posterior inflammation		20/40	20/40	Topical CS	60
6	Topical + systemic CS 20 mg/day	Complete response several relapses: Vitritis OU	Cushing-like syndrome, osteopenia, skin fragility, and CS dependency	MTX	Anterior and intermediate inflammation	Pulmonary embolism	20/20	20/20	Systemic CS 9 mg/day + MTX 10 mg/week	53
7	Topical CS	Vitritis OR peripheral diffuse choroiditis atrophy	No	Systemic CS 40 mg	Vitritis OR persistent		—	—	Subconjunctival injections of triamcinolone	13
8	DXM intravitreal implant	Improvement of CSME	No	No	No inflammation		20/20	20/25	No	15
9	Topical CS	Complete response	No	No	No inflammation				No	19
10	Topical CS	Complete response	No	None	Papilledema	Chest pain	0	20/20	No	11
11	Topical CS	Complete response	No	Dexamethasone intravitreal implant	Recurrent CSME		20/50	20/25		40

CSME = Macular edema, OD = right eye, OS = left eye, OU = both eyes, MFC = multifocal choroiditis, ERM = epiretinal membrane, CT = computed tomography, MTX = methotrexate, and CS = corticosteroids.

Table 3: Comparison of postprocedure patients with control patients: demographic characteristics and ophthalmic, laboratory, and radiologic features.

	Patients with ocular surgery ($n = 11$)	Controls ($n = 44$)	P value
Median age at diagnosis (years)	69.7	52.7	**0.004**
Females	11	32	**0.05**
Ethnicity Cau/Afr/North-Afr/As	10/1/0/0	35/1/7/1	0.33
Ophthalmologic findings			
Unilateral/bilateral/unknown	5/6/0	11/32/1	0.42
Granulomatous	9	20	0.07
Synechiae	1	20	**0.05**
Elevated intraocular pressure	1	2	0.26
Retinal vasculitis	2	5	0.50
Macular edema	8	18	0.16
Papilledema	2	6	0.51
Multifocal choroiditis	3	14	0.999
Other ophthalmic features at diagnosis	3	5	0.33
Other systemic features at diagnosis	2	11	1
Other systemic features during course	0	6	0.22
Chest imaging			
X-ray staging I/II/III/IV (scadding)	7/1/3/0	23/17/3/1	0.08
Serum markers			
Elevated ACE	7	18	0.65
Elevated lysozyme	6	22	0.999
Treatment and outcome			
Topical steroids	8	35	0.27
Systemic steroids	6	25	0.27
Immunosuppressants	1	12	0.12
Evolution to remission	5	13	0.76

Cau = Caucasian, Afr = African, North-Afr = North African, As = Asian, and ACE = angiotensin-converting enzyme.

inclusions, is also an important limitation that will require further studies to confirm our findings.

5. Conclusions

We describe herein the first series of postophthalmic procedure sarcoid uveitis. The major message is that sarcoid uveitis has similar characteristics (demography, course, and outcome) in patients with or without ophthalmic procedure. As a consequence, ophthalmic intervention should be seen as a potential trigger of latent sarcoidosis, especially in older Caucasian females.

Conflicts of Interest

The authors declare that they have no conflicts of interest.

References

[1] N. Okhravi, H. M. A. Towler, and S. L. Lightman, "Cataract surgery in patients with uveitis," *Eye*, vol. 14, no. 5, pp. 689-690, 2000.

[2] Endophthalmitis Vitrectomy Study Group, "Results of the endophthalmitis vitrectomy study. A randomized trial of immediate vitrectomy and of intravenous antibiotics for the treatment of postoperative bacterial endophthalmitis," *Archives of Ophthalmology*, vol. 113, no. 12, pp. 1479–1496, 1995.

[3] S. R. Irvine, "A newly defined vitreous syndrome following cataract surgery," *American Journal of Ophthalmology*, vol. 36, no. 5, pp. 599–619, 1953.

[4] X. K. Chu and C.-C. Chan, "Sympathetic ophthalmia: to the twenty-first century and beyond," *Journal of Ophthalmic Inflammation and Infection*, vol. 3, no. 1, p. 49, 2013.

[5] M. C. Monson, N. Mamalis, and R. J. Olson, "Toxic anterior segment inflammation following cataract surgery," *Journal of Cataract & Refractive Surgery*, vol. 18, no. 2, pp. 184–189, 1992.

[6] A. C. Breebaart, R. M. Nuyts, E. Pels, H. F. Edelhauser, and F. D. Verbraak, "Toxic endothelial cell destruction of the cornea after routine extracapsular cataract surgery," *Archives of Ophthalmology*, vol. 108, no. 8, pp. 1121–1125, 1990.

[7] M. C. Iannuzzi, B. A. Rybicki, and A. S. Teirstein, "Sarcoidosis," *New England Journal of Medicine*, vol. 357, no. 21, pp. 2153–2165, 2007.

[8] G. Hillerdal, E. Nöu, K. Osterman, and B. Schmekel, "Sarcoidosis: epidemiology and prognosis. A 15-year European study," *American Review of Respiratory Disease Return*, vol. 130, no. 1, pp. 29–32, 1984.

[9] S. Abad, V. Meyssonier, J. Allali et al., "Association of peripheral multifocal choroiditis with sarcoidosis: a study of thirty-seven patients," *Arthritis Care & Research*, vol. 51, no. 6, pp. 974–982, 2004.

[10] Y. Jamilloux, L. Kodjikian, C. Broussolle, and P. Sève, "Sarcoidosis and uveitis," *Autoimmunity Reviews*, vol. 13, no. 8, pp. 840–849, 2014.

[11] B. A. Henderson, J. Y. Kim, C. S. Ament, Z. K. Ferrufino-Ponce, A. Grabowska, and S. L. Cremers, "Clinical pseudophakic cystoid macular edema: risk factors for development and duration after treatment," *Journal of Cataract & Refractive Surgery*, vol. 33, no. 9, pp. 1550–1558, 2007.

[12] D. A. Jabs, R. B. Nussenblatt, J. T. Rosenbaum, and Standardization of Uveitis Nomenclature (SUN) Working Group, "Standardization of uveitis nomenclature for reporting clinical data. Results of the first international workshop," *American Journal of Ophthalmology*, vol. 140, no. 3, pp. 509–516, 2005.

[13] Y. A. Akova and C. S. Foster, "Cataract surgery in patients with sarcoidosis-associated uveitis," *Ophthalmology*, vol. 101, no. 3, pp. 473–479, 1994.

[14] S. Mehta, M. M. Linton, and J. H. Kempen, "Outcomes of cataract surgery in patients with uveitis: a systematic review and meta-analysis," *American Journal of Ophthalmology*, vol. 158, no. 4, pp. 676.e7–692.e7, 2014.

[15] M. O. M. Wong, J. W. Y. Lee, B. N. K. Choy, J. C. H. Chan, and J. S. M. Lai, "Systematic review and meta-analysis on the efficacy of selective laser trabeculoplasty in open-angle glaucoma," *Survey of Ophthalmology*, vol. 60, no. 1, pp. 36–50, 2015.

[16] E. Karahan, D. Er, and S. Kaynak, "An overview of Nd:YAG laser capsulotomy," *Medical Hypothesis, Discovery and Innovation in Ophthalmology*, vol. 3, no. 2, pp. 45–50, 2014.

[17] D. Valeyre, A. Prasse, H. Nunes, Y. Uzunhan, P.-Y. Brillet, and J. Müller-Quernheim, "Sarcoidosis," *The Lancet*, vol. 383, no. 9923, pp. 1155–1167, 2014.

[18] E. S. Chen, Z. Song, M. H. Willett et al., "Serum amyloid a regulates granulomatous inflammation in sarcoidosis through toll-like receptor-2," *American Journal of Respiratory and Critical Care Medicine*, vol. 181, no. 4, pp. 360–373, 2010.

[19] J. E. E. Yager, A. F. Hernandez, C. Steenbergen et al., "Recurrence of cardiac sarcoidosis in a heart transplant recipient," *Journal of Heart and Lung Transplantation*, vol. 24, no. 11, pp. 1988–1990, 2005.

[20] A. Heyll, G. Meckenstock, C. Aul et al., "Possible transmission of sarcoidosis via allogeneic bone marrow transplantation," *Bone Marrow Transplantation*, vol. 14, no. 1, pp. 161–164, 1994.

[21] R. Morita, S. Hashino, K. Kubota et al., "Donor cell-derived sarcoidosis after allogeneic BMT," *Bone Marrow Transplantation*, vol. 43, no. 6, pp. 507-508, 2008.

[22] B. Bodaghi, V. Touitou, C. Fardeau, C. Chapelon, and P. LeHoang, "Ocular sarcoidosis," *La Presse Médicale*, vol. 41, no. 6, pp. e349–e354, 2012.

[23] N. P. Jones, "The manchester uveitis clinic: the first 3000 patients-epidemiology and casemix," *Ocular Immunology and Inflammation*, vol. 23, no. 2, pp. 118–126, 2015.

[24] P. Ungprasert, E. M. Carmona, J. P. Utz, J. H. Ryu, C. S. Crowson, and E. L. Matteson, "Epidemiology of sarcoidosis 1946-2013: a population-based study," *Mayo Clinic Proceedings*, vol. 91, no. 2, pp. 183–188, 2016.

[25] M. Evans, O. Sharma, L. LaBree, R. E. Smith, and N. A. Rao, "Differences in clinical findings between Caucasians and African Americans with biopsy-proven sarcoidosis," *Ophthalmology*, vol. 114, no. 2, pp. 325.e1–333.e1, 2007.

[26] A. Karma, E. Huhti, and A. Poukkula, "Course and outcome of ocular sarcoidosis," *American Journal of Ophthalmology*, vol. 106, no. 4, pp. 467–472, 1988.

[27] Y. Yonekawa and I. K. Kim, "Pseudophakic cystoid macular edema," *Current Opinion in Ophthalmology*, vol. 23, no. 1, pp. 26–32, 2012.

[28] S. Guo, S. Patel, B. Baumrind et al., "Management of pseudophakic cystoid macular edema," *Survey of Ophthalmology*, vol. 60, no. 2, pp. 123–137, 2015.

[29] M. Drancourt, F. Fenollar, D. Denis, and D. Raoult, "Postoperative panophthalmitis caused by whipple disease," *Emerging Infectious Diseases*, vol. 15, no. 5, pp. 825–827, 2009.

[30] F. Damico, S. Kiss, and L. H. Young, "Sympathetic ophthalmia," *Seminars in Ophthalmology*, vol. 20, no. 3, pp. 191–197, 2005.

[31] C. C. Chan, D. Benezra, M. M. Rodrigues et al., "Immunohistochemistry and electron microscopy of choroidal infiltrates and Dalen-Fuchs nodules in sympathetic ophthalmia," *Ophthalmology*, vol. 92, no. 4, pp. 580–590, 1985.

[32] D. G. James, R. Anderson, D. Langley, and D. Ainslie, "Ocular sarcoidosis," *British Journal of Ophthalmology*, vol. 48, pp. 461–470, 1964.

[33] C. Febvay, L. Kodjikian, D. Maucort-Boulch et al., "Clinical features and diagnostic evaluation of 83 biopsy-proven sarcoid uveitis cases," *British Journal of Ophthalmology*, vol. 99, no. 10, pp. 1372–1376, 2015.

[34] A. D. Birnbaum, F. S. Oh, A. Chakrabarti, H. H. Tessler, and D. A. Goldstein, "Clinical features and diagnostic evaluation of biopsy-proven ocular sarcoidosis," *Archives of Ophthalmology*, vol. 129, no. 4, pp. 409–413, 2011.

17

Phenotypic Variation in a Four-Generation Family with Aniridia Carrying a Novel *PAX6* Mutation

Grace M. Wang,[1] Lev Prasov,[1] Hayder Al-Hasani,[1,2] Colin E. R. Marrs,[1] Sahil Tolia,[1] Laurel Wiinikka-Buesser,[1] Julia E. Richards,[1,2] and Brenda L. Bohnsack[1]

[1]*Department of Ophthalmology and Visual Sciences, W.K. Kellogg Eye Center, The University of Michigan, Ann Arbor, MI 48105, USA*
[2]*Department of Epidemiology, The University of Michigan, Ann Arbor, MI 48109, USA*

Correspondence should be addressed to Brenda L. Bohnsack; brendabo@med.umich.edu

Academic Editor: Jesús Pintor

Aniridia is a congenital disease that affects almost all eye structures and is primarily caused by loss-of-function mutations in the *PAX6* gene. The degree of vision loss in aniridia varies and is dependent on the extent of foveal, iris, and optic nerve hypoplasia and the presence of glaucoma, cataracts, and corneal opacification. Here, we describe a 4-generation family in which 7 individuals across 2 generations carry a novel disease-causing frameshift mutation (NM_000280.4(PAX6):c.565TC>T) in *PAX6*. This mutation results in an early stop codon in exon 8, which is predicted to cause nonsense-mediated decay of the truncated mRNA and a functionally null *PAX6* allele. Family members with aniridia showed differences in multiple eye phenotypes including iris and optic nerve hypoplasia, congenital and acquired corneal opacification, glaucoma, and strabismus. Visual acuity ranged from 20/100 to less than 20/800. Patients who required surgical intervention for glaucoma or corneal opacification had worse visual outcomes. Our results show that family members carrying a novel *PAX6* frameshift mutation have variable expressivity, leading to different ocular comorbidities and visual outcomes.

1. Introduction

Familial aniridia is a congenital disease caused by autosomal dominant mutations in the *PAX6* gene that disrupt the development and function of almost all eye structures [1, 2]. While aniridia is named for iris hypoplasia, a feature of the trait that is often readily evident without a specialized examination, the main causes of early visual impairment are optic nerve and foveal hypoplasia. Further, many affected individuals suffer progressive vision loss due to glaucoma or limbal stem cell deficiency. The severity of visual impairment and phenotypic expression in affected individuals varies [3–5].

The *PAX6* gene, located on chromosome 11p13, encodes a transcription factor that is vital for ocular development [6, 7]. *PAX6* is expressed in the surface ectoderm and neural ectoderm during early eye development and is essential for the specification and differentiation of the cornea, lens, ciliary body, retina, and optic nerve [8–16]. To date, 221 mutations in *PAX6* have been reported; most are associated with aniridia, though some mutations are associated with other ocular diseases such as coloboma, morning glory disc anomaly, anterior segment dysgenesis, and cataract with late-onset corneal dystrophy (ClinVar: PAX6[gene]) [2–6, 17–37]. Due to its gene-dosage effect, decreased protein function or expression of a single copy of *PAX6* results in characteristic ocular malformations [11, 17, 20, 38]. While aniridia can be sporadic, the mode of inheritance for the familial form is considered autosomal dominant; however, unlike classical autosomal dominance, PAX6 inheritance shows two phenotypes associated with the different genotypic combinations. Specifically, the presence of one defective copy of PAX6 results in ocular malformations, but mutations in both copies of *PAX6* cause ocular phenotypes that are more severe (e.g., anophthalmia) and brain abnormalities that are incompatible with life [6, 39, 40]. Differences in expressivity are seen when comparing one *PAX6* mutation to another. However, studies have reported that even within families carrying the same mutation, individuals may have different ocular findings [3, 5, 24, 35]. In the current study, we describe the relationships and detailed phenotypes in a 4-generation family in which individuals affected with aniridia carry a novel loss-of-function *PAX6* frameshift mutation. Our findings confirm that significant intrafamily phenotypic variability occurs among individuals carrying the same *PAX6* mutation.

2. Methods

This study was approved by the University of Michigan Institutional Review Board and complied with the US Health Insurance Portability and Accountability Act of 1996 and the Declaration of Helsinki. Informed consent was obtained either from participating individuals or from parents of minor patients. A retrospective chart review was performed on a family that had four generations of individuals affected by aniridia. The following data were collected: age, sex, ocular diagnoses, and history of intraocular surgeries. Visual acuities, anterior segment and fundus examinations, intraocular pressures (IOP), refraction, strabismus examination, and ocular medications were recorded from the last examination. Visual acuity was determined by Snellen or Allen figure optotypes in adults and verbal children. Teller visual acuity cards with conversion to Snellen equivalent were used in preverbal children. Anterior and posterior segment exams were performed using slit lamp biomicroscopy and indirect ophthalmoscopy. IOPs were obtained by Goldmann applanation, Tono-Pen (Reichert, Depew, NY, USA) or iCare (Revenio, Vantaa, Finland) tonometry.

2.1. PAX6 Mutation Screening. Genomic DNA was extracted from buccal epithelial cells obtained by swabs or mouthwash samples of the recruited individuals using the DNeasy kit (Qiagen, Hilden, Germany). Eleven exons of the *PAX6* coding region were amplified from genomic DNA by polymerase chain reaction (PCR) using AmpliTaq Gold polymerase (Applied Biosystems, Foster City, CA, USA). PCR primers and conditions are listed in Table 1. PCR cycling conditions were as follows: denaturation at 94°C for 10 minutes then amplification with 36 cycles of denaturation at 94°C for 30 seconds, annealing at 60°C for 30 seconds, and extension at 72°C for 1 minute, with a final extension at 72°C for 10 minutes. PCR products were verified by the size of amplicons on a 1% agarose gel electrophoresis, diluted, and sequenced via Sanger dideoxynucleotide partial chain termination sequencing on an ABI3730 DNA Analyzer (Applied Biosystems) at the University of Michigan DNA Sequencing Core. All exons were sequenced with the same primers used for amplification, except exon 8 for which the following primer was additionally used: 5′- AGGCTGTCG GGATATAATGC-3′. All variants were compared to high-quality sequence reads in the Exome Aggregation Consortium (ExAC) database. Segregation was confirmed by screening DNA from all available affected and unaffected individuals in the family.

3. Results

Seven related patients affected with familial aniridia were identified and recruited for this study. There were 3 female and 4 male patients and the ages ranged from 2 to 31 years. Based on information obtained by family history, a 4-generation pedigree was constructed, which included a total of 13 affected individuals (Figure 1). The clinical findings for the 7 patients in which genetic analysis was performed are described in Table 2.

3.1. Patient III-5. Patient III-5 is a 29-year-old male with no previous history of glaucoma or ocular surgeries. He has no history of diabetes or other metabolic abnormalities. At the time of his last examination, his best-corrected visual acuity was 20/150 in each eye individually and 20/100 binocularly. IOPs were 23 mmHg in the right eye and 19 mmHg in the left eye. Slit lamp biomicroscopy of both eyes showed mild corneal pannuses, hypoplastic irides with small remnant stumps, and visually insignificant cortical cataracts. Funduscopic examination revealed bilateral foveal hypoplasia and optic nerve hypoplasia. The cup to disc ratio in the right eye was 0.1 and in the left eye was 0.3. The patient had bilateral small amplitude and high-velocity horizontal nystagmus with no relative null point, and he was orthophoric.

3.2. Patient IV-1. Patient IV-1 is the 3-year-old son of patient III-5. He has a body mass index of 23.7 kg/m^2 and to date has no history of diabetes or other metabolic problems. Unlike his father, he was diagnosed with glaucoma at 4 months of age and underwent placement of a Baerveldt101-350 glaucoma drainage device (Abbott Medical Optics, Santa Ana, CA, USA) in his left eye at 6 months of age and in his right eye at 9 months of age. He also underwent bilateral medial rectus recessions for esotropia at 2 years of age. At his last examination, his best-corrected visual acuity was 20/200 in each eye and binocularly. The patient was not on any glaucoma medications, and IOPs were 13 mmHg in the right eye and 14 mmHg in the left eye. Slit lamp examination of each eye showed a superotemporal glaucoma drainage device with an overlying bleb. The tube in each eye was oriented vertically along the temporal zonules and was not touching the cornea or lens. The corneas were clear with minimal pannuses, the irides were hypoplastic with small remnant stumps, and the lenses were clear. Fundoscopic examination showed foveal and optic nerve hypoplasia. The optic nerves had a cup to disc ratio of 0.0 in each eye. Cycloplegic refraction was $+1.00 + 1.00 \times 90$ in the right eye and $+1.00 + 1.00 \times 80$ in the left eye. Like his father, the patient had bilateral small amplitude and high-velocity horizontal nystagmus with no relative null point, and he was orthophoric in all gazes.

3.3. Patient III-8. Patient III-8 is a 31-year-old woman who is a first cousin of patient III-5. She has a history of type 1 diabetes mellitus that was diagnosed at 5 years of age and has been on an insulin pump since 2009. Her last hemoglobin A1C was 7.7% and her current body mass index was 47.8 kg/m^2. She also has a history of hypothyroidism, which is well-controlled on levothyroxine. She underwent cataract

Table 1: PCR primer sequences.

Exon	Forward primer	Chromosomal coordinates*	Reverse primer	Chromosomal coordinates*	Fragment size
4	TTCCAGTACTTTGTTTCAAGCCCC	chr11:31,806,650-31,806,673	AAACTCGGGCGGGCTGTTCTTAAG	chr11:31,806,160-31,806,183	514 bp
5	CCTCTTCACTCTGCTCTCTT	chr11:31,802,874-31,802,893	ATGAAGAGAGGGCGTTGAGA	chr11:31,802,637-31,802,656	258 bp
5a	TGAAAGTATCATCATATTTGTAG	chr11:31,801,999-31,802,021	GGGAAGTGGACAGAAAACCA	chr11:31,801,785-31,801,804	237 bp
6	TGAAAGTATCATCATATTTGTAG	chr11:31,801,999-31,802,021	AGGAGAGAGCATTGGGCTTA	chr11:31,801,507-31,801,526	515 bp
7	CAGGAGACACTACCATTTGG	chr11:31,800,880-31,800,899	CAGGCCTTCAAATGCAGTCTCACC	chr11:31,800,557-31,800,580	343 bp
8	GGGAATGTTTTGGTGAGGCT	chr11:31,794,891-31,794,910	CAAAGGGCCCTGGCTAAATT	chr11:31,794,540-31,794,559	371 bp
9	GTAGTTCTGGCACAATATGG	chr11:31,794,136-31,794,155	GTACTCTGTACAAGCACCTC	chr11:31,793,950-31,793,969	206 bp
10	GTAGACACAGTGCTAACCTG	chr11:31,793,820-31,793,839	CCCGGAGCAAACAGGTTTAA	chr11:31,793,597-31,793,616	243 bp
11	TTAAACCTGTTTGCTCCGGG	chr11:31,793,597-31,793,616	AGTGCGAAAAGCTCTCAAGGGTGC	chr11:31,793,326-31,793,349	291 bp
12	GCTGTGTGATGTGTTCCTCA	chr11:31,790,891-31,790,910	TTTCCCTTTTCAATCCCCATCCCC	chr11:31,790,566-31,790,589	345 bp
13	CATGTCTGTTTCTCAAAGGGA	chr11:31,790,055-31,790,075	CCCCAGTGGTACAATACAGGACAC	chr11:31,789,782-31,789,805	294 bp

*UCSC human genome, hg38 accessed 9/10/2017. In a 25 μL PCR reaction for each coding exon, 0.3 μL of AmpliTaq Gold (Applied Biosystems), with 2 μL of 25 mM MgCl2, 0.2 of 25 mM dinucleotide triphosphate, and 0.5 μL of 25 mM primers were used. For exon 4, we used 5 μL of Q-solution (Qiagen) and changed MgCl2 volume to to 2.5 μL and accounted for this from the water to keep the reaction volume at 25 μL. In all of the amplicons, genomic DNA was denatured at 94°C for 10 minutes then amplified by 36 cycles of 94°C denaturation for 30 seconds, 60°C annealing for 30 seconds, and 72°C extension for 1 minute with final extension of 72°C for 10 minutes.

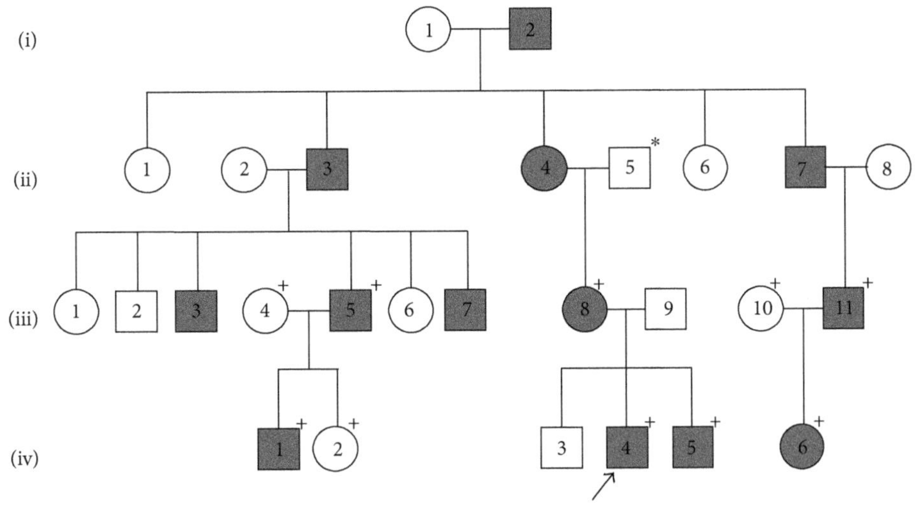

FIGURE 1: Four-generation family with familial aniridia. Pedigree of a four-generation family in which 13 individuals were affected with familial aniridia (gray circles and gray squares). The plus sign (+) denotes individuals who underwent *PAX6* sequencing and affected individuals with genetic confirmation of the novel frameshift mutation PAX6 p.Ile190SerfsTer17. The arrow indicates the proband. The star (*) indicates a family member with reported aniridia.

extraction with intraocular lens placement in both eyes when she was 15 years old. At 20 years of age, she was diagnosed with glaucoma, which has been managed medically with use of timolol and dorzolamide. She also has a history of a V-pattern exotropia for which she underwent bilateral lateral rectus recessions at 2 years of age and bilateral medial rectus resections and bilateral inferior oblique recessions at 2.5 years of age. She then developed a consecutive esotropia and underwent bilateral medial rectus recessions with inferior transpositions and left inferior oblique anteriorization at 7 years of age. At her last examination, her best-corrected visual acuity was 20/125 in the right eye and 20/200 in the left eye and her IOPs by Goldmann applanation were 14 mmHg in the right eye and 17 mmHg in the left eye. Slit lamp examination showed corneal epithelial irregularities and pannus with neovascularization in both eyes (arrows, Figure 2(a)). The irides were hypoplastic with small remnant stumps (arrowheads, Figure 2(a)). Fundoscopic examination showed foveal hypoplasia. The optic nerves were hypoplastic and had a cup to disc ratio of 0.4 in the right eye and 0.5 in the left eye. Refraction was $-2.25+4.00\times160$ in the right eye and $-1.50+2.50\times85$ in the left eye. She had horizontal high-velocity nystagmus of both eyes and a V-pattern exotropia. Per patient and family report, both of her parents had aniridia (II-4 and II-5).

3.4. Patient IV-4. Patient IV-4 is the 10-year-old son of patient III-8 and second cousin of patient IV-1. His last body mass index was 23.8 kg/m^2 and to date has no history of diabetes or other metabolic abnormalities. He was diagnosed with glaucoma at 5 years of age and underwent placement of Baerveldt 101-350 glaucoma drainage devices in both eyes at 6 years of age. He also has a history of a V-pattern esotropia and bilateral medial rectus recessions with half tendon infraplacement. Further, bilateral inferior oblique partial anteriorization was performed at 3 years of age. At his last examination, his best-corrected visual acuity was 20/300 in the right eye, 20/250 in the left eye, and 20/200 binocularly. IOPs were 14 mmHg in the right eye and 17 mmHg in the left eye on timolol and dorzolamide in both eyes. Slit lamp examination showed superotemporal glaucoma drainage devices with overlying blebs. The tubes were in the anterior chamber, oriented vertically along the temporal zonules without corneal or lens touch. Both corneas had 360 degrees of pannus with neovascularization (arrows, Figure 2(b)). In the right eye, the pannus extended into the visual axis and had underlying corneal stromal haze. The irides were hypoplastic with short remnant stumps (arrowheads, Figure 2(b)). There were mild cortical and posterior subcapsular cataracts that were not visually significant. Fundoscopic examination showed optic nerve and foveal hypoplasia. The optic nerves had a cup to disc ratio of 0.8 and 0.6 for the right and left eye, respectively. Cycloplegic refraction was −3.50 in the right eye and −3.00 in the left eye. He had bilateral moderate amplitude and moderate velocity horizontal nystagmus with no null point, and he showed a 50 prism diopter exotropia.

3.5. Patient IV-5. Patient IV-5 is the 3-year-old son of patient III-8, brother of patient IV-4, and second cousin of patient IV-1. He has no history of diabetes or metabolic abnormalities. He was diagnosed with glaucoma at 2 years of age and has been medically managed with timolol and dorzolamide in both eyes. At his last examination, visual acuity by Teller Acuity cards was estimated to be 20/380 in each eye individually and 20/260 binocularly. IOPs were 20 mmHg in the right eye and 15 mmHg in the left eye. Slit lamp examination showed clear corneas without pannuses, and hypoplastic irides were very small remnant stumps. There was a focal cortical cataract in the right eye that was not visually significant. Fundoscopic examination showed foveal hypoplasia in both eyes. The optic nerves had no cupping or evidence of hypoplasia. The patient has a small amplitude, has high-velocity horizontal nystagmus with a null point in left gaze, and has a 45 prism diopter exotropia.

Table 2: Summary of clinical findings.

Patient	VA	Initial anterior segment findings	Initial posterior segment findings	IOP (mmHg) glaucoma meds	Glaucoma diagnosis (Dx) and glaucoma surgeries	Other ocular surgeries
III-5	OD: 20/150 OS: 20/150 OU: 20/100	Corneal pannuses Hypoplastic irides Cortical cataracts	Foveal hypoplasia Optic nerve Hypoplasia	OD: 23 OS: 19 No meds	No glaucoma	OD: none OS: none
IV-1	OD: 20/200 OS: 20/200 OU: 20/200	Corneal pannuses Hypoplastic irides	Foveal hypoplasia Optic nerve Hypoplasia	OD: 13 OS: 14 No meds	Glaucoma Dx @ 0.3 years OD: s/p Baerveldt 101-350 OS: s/p Baerveldt 101-350	Strabismus: s/p bilateral medial rectus recessions
III-8	OD: 20/125 OS: 20/200	Corneal epithelial irregularities and pannus with neovascularization Hypoplastic irides	Foveal hypoplasia Optic Nerve hypoplasia	OD: 14 OS: 17 Timolol Dorzolamide	Glaucoma Dx @ 20 years No glaucoma surgeries	OD: s/p ECCE-IOL OS: s/p ECCE-IOL Strabismus: s/p bilateral lateral rectus Recessions, s/p Bilateral Inferior Oblique Recessions, s/p Bilateral Medial Rectus Recessions with Inferior Transpositions, s/p Left Inferior Oblique Anteriorization
IV-4	OD: 20/300 OS: 20/250 OU: 20/200	Corneal pannus Cortical and posterior subcapsular cataracts	Foveal hypoplasia Optic nerve Hypoplasia	OD: 14 OS: 17 Timolol Dorzolamide	Glaucoma Dx @ 5 years OD: s/p Baerveldt 101-350 OS: s/p Baerveldt 101-350	Strabismus: s/p bilateral medial rectus recessions with half tendon infraplacement, s/p bilateral inferior oblique partial anteriorization
IV-5	OD: 20/380 OS: 20/380 OU: 20/260	Hypoplastic irides Focal cataract OD	Foveal hypoplasia	OD: 20 OS: 15 Timolol Dorzolamide	Glaucoma Dx @ 2 years No glaucoma surgeries	OD: none OS: none
III-11	OD: CF @ 1 ft OS: CF @ 1 ft	Peters anomaly Partial hypoplastic irides	Foveal hypoplasia	OD: 20 OS: 15 Timolol	Glaucoma Dx @ 6 years OD: none OS: s/p trabeculectomy with mitomycin $C \times 2$, s/p cyclophotocoagulation $\times 2$	OD: s/p penetrating keratoplasty OS: s/p ECCE, s/p superficial keratectomy, s/p penetrating keratoplasty
IV-6	OD: 20/150 OS: 20/100	Corneal pannuses Hypoplastic irides Posterior subcapsular cataracts	Foveal hypoplasia	OD: unable OS: unable	No glaucoma	OD: none OS: none

ECCE: extracapsular cataract extraction; IOL: intraocular lens; CF: counting fingers.

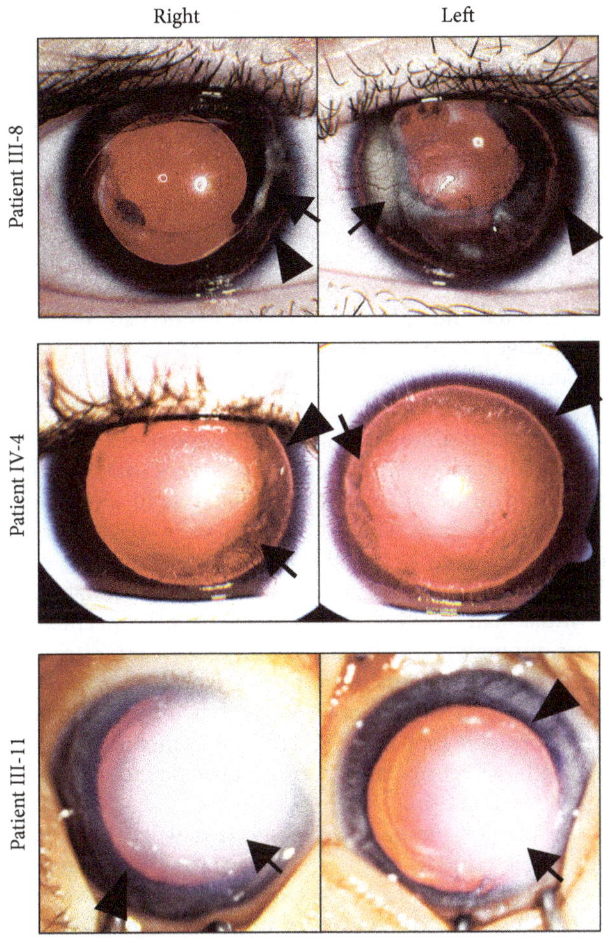

Figure 2: Phenotypic variations in individuals with *PAX6* p.Ile190SerfsTer17. mutation. Anterior segment photographs of the right and left eyes of individuals with the *PAX6* NM_000280.4(PAX6):c.565TC>T frameshift mutation showed phenotypic variation. Patient III-8 (a) at 31 years of age had almost complete iris hypoplasia with small remnant stumps (arrowheads), intraocular lenses, and corneal pannuses with neovascularization (arrows) in both eyes. In the left eye, the corneal pannus was associated with underlying stromal scarring. Patient IV-4 (b) at 5 years of age, prior to placement of glaucoma drainage devices, had corneal pannuses with neovascularization (arrows) and corneal epithelial irregularities in both eyes. Patient IV-4 also had almost complete iris hypoplasia with small remnant stumps (arrowheads) in both eyes. Patient III-11 (c) at 2 months of age, prior to penetrating keratoplasty, had bilateral central corneal opacities consistent with Peters anomaly (arrows) with the opacity of the right eye much denser than the left eye. However, patient III-11 exhibited only partial iris hypoplasia (arrowheads) in both eyes.

His cycloplegic refraction was $-3.50+2.00\times120$ in the right eye and $-3.50+2.00\times60$ in the left eye.

3.6. Patient III-11. Patient III-11 is a 29-year-old male who is first cousins with patient III-4 and patient III-8. He has no history of diabetes or metabolic abnormalities. His ocular history is notable for bilateral Peters anomaly and partial iris hypoplasia (Figure 2(c)). At 2 months of age, he underwent penetrating keratoplasty of the right eye, which subsequently became vascularized and was not replaced due to poor visual potential. In the left eye, he underwent extracapsular cataract extraction at 2 years of age. He developed glaucoma of the left eye, which necessitated 2 trabeculectomies with mitomycin C at 6 years of age and 2 treatments of cyclophotocoagulation at 7 years of age. The left cornea underwent a superficial keratectomy for band keratopathy at 9 years of age and then penetrating keratoplasty at 11 years of age. The left corneal graft was complicated by persistent epithelial defects and by 20 years of age, the graft had failed and the patient did not desire repeat penetrating keratoplasty. At his last examination, he was not able to see the 20/800 optotypes and was only able to detect the number of fingers held at 1 foot in front of each eye. IOPs were 20 mmHg in the right eye and 15 mmHg in the left eye on timolol. Slit lamp examination on the right showed a corneal graft with central and inferior conjunctivalization, hypoplastic iris, and white cataract. The left eye had a corneal graft with diffuse stromal thickening, band keratopathy, and 360 degrees of pannus and hypoplastic iris. Neither eye had a view to the fundus.

3.7. Patient IV-6. Patient IV-6 is a 5-year-old daughter of patient III-11 and second cousin to patients IV-1, IV-4, and IV-5 and has no history of diabetes or metabolic abnormalities. Further, she has no history of glaucoma or previous ocular surgeries. At her last examination, her best-corrected visual acuity was 20/150 in the right eye and 20/100 in the left eye. She was unable to tolerate IOP testing, but both eyes were soft by digital palpation. Slit lamp examination of both eyes showed mild corneal pannuses, small remnant iris stumps, and trace visually insignificant posterior subcapsular cataracts. Fundoscopic examination showed foveal hypoplasia and normal optic nerves with cup to disc ratios of 0.2 in both eyes. Cycloplegic refraction was $+0.2\ 5+4.25\times102$ in the right eye and $+1.25+5.00\times70$ in the left eye. She had a 9 prism diopter esotropia and horizontal nystagmus of both eyes.

3.8. PAX6 Mutational Analysis. The paired homeobox gene PAX6 gene on chromosome 11p13 comprises two major splice forms, with a total of 14 exons, including 11 coding exons. *PAX6* gene sequencing was performed on all seven patients in this study, and three unaffected family members A novel frameshift mutation from a single nucleotide deletion (NM_000280.4(PAX6):c.565TC>T) was found to perfectly segregate in all seven patients with aniridia and was absent in family members without aniridia (Figure 3). Individual III-8 was found to carry a single *PAX6* mutation presumably inherited from her mother, despite the reported history that both of her parents had aniridia. This frameshift mutation p.Ile190SerfsTer17 in exon 8 of *PAX6* is predicted to cause an early stop codon and a functionally null *PAX6* allele. This mutation was not found in the ClinVar or ExAC databases.

4. Discussion

The ocular phenotypes associated with *PAX6* mutations underscore the essential role of *PAX6* in eye development.

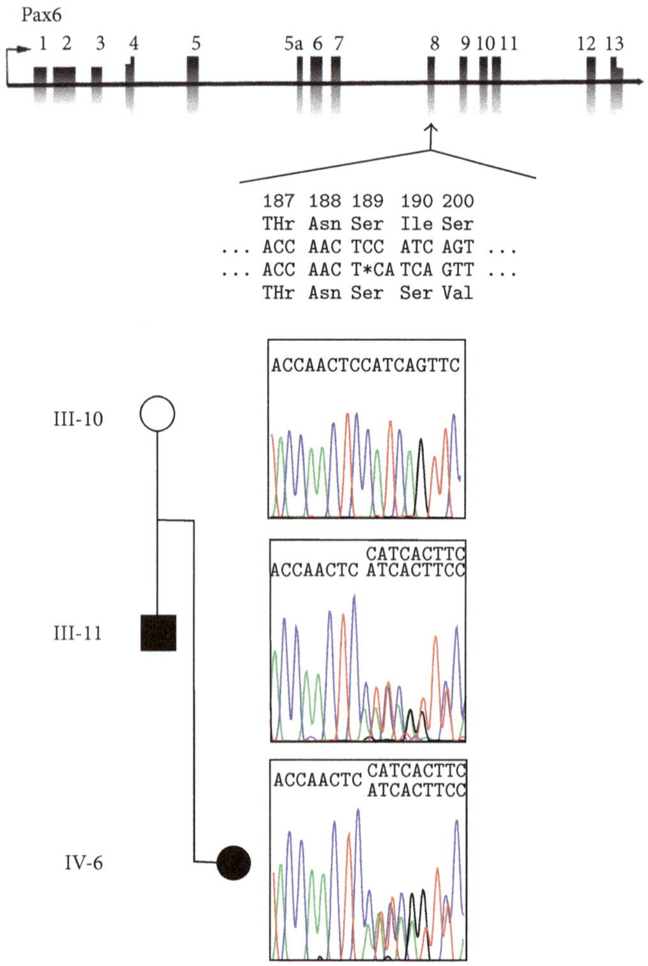

Figure 3: Sequencing confirming *PAX6* frameshift mutation. Schematic of *PAX6* gene shows the location of the NM_000280.4(PAX6):c.565TC>T frameshift mutation and its effect on the coding protein. The Sanger chromatogram traces show transmission of the mutation from father (III-11) to daughter (IV-6) in one branch of the family and absence of the mutation in the unaffected mother (III-10).

The "classic" presentation of aniridia includes iris, optic nerve, and foveal hypoplasia and congenital cataracts with progressive corneal opacification due to limbal stem cell deficiency [1, 20, 41]. In addition, approximately 50% of affected individuals have glaucoma secondary to anterior rotation of the iris root and/or inherent goniotrabeculodysgenesis [26, 32, 38, 42, 43]. However, there is a phenotypic spectrum associated with *PAX6* mutations, which can include some to all of the abovementioned ophthalmic findings as well as congenital corneal opacification (Peters anomaly), anterior segment dysgenesis, and colobomas [4, 6, 17, 20, 25, 32, 34].

PAX6 is a transcription factor, which has 2 DNA-binding domains, a long paired domain, and a homeodomain [44]. Disease-causing mutations span the *PAX6* coding sequence and regulatory regions. Missense mutations are associated with milder phenotypes such as isolated congenital cataracts, anterior segment dysgenesis, and colobomas [2, 6, 27, 32, 34, 45]. In contrast, large deletions and mutations that cause premature stop codons are associated with aniridia. We identified a novel frameshift mutation (NM_000280.4(PAX6):c.565TC>T) from a single nucleotide deletion in exon 8, which encodes the initial homeodomain sequence. It is hypothesized that truncated mutant *PAX6* mRNA is degraded through nonsense-mediated decay prior to translation [42, 43]. Thus, it is predicted to be a complete loss of a function *PAX6* allele, consistent with the aniridia phenotype.

In the current study, we present an example of phenotypic variation in a 4-generation family with aniridia. Of the 7 affected individuals who were genotyped, the visual acuity ranged from 20/100 to worse than 20/800. Within our family, all affected individuals had foveal hypoplasia, which is the main cause of visual impairment. Six of the 7 individuals had almost complete iris hypoplasia. Two individuals had progressive corneal irregularities with significant pannus and corneal neovascularization, due to severe limbal stem cell deficiency. Five individuals were diagnosed with glaucoma between 4 months and 20 years of age, and 3 required surgery to obtain IOP control. Most notably, one individual had bilateral congenital corneal opacifications (Peters anomaly), which resulted in poor vision after failed corneal transplantation in both eyes. These results indicate that the same *PAX6* mutation can yield a wide range of ocular phenotypes and that more severe visual impairment correlated with glaucoma and corneal opacification, requiring surgical intervention.

The phenotypic variation associated with *PAX6* mutations may be due to differences in genetic background that affect the expression of *PAX6* coregulators and downstream targets. *PAX6* encodes a transcription factor that is an early marker of neural epithelium and demarcates specific domains of the developing central nervous system. Within the neural epithelial-derived optic vesicle, animal studies have demonstrated that *Pax6* acts together with additional transcription factors such as *Pax2*, *Six6*, *Gsx2*, *Pax5*, and *Lhx2* to regulate invagination to form the bilayered cup that will become the retina, retinal pigmented epithelium, and iris pigmented epithelium [8, 10, 12, 46]. Further, *Pax6* is specifically expressed in the lens placode through a combination of activation by *Sox2*, *Oct-1*, and *Foxe3* in the surface ectoderm and inhibition by TGFβ and Wnt signaling in the periocular neural crest [47–51]. Together, these signaling pathways stimulate separation of the lens vesicle from the overlying surface ectoderm and neural crest migration into the anterior segment. Minor alterations in expression or function of these additional signaling pathways and coregulators through single nucleotide polymorphism variants may exacerbate or mitigate the effect of a *PAX6* mutation during different processes of eye development.

Transcriptional and epigenetic regulation also alter the function of *PAX6*, which may result in different ocular phenotypes. The *PAX6* locus is complex and is regulated by three promoters. The P0 and P1 promoters drive expression of the *Pax6* transcript and the alternatively spliced *Pax6(5a)* variant, while the internal Pα promotor encodes truncated Pax6 p32 proteins that lack the DNA-binding paired domain [52, 53]. The specific regulation of the Pα promoter and the function of these truncated proteins have yet to be determined. In addition, the paired domain of *Pax6(5a)* has a different DNA-binding capacity, and this variant primarily plays a role in iris formation [54]. Stochastic events, which may differentially regulate the transcription and activity of *Pax6* and the *Pax6(5a)* variant, may influence phenotype. Further, epigenetic alteration of *PAX6* regulates DNA binding, transcriptional activation, and protein degradation. For example, posttranslational sumoylation of the Pax6 p32 protein by SUMO-1 enhances DNA-binding activity of the homeodomain and increases transcriptional activation of target proteins [55]. In contrast, Trim11, a ubiquitin E3 ligase decreases *PAX6* activity by tagging the protein for degradation by the proteasome [56]. In addition, the DNA-binding activity of the *PAX6* homeobox domain is modified by histone variants such as *H3K4me1*, *H3K27ac*, *H3K4m3*, and *H3K37me3* [57]. Thus, *PAX6* transcription and protein function are regulated at multiple levels, all of which are targets for differential expression and activity in the functional copy of PAX6. These may account for the phenotypic variability in the ocular findings associated with dominantly inherited *PAX6* null mutations.

In addition to its role in ocular development, *PAX6* has been shown to regulate pancreatic islet cell development [58, 59]. The clinical implications of *PAX6* mutations on glucose tolerance are unclear as published studies include few patients and show conflicting results [60, 61]. In our study, only 1 patient had a history of type 1 diabetes, while the remainder of the individuals had no history of glucose intolerance. Additional studies, which include a larger number of individuals with aniridia, are required to better understand whether *PAX6* mutations also have phenotypic variability in regards to glucose regulation.

In the current study, we describe a novel disease-causing frameshift mutation (NM_000280.4(PAX6):c.565TC>T) in *PAX6* in a 4-generation family affected with aniridia. Family members with aniridia showed phenotypic variation and differences in visual outcomes that correlated with surgical intervention for glaucoma or corneal opacification. Further studies which investigate modifications and interactions of *PAX6* are required for better understanding of the phenotypic variations in aniridia.

5. Conclusions

We describe a novel disease-causing frameshift mutation (NM_000280.4(PAX6):c.565TC > T) in *PAX6* which showed phenotypic variation in a 4-generation family. Differences in ocular comorbidities resulted in a range of visual outcomes in affected individuals.

Disclosure

A portion of this manuscript was presented at the 2017 Annual Meeting of the American Association of Pediatric Ophthalmology and Strabismus and published with the meeting abstracts in J AAPOS [62]. The authors alone are responsible for the content and writing of this article.

Conflicts of Interest

The authors report no conflicts of interest.

Acknowledgments

This study is funded in part by Research to Prevent Blindness and a grant from the Public Health Genetics Certificate Program of the University of Michigan School of Public Health.

References

[1] S. C. Brauner, D. S. Walton, and T. C. Chen, "Aniridia," *International Ophthalmology Clinics*, vol. 48, no. 2, pp. 79–85, 2008.

[2] A. Cvekl and P. Callaerts, "Pax6: 25th anniversary and more to learn," *Experimental Eye Research*, vol. 156, pp. 10–21, 2017.

[3] S. K. Dubey, N. Mahalaxmi, P. Vijayalakshmi, and P. Sundaresan, "Mutational analysis and genotype-phenotype correlations in southern Indian patients with sporadic and familial aniridia," *Molecular Vision*, vol. 21, pp. 88–97, 2015.

[4] M. Hingorani, K. A. Williamson, A. T. Moore, and V. van Heyningen, "Detailed ophthalmologic evaluation of 43 individuals with PAX6 mutations," *Investigative Ophthalmology & Visual Science*, vol. 50, no. 6, p. 2581, 2009.

[5] T. Yokoi, S. Nishina, M. Fukami et al., "Genotype-phenotype correlation of PAX6 gene mutations in aniridia," *Human Genome Variation*, vol. 3, no. 1, article 15052, 2016.

[6] T. Glaser, L. Jepeal, J. G. Edwards, S. R. Young, J. Favor, and R. L. Maas, "PAX6 gene dosage effect in a family with congenital cataracts, aniridia, anophthalmia and central nervous system defects," *Nature Genetics*, vol. 7, no. 4, pp. 463–471, 1994.

[7] T. Glaser, D. S. Walton, and R. L. Maas, "Genomic structure, evolutionary conservation and aniridia mutations in the human PAX6 gene," *Nature Genetics*, vol. 2, no. 3, pp. 232–239, 1992.

[8] R. Ashery-Padan, T. Marquardt, X. Zhou, and P. Gruss, "Pax6 activity in the lens primordium is required for lens formation and for correct placement of a single retina in the eye," *Genes & Development*, vol. 14, no. 21, pp. 2701–2711, 2000.

[9] N. Bäumer, T. Marquardt, A. Stoykova, R. Ashery-Padan, K. Chowdhury, and P. Gruss, "Pax6 is required for establishing naso-temporal and dorsal characteristics of the optic vesicle," *Development*, vol. 129, no. 19, pp. 4535–4545, 2002.

[10] M. V. Canto-Soler and R. Adler, "Optic cup and lens development requires Pax6 expression in the early optic vesicle during a narrow time window," *Developmental Biology*, vol. 294, no. 1, pp. 119–132, 2006.

[11] N. Davis, C. Yoffe, S. Raviv et al., "Pax6 dosage requirements in iris and ciliary body differentiation," *Developmental Biology*, vol. 333, no. 1, pp. 132–142, 2009.

[12] J. C. Grindley, D. R. Davidson, and R. E. Hill, "The role of Pax-6 in eye and nasal development," *Development*, vol. 121, no. 5, pp. 1433–1442, 1995.

[13] R. E. Hill, J. Favor, B. L. M. Hogan et al., "Mouse small eye results from mutations in a paired-like homeobox-containing gene," *Nature*, vol. 354, no. 6354, pp. 522–525, 1991.

[14] B. L. Hogan, E. M. Hirst, G. Horsburgh, and C. M. Hetherington, "Small eye (Sey): a mouse model for the analysis of craniofacial abnormalities," *Development*, vol. 103, pp. 115–119, 1988.

[15] M. Kroeber, N. Davis, S. Holzmann et al., "Reduced expression of Pax6 in lens and cornea of mutant mice leads to failure of chamber angle development and juvenile glaucoma," *Human Molecular Genetics*, vol. 19, no. 17, pp. 3332–3342, 2010.

[16] S. Nornes, M. Clarkson, I. Mikkola et al., "Zebrafish contains two Pax6 genes involved in eye development," *Mechanisms of Development*, vol. 77, no. 2, pp. 185–196, 1998.

[17] N. Azuma, Y. Yamaguchi, H. Handa et al., "Mutations of the PAX6 gene detected in patients with a variety of optic-nerve malformations," *The American Journal of Human Genetics*, vol. 72, no. 6, pp. 1565–1570, 2003.

[18] F. Bayrakli, I. Guney, Y. Bayri et al., "A novel heterozygous deletion within the 3′ region of the PAX6 gene causing isolated aniridia in a large family group," *Journal of Clinical Neuroscience*, vol. 16, no. 12, pp. 1610–1614, 2009.

[19] S. Bhatia, H. Bengani, M. Fish et al., "Disruption of autoregulatory feedback by a mutation in a remote, ultraconserved PAX6 enhancer causes aniridia," *The American Journal of Human Genetics*, vol. 93, no. 6, pp. 1126–1134, 2013.

[20] A. Brown, M. McKie, V. van Heyningen, and J. Prosser, "The human PAX6 mutation database," *Nucleic Acids Research*, vol. 26, no. 1, pp. 259–264, 1998.

[21] P. Chen, X. Zang, D. Sun et al., "Mutation analysis of paired box 6 gene in inherited aniridia in northern China," *Molecular Vision*, vol. 19, pp. 1169–1177, 2013.

[22] F. Cheng, W. Song, Y. Kang, S. Yu, and H. Yuan, "A 556 kb deletion in the downstream region of the PAX6 gene causes familial aniridia and other eye anomalies in a Chinese family," *Molecular Vision*, vol. 17, pp. 448–455, 2011.

[23] A. V. D'Elia, L. Pellizzari, D. Fabbro et al., "A deletion 3′ to the PAX6 gene in familial aniridia cases," *Molecular Vision*, vol. 13, pp. 1245–1250, 2007.

[24] I. De Becker, M. Walter, and L.-P. Noel, "Phenotypic variations in patients with a 1630 A>T point mutation in the PAX6 gene," *Canadian Journal of Ophthalmology*, vol. 39, no. 3, pp. 272–278, 2004.

[25] M. Sarfarazi, R. R. McInnes, E. F. Percin et al., "Human microphthalmia associated with mutations in the retinal homeobox gene CHX10," *Nature Genetics*, vol. 25, no. 4, pp. 397–401, 2000.

[26] E. Gramer, C. Reiter, and G. Gramer, "Glaucoma and frequency of ocular and general diseases in 30 patients with aniridia: a clinical study," *European Journal of Ophthalmology*, vol. 22, no. 1, pp. 104–110, 2018.

[27] I. M. Hanson, J. M. Fletcher, T. Jordan et al., "Mutations at the PAX6 locus are found in heterogeneous anterior segment malformations including Peters' anomaly," *Nature Genetics*, vol. 6, no. 2, pp. 168–173, 1994.

[28] Y. Kang, Y. Lin, X. Li et al., "Mutation analysis of PAX6 in inherited and sporadic aniridia from northeastern China," *Molecular Vision*, vol. 18, pp. 1750–1754, 2012.

[29] J. D. Lauderdale, J. S. Wilensky, E. R. Oliver, D. S. Walton, and T. Glaser, "3′ deletions cause aniridia by preventing PAX6 gene expression," *Proceedings of the National Academy of Sciences of the United States of America*, vol. 97, no. 25, pp. 13755–13759, 2000.

[30] Y. Lin, X. Liu, S. Yu et al., "PAX6 analysis of two sporadic patients from southern China with classic aniridia," *Molecular Vision*, vol. 18, pp. 2190–2194, 2012.

[31] S. H. Park, M. S. Kim, H. Chae, Y. Kim, and M. Kim, "Molecular analysis of the PAX6 gene for congenital aniridia in the Korean population: identification of four novel mutations," *Molecular Vision*, vol. 18, pp. 488–494, 2012.

[32] J. Prosser and V. van Heyningen, "PAX6 mutations reviewed," *Human Mutation*, vol. 11, no. 2, pp. 93–108, 1998.

[33] D. O. Robinson, R. J. Howarth, K. A. Williamson, V. van Heyningen, S. J. Beal, and J. A. Crolla, "Genetic analysis of chromosome 11p13 and the PAX6 gene in a series of 125 cases referred with aniridia," *American Journal of Medical Genetics Part A*, vol. 146A, no. 5, pp. 558–569, 2008.

[34] I. Tzoulaki, I. M. S. White, and I. M. Hanson, "PAX6 mutations: genotype-phenotype correlations," *BMC Genetics*, vol. 6, no. 1, p. 27, 2005.

[35] A. Wawrocka, B. Budny, S. Debicki, A. Jamsheer, A. Sowinska, and M. R. Krawczynski, "PAX6 3′ deletion in a family with aniridia," *Ophthalmic Genetics*, vol. 33, no. 1, pp. 44–48, 2011.

[36] N. Weisschuh, B. Wissinger, and E. Gramer, "A splice site mutation in the PAX6 gene which induces exon skipping causes autosomal dominant inherited aniridia," *Molecular Vision*, vol. 18, pp. 751–757, 2012.

[37] X. Zhang, P. Wang, S. Li, X. Xiao, X. Guo, and Q. Zhang, "Mutation spectrum of PAX6 in Chinese patients with aniridia," *Molecular Vision*, vol. 17, pp. 2139–2147, 2011.

[38] H. Kokotas and M. B. Petersen, "Clinical and molecular aspects of aniridia," *Clinical Genetics*, vol. 77, no. 5, pp. 409–420, 2010.

[39] B. Schmidt-Sidor, K. Szymańska, K. Williamson et al., "Malformations of the brain in two fetuses with a compound heterozygosity for two PAX6 mutations," *Folia Neuropathologica*, vol. 47, no. 4, pp. 372–382, 2009.

[40] B. D. Solomon, D. E. Pineda-Alvarez, J. Z. Balog et al., "Compound heterozygosity for mutations inPAX6in a patient with complex brain anomaly, neonatal diabetes mellitus, and microophthalmia," *American Journal of Medical Genetics. Part A*, vol. 149A, no. 11, pp. 2543–2546, 2009.

[41] M. Hingorani, I. Hanson, and V. van Heyningen, "Aniridia," *European Journal of Human Genetics*, vol. 20, no. 10, pp. 1011–1017, 2012.

[42] H. Lee, R. Khan, and M. O'Keefe, "Aniridia: current pathology and management," *Acta Ophthalmologica*, vol. 86, no. 7, pp. 708–715, 2008.

[43] L. B. Nelson, G. L. Spaeth, T. S. Nowinski, C. E. Margo, and L. Jackson, "Aniridia: a review," *Survey of Ophthalmology*, vol. 28, no. 6, pp. 621–642, 1984.

[44] C. C. T. Ton, H. Hirvonen, H. Miwa et al., "Positional cloning and characterization of a paired box- and homeobox-containing gene from the aniridia region," *Cell*, vol. 67, no. 6, pp. 1059–1074, 1991.

[45] I. Hanson, A. Churchill, J. Love et al., "Missense mutations in the most ancient residues of the PAX6 paired domain underlie a spectrum of human congenital eye malformations," *Human Molecular Genetics*, vol. 8, no. 2, pp. 165–172, 1999.

[46] H. M. Reza, Y. Takahashi, and K. Yasuda, "Stage-dependent expression of Pax6 in optic vesicle/cup regulates patterning genes through signaling molecules," *Differentiation*, vol. 75, no. 8, pp. 726–736, 2007.

[47] A. Bhinge, J. Poschmann, S. C. Namboori et al., "MiR-135b is a direct PAX6 target and specifies human neuroectoderm by inhibiting TGF-β/BMP signaling," *The EMBO Journal*, vol. 33, no. 1, pp. 1271–1283, 2014.

[48] A. Blixt, H. Landgren, B. R. Johansson, and P. Carlsson, "Foxe3 is required for morphogenesis and differentiation of the

anterior segment of the eye and is sensitive to Pax6 gene dosage," *Developmental Biology*, vol. 302, no. 1, pp. 218–229, 2007.

[49] T. Grocott, S. Johnson, A. P. Bailey, and A. Streit, "Neural crest cells organize the eye via TGF-β and canonical Wnt signalling," *Nature Communications*, vol. 2, p. 265, 2011.

[50] Y. Kamachi, M. Uchikawa, A. Tanouchi, R. Sekido, and H. Kondoh, "Pax6 and SOX2 form a co-DNA binding partner complex that regulates initiation of lens development," *Genes & Development*, vol. 15, no. 10, pp. 1272–1286, 2001.

[51] Y. Ma, K. Certel, Y. Gao et al., "Functional interactions between drosophila bHLH/PAS, Sox, and POU transcription factors regulate CNS midline expression of the slit gene," *The Journal of Neuroscience*, vol. 20, no. 12, pp. 4596–4605, 2000.

[52] C. Carrière, S. Plaza, J. Caboche et al., "Nuclear localization signals, DNA binding, and transactivation properties of quail Pax-6 (Pax-QNR) isoforms," *Cell Growth & Differentiation*, vol. 6, no. 12, pp. 1531–1540, 1995.

[53] P. X. Xu, X. Zhang, S. Heaney, A. Yoon, A. M. Michelson, and R. L. Maas, "Regulation of Pax6 expression is conserved between mice and flies," *Development*, vol. 126, no. 2, pp. 383–395, 1999.

[54] S. Singh, R. Mishra, N. A. Arango, J. M. Deng, R. R. Behringer, and G. F. Saunders, "Iris hypoplasia in mice that lack the alternatively spliced Pax6(5a) isoform," *Proceedings of the National Academy of Sciences of the United States of America*, vol. 99, no. 10, pp. 6812–6815, 2002.

[55] Q. Yan, L. Gong, M. Deng et al., "Sumoylation activates the transcriptional activity of Pax-6, an important transcription factor for eye and brain development," *Proceedings of the National Academy of Sciences of the United States of America*, vol. 107, no. 49, pp. 21034–21039, 2010.

[56] T. C. Tuoc and A. Stoykova, "Trim11 modulates the function of neurogenic transcription factor Pax6 through ubiquitin-proteosome system," *Genes & Development*, vol. 22, no. 14, pp. 1972–1986, 2008.

[57] J. Sun, S. Rockowitz, Q. Xie, R. Ashery-Padan, D. Zheng, and A. Cvekl, "Identification of in vivo DNA-binding mechanisms of Pax6 and reconstruction of Pax6-dependent gene regulatory networks during forebrain and lens development," *Nucleic Acids Research*, vol. 43, no. 14, pp. 6827–6846, 2015.

[58] M. Sander, A. Neubuser, J. Kalamaras, H. C. Ee, G. R. Martin, and M. S. German, "Genetic analysis reveals that PAX6 is required for normal transcription of pancreatic hormone genes and islet development," *Genes & Development*, vol. 11, no. 13, pp. 1662–1673, 1997.

[59] L. St-Onge, B. Sosa-Pineda, K. Chowdhury, A. Mansouri, and P. Gruss, "Pax6 is required for differentiation of glucagon-producing alpha-cells in mouse pancreas," *Nature*, vol. 387, no. 6631, pp. 406–409, 1997.

[60] T. Yasuda, Y. Kajimoto, Y. Fujitani et al., "PAX6 mutation as a genetic factor common to aniridia and glucose intolerance," *Diabetes*, vol. 51, no. 1, pp. 224–230, 2002.

[61] L. Hergott-Faure, S. Borot, C. Kleinclauss, M. Abitbol, and A. Penfornis, "Pituitary function and glucose tolerance in a family with a PAX6 mutation," *Annales d'endocrinologie*, vol. 73, no. 6, pp. 510–514, 2012.

[62] G. M. Wang, L. Prasov, J. Richards, and B. L. Bohnsack, "Phenotypic variation in a four-generation family with aniridia carrying a novel PAX6 mutation," *Journal of AAPOS*, vol. 21, no. 4, pp. e36–e37, 2017.

18

Poor Sleep Quality is the Risk Factor for Central Serous Chorioretinopathy

Yuying Ji, Miaoling Li, Xiongze Zhang, Yuting Peng, and Feng Wen

State Key Laboratory of Ophthalmology, Zhongshan Ophthalmic Center, Sun Yat-sen University, 54 South Xianlie Road, Guangzhou 510060, China

Correspondence should be addressed to Feng Wen; wenfeng208@foxmail.com

Academic Editor: Enrico Peiretti

Purpose. Whether sleep disturbance is related with central serous chorioretinopathy (CSC) is still in controversy. This study is designed to investigate sleep status in CSC using definite and well-established methods. *Methods.* A total of 134 CSC patients and 134 age- and sex-matched normal controls were recruited in the study. Demographic data were collected through a questionnaire. Body mass index (BMI) was calculated by weight divided by height squared. The Pittsburgh Sleep Quality Index (PSQI) and Epworth Sleepiness Scale (ESS) were administered to all subjects to assess the sleep quality and daytime sleepiness, respectively. Depression Anxiety Stress Scales 21-item version (DASS-21) was also used to evaluate the emotion status as a positive control. Poor sleep quality was defined as PSQI > 5 and sleep apnea tendency as ESS > 10. Positive criteria scores were ≥10 for depression, ≥8 for anxiety, and ≥15 for stress. *Results.* There was no significant difference of BMI between the two groups ($p = 0.075$). The prevalence of poor sleep quality (58.2% versus 23.9%; $p < 0.001$) in CSC patients was significantly higher than normal. Specifically, CSC patients presented worse performance in certain components of sleep quality, that is, sleep latency, sleep duration, and sleep efficiency. More participants had stress (23.9% versus 3%, $p < 0.001$), depression (25.4% versus 10.4%; $p = 0.001$), and anxiety (28.4% versus 14.9%; $p = 0.008$) emotions in CSC than that in normal. No significant difference was observed in sleep apnea tendency. Through logistic regression analysis, CSC patients were more likely to be in poor sleep quality ($p < 0.001$; OR 3.608 (2.071–6.285)) and stress emotion ($p = 0.002$, OR 6.734 (1.997–22.711)). *Conclusion.* Poor sleep quality is risk factor for CSC patients. Attention of sleep quality should be paid when treating them.

1. Introduction

Central serous chorioretinopathy (CSC) is a common disorder characterized by serous retinal detachment (SRD) and/or retinal pigment epithelial detachment and often associated with subretinal fluid leakage [1, 2]. It ranks the fourth among the nonsurgical posterior segment diseases [3]. Several independent studies have reported that it occurs most frequently in mid-age with the peak age around 45 years old and a male preponderance [4, 5]. The exact mechanism of CSC is still unknown. Certain events have been reported to be risk factors for CSC, such as stress [6], type A behavior [7], hypertension [8], sleep disturbance [9, 10], or sleep apnea [11, 12]. However, whether sleep disturbance is associated with CSC is in controversy, and sometimes it is confused with sleep apnea. In order to have a better understanding and guidance for the cause and treatment of the disease, we conducted this survey to collect sleep situation of CSC patients and analyze their association with the disease.

2. Materials and Methods

2.1. Compliance. The study procedure was approved by the Ethics Committee of the Zhongshan Ophthalmic Center, Sun Yat-sen University. The protocol was conducted according to the Declaration of Helsinki. After explaining the purpose and procedure of the study, all the subjects signed the written informed consent.

2.2. Inclusion and Exclusion Criteria. Treatment-naive CSC patients were enrolled from the outpatient in the Zhongshan Ophthalmic Center. They all underwent physical examination including height, weight, and blood pressure. Ophthalmic examinations were taken in all the CSC patients, including visual acuity, slit-lamp biomicroscopy, direct ophthalmoscopy, color fundus image, and fundus fluorescence angiography (FFA, FFA 450 plus, Zeiss, Germany).

An inclusion criterion for acute CSC was focal serous retinal detachment involving macula with one or more leakage in FFA within 6 months. For chronic patients, inclusion criteria were persistent subretinal fluid involving macula for at least 6 months or serous retinal detachment with diffuse atrophy and decompensation of retinal pigment epithelium (RPE) (also referred to as diffuse retinal pigment epitheliopathy) with/without gradual, indistinct RPE leakage on FFA [2, 13, 14].

Volunteers enrolled from oral and poster advertisements around our hospital were included as the control group. They were age and sex matched at a ratio of 1 : 1. They all underwent ophthalmic examinations including visual acuity, slit-lamp biomicroscopy, and direct ophthalmoscopy to rule out the ophthalmic diseases. Physical examination including height, weight, and blood pressure was taken in all the participants.

Participants with other fundus diseases such as rhegmatogenous retinal detachment, choroidal neovascularization, polypoidal choroidal vasculopathy (PCV), retinal vein occlusion, diabetic retinopathy, Vogt–Koyanagi–Harada, optic disc pit, and scleritis were excluded. Participants with a history of trauma or surgery within one month were also excluded. Participants with hypertension (when systolic pressure was consistently greater than 140 mmHg or when diastolic pressure was consistently 90 mmHg or more) and alcohol, tobacco, or steroid using history were also excluded.

Finally, a total of 134 CSC patients and 134 age- and sex-matched controls were included in our study.

2.3. Criteria for Evaluations. Body mass index (BMI) was calculated using the formula in which weight in kilograms is divided by height in meters squared. Participants were divided into four groups (underweight, healthy, overweight, and obese) according to the BMI score. Underweight was defined as BMI score <18.5, healthy was 18.5 to 24.99, overweight was 25.0 to 29.99, and obese was 30 or higher.

2.3.1. PSQI. The Pittsburgh Sleep Quality Index (PSQI) is a self-report questionnaire that assesses sleep quality over a 1-month time interval [15], developed by researchers in the University of Pittsburgh (http://www.psychiatry.pitt.edu/node/8240). The PSQI was intended to be a standardized sleep questionnaire for clinicians and researchers. The PSQI has well-established reliability and validity and is widely used in clinical research. The measure consists of 19 individual items designed to assess seven components of sleep: subjective sleep quality, sleep latency, sleep duration, habitual sleep efficiency, sleep disturbances, use of sleeping medication, and daytime dysfunction. These items generate a global score with a range of 0–21. More global sleep score indicated poorer sleep quality. A global sleep score above 5 (not including 5) was defined as poor sleep quality in our study.

2.3.2. ESS. The Epworth Sleepiness Scale (ESS) is a scale introduced in 1991 in Australia. The scale was designed to measure daytime sleepiness and was helpful in diagnosing sleep disorders [16]. The questionnaire described eight different situations in daily life and asked the subject to rate his or her probability of falling asleep on a scale of increasing possibility from 0 to 3. The cumulative score in eight questions was the total score. A number below 10 was considered to be normal and above 10 indicated a tendency for sleep apnea.

2.3.3. Emotion Status Evaluation. Stress was thought to be closely related with CSC. So, we used Depression Anxiety Stress Scales 21-item version (DASS-21) to evaluate the emotion status as a positive control. DASS, developed by Lovibond and Lovibond [17], was made up of 42 self-report items designed to measure the three related negative emotional states of depression, anxiety, and tension/stress. The DASS-21 was a short version of DASS that contains a 21-question assessment and had the same internal consistency and concurrent validity as DASS. It included seven questions. The scores were calculated by adding up the scores for each item in the section. Each of these was rated on a four-point Likert Scale of frequency or severity of the participants' experiences over the last week with the intention of emphasizing states over traits. These scores ranged from 0, meaning that the client believed the item "did not apply to them at all," to 3 meaning that the client considered the item to "apply to them very much or most of the time." The definition of positive in emotion was 10 and above for depression, 8 and above for anxiety, 15 and above for stress.

2.4. Survey Quality Control. All the investigators were medical professionals. They were trained about the survey components and the survey process. Participants filled in the questionnaire by themselves. Investigators supervised the circumstances and the time. After the survey was done, investigators made sure that participants had already answered all the questions. If there were any obvious mistakes and omit options, investigators pointed out and explained to participants to help complete the survey.

2.5. Statistical Analysis. The SPSS 22.0 software (SPSS Inc., Chicago, IL, USA) was used to perform the statistical analysis. The continuous variables were expressed in the form mean ± standard deviation in normal distributed sample and in frequency and percentage form in non-normally distributed sample. The independent *t*-test and Mann–Whitney *U* test were used for the comparison of continuous variables. The chi-square test and Kruskal–Wallis *H* test were used to compare the categorical variables. Pearson correlation analysis was used to evaluate the relationship between PSQI and DASS-21 scores. Logistic regression analysis was used to compare the risk factors between CSC and normal controls. $p < 0.05$ was considered to be statistically significant.

According to the positive rates in CSC patients and normal controls, the set of alpha was 0.01, permissible error was less than 0.01, the sample size should be larger than 133 to estimate the differences.

3. Results

The demographic data of 134 CSC patients and 134 normal controls are shown in Table 1. Participants were predominantly male with a mean age of 44.57 ± 6.29 years for CSC patients and 44.36 ± 5.83 for normal controls ($p = 0.777$). The mean BMI is 22.51 ± 2.38 for CSC patients and 22.32 ± 2.80 for controls with an insignificant difference ($p = 0.075$).

Among all the participants, 20 CSC patients and 16 normal controls had gone to bed after 24:00, with the last one at 2 a.m. in the morning. Ten CSC patients and 10 normal controls had got up early in the morning; the earliest is around 4 a.m. in the morning. As shown in Table 1, no differences were observed in the distribution of sleep and wake up time between CSC patients and normal controls ($p = 0.161$ for sleep time; $p = 0.333$ for wake up time).

The PSQI, ESS, and DASS scale results are shown in Table 2. According to the cutoff criterion, 58.2% of CSC patients and 23.9% of normal controls had poor sleep quality. There were 23.9% of CSC patients and only 3% of normal controls who were in stress emotion. The percentage of poor sleep quality and stress emotion in CSC patients was significantly higher than that in normal controls ($p < 0.001$). There were also more participants who had depression and anxiety emotion in CSC than in normal controls with a statistically different p value ($p = 0.001$ for depression, $p = 0.008$ for anxiety). No significant difference was observed in sleep apnea tendency between two groups. Through Pearson correlation analysis, a positive correlation existed between PSQI and DASS-21 scores in both groups, as shown in Table 3.

The details in four out of seven subscale dimensions of PSQI are shown in Table 4. Compared with controls, CSC patients reported more percentage in bad subjective sleep quality ($p < 0.001$), longer time of sleep latency ($p < 0.001$), shorter sleep duration ($p < 0.001$), and less sleep efficiency ($p < 0.001$), indicating they were worse sleepers than normal controls.

Table 5 shows the results of logistic regression analysis. It showed that CSC patients were more likely to be in poor sleep quality ($p < 0.001$; OR 3.608 (2.071–6.285)) and stress emotion ($p = 0.002$; OR 6.734 (1.997–22.711)). But depression did not increase the risk ($p = 0.378$; OR 1.563 (0.579–4.218)) neither did the anxiety ($p = 0.390$; OR 0.669 (0.267–1.673)).

4. Discussion

Our case-control study involving a relatively large sample size reveals that CSC patients performed worse in sleep function and emotion regulation in China, suggesting that poor sleep quality and stress are risk factors for CSC. But sleep apnea is not associated with CSC.

Our findings expand the observations of sleep status in CSC patients. Setrouk et al. [18] conducted a retrospective case-control study, and there was no significant difference in

Table 1: Comparison between CSC patients and normal controls.

	CSC ($n = 134$)	Control ($n = 134$)	p
Age (mean ± standard deviation)	44.57 ± 6.29	44.36 ± 5.83	0.777 (independent t-test)
Sex			
Male	110 (82.1%)	110 (82.1%)	1 (chi-square test)
Female	24 (17.9)	24 (17.9)	
BMI	22.51 ± 2.38	22.32 ± 2.80	0.075 (Kruskal–Wallis H test)
Underweight	6 (4.5%)	8 (5.97%)	
Healthy	106 (79.1%)	114 (85.07%)	
Overweight	22 (16.4%)	12 (8.96%)	
Sleep time			
20:00–21:00	4 (2.99%)	10 (7.46%)	0.161 (Kruskal–Wallis H test)
21:01–24:00	110 (82.10%)	108 (80.60%)	
0:01–2:00	20 (14.93%)	16 (11.94%)	
Wake up time			
4:00–5:00	10 (7.46%)	10 (7.46%)	0.333 (Kruskal–Wallis H test)
5:01–9:00	118 (88.06%)	112 (83.58%)	
9:01–10:00	6 (4.48%)	12 (8.96%)	

CSC, central serous chorioretinopathy; BMI, body mass index.

Table 2: Sleep and emotion status in CSC patients and controls.

	Results	Score	CSC	Control	p (chi-square test)
PSQI	–	≤5	56 (41.8%)	102 (76.1%)	**<0.001**
	+	>5	78 (58.2%)	32 (23.9%)	
ESS	–	≤10	120 (89.6%)	122 (91.0%)	0.680
	+	>10	14 (10.4%)	12 (9.0%)	
Depression	–	<10	100 (74.6%)	120 (89.6%)	0.001
	+	≥10	34 (25.4%)	14 (10.4%)	
Anxiety	–	<8	96 (71.6%)	114 (85.1%)	0.008
	+	≥8	38 (28.4%)	20 (14.9%)	
Stress	–	<15	102 (76.1%)	130 (97.0%)	**<0.001**
	+	≥15	32 (23.9%)	4 (3.0%)	

CSC, central serous chorioretinopathy; PSQI, Pittsburgh Sleep Quality Index; ESS, Epworth Sleepiness Scale.

Table 3: Correlation between PSQI and DASS-21 scores in CSC and control groups (Pearson correlation analysis).

	PSQI (CSC)		PSQI (control)	
	r	p	r	p
Depression	0.350	<0.001	0.529	<0.001
Anxiety	0.235	0.006	0.577	<0.001
Stress	0.369	<0.001	0.588	<0.001

CSC, central serous chorioretinopathy; PSQI, Pittsburgh Sleep Quality.

Table 4: Subscale of sleep features in CSC and controls.

	CSC		Controls		*p*
	n	%	*n*	%	
Subjective sleep quality					
0-very good	14	10.4	30	22.4	
1-fairly good	74	55.2	86	64.2	**<0.001**
2-fairly bad	24	17.9	18	13.4	(Kruskal–Wallis *H* test)
3-very bad	22	16.4	0	0	
Sleep latency >15 min	116	86.6	86	64.2	**<0.001** (chi-square test)
Sleep duration					
>7 h	46	32.8	94	70.1	
6-7 h	42	31.3	28	20.9	**<0.001**
5-6 h	28	20.9	6	4.5	(Kruskal–Wallis *H* test)
<5 h	18	13.4	6	4.5	
Sleep efficiency					
≥85%	66	49.3	110	82.1	
75%–84%	30	22.4	16	11.9	**<0.001**
65%–74%	20	14.9	2	1.5	(Kruskal–Wallis *H* test)
<65%	18	13.4	6	4.5	

CSC, central serous chorioretinopathy.

Table 5: The logistic regression of risk factors in CSC.

	Odds ratio	95% confidence interval	*p* value
PSQI ≥ 5	3.608	2.071–6.285	<0.001
Stress (+)	6.734	1.997–22.711	0.002
Depression (+)	1.563	0.579–4.218	0.378
Anxiety (+)	0.669	0.267–1.673	0.390

CSC, central serous chorioretinopathy; PSQI, Pittsburgh Sleep Quality Index.

PSQI scores between chronic CSC and other patients with a limited sample size of 29. A retrospective study carried out in Korea in 2012 including 113 CSC patients indicated that sleep disturbance defined as "subjects were questioned whether they awoke feeling tired or if they experienced fatigue during the day" was strongly associated with CSC [9]. This definition was indistinct. We use a standard assessment of sleep quality by the PSQI questionnaire, which combined the quality and quantity of sleep, graded sleep according to the scores, and was a validated, reliable tool. Through our study, we find that CSC patients in China had worse sleep quality, especially in dimension of subjective sleep quality, sleep latency, sleep duration, and sleep efficiency. These findings provide more information about CSC patients. In a meta-analysis conducted by Liu et al. [10], three studies used for the "sleep disturbance" were not under the same criteria. Two of the three studies were actually related with sleep apnea, and one study conducted by Brodie et al. [11], as we previous described, had ruled out the obstructive sleep apnea as a risk factor after being adjusted for BMI. The remaining study used a vague definition for "sleep disturbance" as discussed before.

Our study does not evaluate shift work or irregular hours which might have an impact on CSC through circadian disruption [18–20]. But from the sleep and wake up time of our participants, no obvious circadian disruption is observed.

Our study does not suggest that patients with CSC are more likely to have sleep apnea. In a meta-analysis conducted by Wu et al. [21], it was suggested that patients with CSCR is more likely to have sleep apnea. But the diagnostic criteria were not the same in the included six studies. And BMI, a known risk factor for sleep apnea [22, 23], was not investigated in five out of the six studies. When Brodie et al. [11] corrected the BMI, no significant relationship was found between obstructive sleep apnea and CSC. Although sleep apnea is not diagnosed through ESS, scores over 10 are indicating a tendency for sleep apnea. Our result is similar with Brodie's result. This might be attributed to the BMI, an important risk factor for obstructive sleep apnea. Most patients in our study have a normal BMI as the normal controls.

Our study further extends the understanding of emotion status in CSC patients. Data from DASS-21 show that prevalence of depression, anxiety, and stress emotion was significantly higher in CSC patients compared to that in normal controls. Psychological stress and type A behavior were found to be associated with onset of CSC [6, 7]. Furthermore, in recent years, antianxiety drugs [24], psychopharmacologic medication use [25], and stress [19] were found to be risk factors for CSC, and a history of psychiatric illness increased the CSC recurrence risk [26]. The scores and grading in our DASS-21 test provide further evidence from CSC patients' subjective feelings, suggesting that many CSC patients have unhealthy emotions especially the stress.

The cause and effect relationship between sleep, emotion, and CSC is not clear. The following are our speculations. First, glucocorticoid is involved in the development of central serous chorioretinopathy [27]. Increased levels of 24-hour urine corticosteroid and serum cortisol are found in CSC patients [28, 29]. Under certain physiological stress, the adrenal gland secretes glucocorticoid in response to the signal from the hypothalamus and may contribute to the pathogenesis of the disorder [30]. Second, depression will influence the effects of peptides on sleep EEG and hormone secretion [31], and this could explain that there are more patients with the depression emotion than controls. These studies suggest that attention should be paid to patients' emotions and sleep quality when treating CSC patients.

There are some limitations of this study. First, we do not include all the possible risk factors for CSC such as *Helicobacter pylori* and shift work to be more comprehensive. Second, the patients enrolled in this study come from one ophthalmic center, and multicenter analysis will be more persuasive and thorough.

5. Conclusion

The study reveals that poor sleep quality and stress emotion are risk factors for CSC patients in China. It may indicate that attention should be paid to patients' sleep and emotions to achieve better treatment outcome.

Abbreviations

BMI: Body mass index

CSC: Central serous chorioretinopathy
DASS: Depression Anxiety Stress Scales
ESS: Epworth Sleepiness Scale
FFA: Fundus fluorescence angiography
PCV: Polypoidal choroidal vasculopathy
PSQI: Pittsburgh Sleep Quality Index
RPE: Retinal pigment epithelium
SRD: Serous retinal detachment.

Conflicts of Interest

The authors declare that they have no conflicts of interest.

Acknowledgments

This study was supported by the National Natural Science Foundation of China (Grant no. 81470647), the Fundamental Research Funds of State Key Laboratory of Ophthalmology, and the Medical Science Technology Research Funds of Guangdong Province (Grant no. A2016101).

References

[1] A. Daruich, A. Matet, A. Dirani et al., "Central serous chorioretinopathy: recent findings and new physiopathology hypothesis," *Progress in Retinal and Eye Research*, vol. 48, pp. 82–118, 2015.

[2] B. Nicholson, J. Noble, F. Forooghian, and C. Meyerle, "Central serous chorioretinopathy: update on pathophysiology and treatment," *Survey of Ophthalmology*, vol. 58, no. 2, pp. 103–126, 2013.

[3] M. Wang, I. C. Munch, P. W. Hasler, C. Prunte, and M. Larsen, "Central serous chorioretinopathy," *Acta Ophthalmologica*, vol. 86, no. 2, pp. 126–145, 2008.

[4] A. S. Kitzmann, J. S. Pulido, N. N. Diehl, D. O. Hodge, and J. P. Burke, "The incidence of central serous chorioretinopathy in Olmsted county, Minnesota, 1980–2002," *Ophthalmology*, vol. 115, no. 1, pp. 169–173, 2008.

[5] R. Liegl and M. W. Ulbig, "Central serous chorioretinopathy," *Ophthalmologica*, vol. 232, no. 2, pp. 65–76, 2014.

[6] G. S. Gelber and H. Schatz, "Loss of vision due to central serous chorioretinopathy following psychological stress," *American Journal of Psychiatry*, vol. 144, no. 1, pp. 46–50, 1987.

[7] L. A. Yannuzzi, "Type-A behavior and central serous chorioretinopathy," *Retina*, vol. 7, no. 2, pp. 111–131, 1987.

[8] R. Haimovici, S. Koh, D. R. Gagnon, T. Lehrfeld, and S. Wellik, "Risk factors for central serous chorioretinopathy: a case-control study," *Ophthalmology*, vol. 111, no. 2, pp. 244–249, 2004.

[9] Y. Eom, J. Oh, S. W. Kim, and K. Huh, "Systemic factors associated with central serous chorioretinopathy in Koreans," *Korean Journal of Ophthalmology*, vol. 26, no. 4, pp. 260–264, 2012.

[10] B. Liu, T. Deng, and J. Zhang, "Risk factors for central serous chorioretinopathy: a systematic review and meta-analysis," *Retina*, vol. 36, no. 1, pp. 9–19, 2016.

[11] F. L. Brodie, E. S. Charlson, T. S. Aleman et al., "Obstructive sleep apnea and central serous chorioretinopathy," *Retina*, vol. 35, no. 2, pp. 238–243, 2015.

[12] G. F. Yavaş, T. Küsbeci, M. Kaşikci et al., "Obstructive sleep apnea in patients with central serous chorioretinopathy," *Current Eye Research*, vol. 1, no. 39, pp. 88–92, 2013.

[13] F. C. Piccolino, C. M. Eandi, L. Ventre, R. C. R. De La Longrais, and F. M. Grignolo, "Photodynamic therapy for chronic central serous chorioretinopathy," *Retina*, vol. 23, no. 6, pp. 752–763, 2003.

[14] L. A. Yannuzzi, J. S. Slakter, N. E. Gross et al., "Indocyanine green angiography-guided photodynamic therapy for treatment of chronic central serous chorioretinopathy: a pilot study," *Retina*, vol. 23, no. 3, pp. 288–298, 2003.

[15] D. J. Buysse, C. R. Reynolds, T. H. Monk, S. R. Berman, and D. J. Kupfer, "The Pittsburgh Sleep Quality Index: a new instrument for psychiatric practice and research," *Psychiatry Research*, vol. 28, no. 2, pp. 193–213, 1989.

[16] M. W. Johns, "A new method for measuring daytime sleepiness: the Epworth Sleepiness Scale," *Sleep*, vol. 14, no. 6, pp. 540–545, 1991.

[17] P. F. Lovibond and S. H. Lovibond, "The structure of negative emotional states: comparison of the Depression Anxiety Stress Scales (DASS) with the beck depression and anxiety inventories," *Behaviour Research and Therapy*, vol. 33, no. 3, pp. 335–343, 1995.

[18] E. Setrouk, B. Hubault, F. Vankemmel et al., "Circadian disturbance and idiopathic central serous chorioretinopathy," *Graefe's Archive for Clinical and Experimental Ophthalmology*, vol. 254, no. 11, pp. 2175–2181, 2016.

[19] E. Bousquet, M. Dhundass, M. Lehmann et al., "Shift work: a risk factor for central serous chorioretinopathy," *American Journal of Ophthalmology*, vol. 165, pp. 23–28, 2016.

[20] K. J. Wright, R. K. Bogan, and J. K. Wyatt, "Shift work and the assessment and management of shift work disorder (SWD)," *Sleep Medicine Reviews*, vol. 17, no. 1, pp. 41–54, 2013.

[21] C. Y. Wu, T. Riangwiwat, P. Rattanawong, B. Nesmith, and A. Deobhakta, "Association of obstructive sleep apnea with central serous chorioretinopathy and choroidal thickness: a systematic review and meta-analysis," *Retina*, 2018, In press.

[22] T. Young, M. Palta, J. Dempsey, J. Skatrud, S. Weber, and S. Badr, "The occurrence of sleep-disordered breathing among middle-aged adults," *New England Journal of Medicine*, vol. 328, no. 17, pp. 1230–1235, 1993.

[23] P. E. Peppard, T. Young, J. H. Barnet, M. Palta, E. W. Hagen, and K. M. Hla, "Increased prevalence of sleep-disordered breathing in adults," *American Journal of Epidemiology*, vol. 177, no. 9, pp. 1006–1014, 2013.

[24] D. C. Tsai, S. J. Chen, C. C. Huang et al., "Epidemiology of idiopathic central serous chorioretinopathy in Taiwan, 2001–2006: a population-based study," *PLoS One*, vol. 8, no. 6, Article ID e66858, 2013.

[25] M. K. Tittl, R. F. Spaide, D. Wong et al., "Systemic findings associated with central serous chorioretinopathy," *American Journal of Ophthalmology*, vol. 128, no. 1, pp. 63–68, 1999.

[26] A. C. Fok, P. P. Chan, D. S. Lam, and T. Y. Lai, "Risk factors for recurrence of serous macular detachment in untreated patients with central serous chorioretinopathy," *Ophthalmic Research*, vol. 46, no. 3, pp. 160–163, 2011.

[27] E. A. Bouzas, P. Karadimas, and C. J. Pournaras, "Central serous chorioretinopathy and glucocorticoids," *Survey of Ophthalmology*, vol. 47, no. 5, pp. 431–448, 2002.

[28] S. P. Garg, T. Dada, D. Talwar, and N. R. Biswas, "Endogenous cortisol profile in patients with central serous chorioretin-

opathy," *British Journal of Ophthalmology*, vol. 81, no. 11, pp. 962–964, 1997.

[29] R. Haimovici, S. Rumelt, and J. Melby, "Endocrine abnormalities in patients with central serous chorioretinopathy," *Ophthalmology*, vol. 110, no. 4, pp. 698–703, 2003.

[30] N. C. Nicolaides, E. Kyratzi, A. Lamprokostopoulou, G. P. Chrousos, and E. Charmandari, "Stress, the stress system and the role of glucocorticoids," *Neuroimmunomodulation*, vol. 22, no. 1-2, pp. 6–19, 2015.

[31] A. Steiger, M. Dresler, M. Kluge, and P. Schussler, "Pathology of sleep, hormones and depression," *Pharmacopsychiatry*, vol. 46, no. S1, pp. S30–S35, 2013.

19

Manifestation of Clinical Categories of Ocular Graft-versus-Host Disease

Yuan Qiu, Jing Hong, and Rongmei Peng

Department of Ophthalmology, Peking University Third Hospital, Beijing, China

Correspondence should be addressed to Jing Hong; hongjing196401@163.com

Academic Editor: Marta Sacchetti

This study aims at improving the understanding of the subjective symptoms and signs of two different clinical categories of ocular graft-versus-host disease. After reviewing and screening 193 posthematopoietic stem cell transplantation (HSCT) patients of Peking University Third Hospital, we enrolled 148 (21 acute ocular GVHD, 127 chronic ocular GVHD). Patients' subjective symptoms, ocular parameters, and typical ocular signs were collected and evaluated at the same visit. Classic acute ocular GVHD patients had variable levels of conjunctival involvement but few had keratopathy; increased mucus secretion (21 of 21, 100.0%), red eye (19 of 21, 90.5%), and lacrimation (11 of 21, 52.4%) were the characteristic symptoms. The classic chronic ocular group had severe eye dryness and further corneal lesions, including filamentary keratitis, corneal ulcer, and corneal vascularization. Eye dryness (115 of 127, 90.6%), increased fibrous secretion (53 of 127, 41.7%), photophobia (50 of 127, 39.4%), and alacrimia (45 of 127, 35.4%) were the most common symptoms. Although 44.1% (56 of 127) of these patients had a history of acute ocular GVHD episodes, most were overlooked, so they did not receive stepwise evaluation and treatment. Management of ocular GVHD is very challenging and requires cooperation among disciplines.

1. Introduction

Allogeneic hematopoietic stem cell transplantation (allo-HSCT) is a potentially curative treatment for a variety of hematologic malignancies, and indications for HSCT could expand to other blood disorders, such as aplastic anemia, sickle cell disease, and immune disorders [1–3]. More than 25,000 HSCT procedures are performed annually, and the number of transplants and survival rates are increasing worldwide [4, 5].

Graft-versus-host disease (GVHD), an immune-mediated disease caused by complex interactions between donor and recipient immune systems, is a leading cause of morbidity and mortality following HSCT [4, 6, 7]. The 2014 National Institutes of Health Consensus recognized 2 principal categories of GVHD (acute and chronic) according to clinical features rather than the temporal relationship to the time of transplantation. Acute GVHD, which is stimulated by damaged recipient tissue and amplified by donor t-cells, includes the classic manifestations of erythema, maculopapular rash, nausea, vomiting, anorexia, profuse diarrhea, ileus, and cholestatic liver disease. Broad categories of this type of GVHD include classic and late-onset acute GVHD, which occurs within 100 days after transplantation or donor lymphocyte infusion. Chronic GVHD, related to thymic damage and impaired negative selection of autoreactive t-cells, is diagnosed according to at least one diagnostic manifestation or at least one distinctive manifestation plus a pertinent biopsy, laboratory, or other tests (e.g., Schirmer's test) in each organ [6, 8]. The simultaneous presence of features of acute GVHD in patients with chronic GVHD is defined as an overlap syndrome and is classified as a subset of chronic GVHD.

Ocular manifestations can be found in more than 60% of GVHD patients [9]. Dry eye is the most common symptom of GVHD; other distinctive manifestations of chronic ocular GVHD include gritty, cicatricial conjunctivitis, keratoconjunctivitis sicca, and confluent areas of punctate keratopathy [8, 10]. However, these symptoms are inadequate to diagnose ocular GVHD, and reports of other representative subjective symptoms and signs of ocular GVHD are limited.

Thus, physicians are challenged by early recognition and referral of ocular GVHD.

The purpose of this study is to describe, analyze, and compare the characteristics of ocular manifestations of a large cohort of patients with a diagnosis of either acute or chronic ocular GVHD.

2. Materials and Methods

Records of 193 post-HSCT patients who visited Peking University Third Hospital Cornea and Ocular Surface Disease Specialist Clinic from July 2015 to July 2017 were reviewed. Patients who met the following criteria were eligible for the study: (1) diagnosed with ocular GVHD; (2) first visit to ophthalmology clinic; and (3) had not received topical immunosuppressant treatment. Criteria for acute ocular GVHD: (1) recent eye discomfort; (2) classic acute GVHD with skin, GI, or liver involvement; (3) without classic histological or clinical signs of chronic GVHD; and (4) no evidence of infection. Criteria for chronic ocular GVHD: (1) new ocular sicca documented by low Schirmer's test with a mean value of ≤5 mm at 5 minutes or (2) a new onset of keratoconjunctivitis sicca detected by slit lamp exam with mean Schirmer's test values of 6 to 10 mm [6].

We excluded patients with the following criteria: (1) signs of infection, glaucoma, retinopathy, allergy or other immune diseases; (2) with incomplete medical records; or (3) unable to be followed and interviewed in the clinic. The study was approved by the Peking University Third Hospital Medical Science Research Ethics Committee (protocol number: M2017275) and conducted in accordance with the Helsinki Declaration; all participants or their guardians provided written consent.

2.1. Outcome Measures

(1) Data were collected on patients' demographic and transplant characteristics, such as age, gender, primary diseases for which HSCT was performed, donor-to-recipient information, systemic GVHD, and conditioning regimens.

(2) *Patients' major symptoms*: patients' symptoms were evaluated with a special designed questionnaire which included 11 common subjective ocular discomforts (they were increased eye discharge, eye dryness, red eye, foreign body sensation, fluctuating vision, photophobia, burning sensation, lacrimation, alacrimia, edema of eyelids or conjunctiva, and ocular fatigue) at their first visit. The severity of each symptom was graded on a scale of 0 to 4, where 0 indicated none of the time; 1, some of the time; 2, half of the time; 3, most of the time; and 4, all of the time. Patients were asked to grade each symptom according to their present and previous initial discomfort feelings, respectively. We chose symptoms scored ≥3 as major ones for each patient in the study. The questionnaire also included essential time intervals (e.g., latency, i.e., interval from transplant to initial ocular symptoms, time interval between initial symptoms and first visit, and interval between transplant and first visit).

(3) *Objective ocular examinations*: during each patient's first visit to the ophthalmology clinic, we collected the following ocular parameters: (1) best observed vision acuity (measured in logMAR); (2) intraocular pressure (measured with noncontact tonometer); (3) corneal fluorescein staining score (following the consensus on clinical diagnosis and treatment of dry eye in China, cornea was divided into four quadrants; then for each quadrant, no corneal epithelium stained scored 0, 1–30 stained points scored 1, >30 stained points without fusion scored 2, and punctate keratopathy fusion and/or corneal filiform paraphyte and/or corneal ulcer scored 3; final score for each eye is the sum of each quadrant's score) [11]; (4) fluorescein tear film break-up time (TBUT); (5) Schirmer's test score without anesthesia; and (6) conjunctival disease grade (acute GVHD: conjunctival hyperemia, stage I; hyperemia with chemosis and/or serosanguineous exudates, stage II; pseudomembranous conjunctivitis, stage III; and pseudomembranous conjunctivitis with corneal epithelial sloughing, stage IV) [12].

2.2. Statistical Analysis. Data were summarized as mean ± SD or as counts and proportions. We compared demographic, transplant characteristics, and objective ocular examination parameters of chronic and acute GVHD patients using independent sample T-test and Mann–Whitney U test. The chi-square test was used to compare frequencies of different symptoms between the two groups. A two-sided P value less than 0.05 was considered statistically significant.

3. Results

3.1. Patients' Demographics. Records of 193 consecutive post-allo-HSCT patients examined in the Department of Ophthalmology, Peking University Third Hospital, Beijing, were reviewed, and after screening, 148 patients were enrolled in the study (Figure 1). According to diagnostic criteria described above, patients were categorized into acute (21 of 148, 14.2%) or chronic (127 of 148, 85.8%) ocular GVHD groups. The demographics and transplant characteristics, shown in Table 1, were similar between the two groups ($P > 0.05$).

3.2. Subjective Symptom Questionnaire

3.2.1. Acute Ocular GVHD Group. In our study, 21 patients were diagnosed with acute ocular GVHD. Mean latency from transplant to initial ocular symptoms was 8.0 ± 5.0 months; mean interval between transplantation and first visit was 8.6 ± 5.4 months. All patients, 21 of 21 (100%), visited ophthalmologists within 2 months of sensing initial ocular discomfort. The ocular symptoms reported at first visits were similar to their initial symptoms.

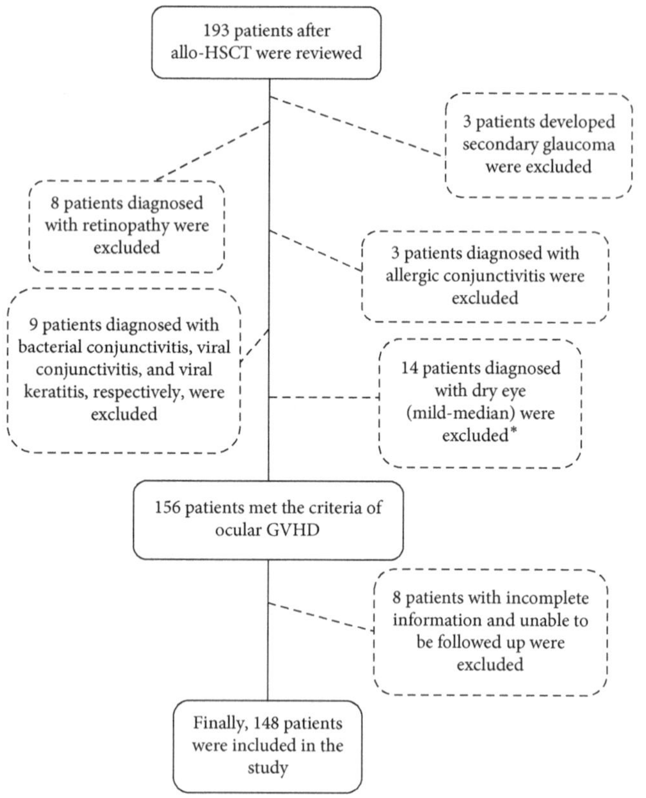

FIGURE 1: Flow diagram of patient selection. *These patients reported onset of dry eye symptoms, including irritation, burning sensation, dryness, or foreign body sensation that required treatment with frequent topical lubricants. However, signs of ocular surface abnormalities including decreased Schirmer's test (≤5 mm), tear break-up time (≤5 seconds), presence of conjunctivitis, and corneal fluorescein staining were absent.

This group reported increased eye discharge (21 of 21, 100.0%), red eye (19 of 21, 90.5%), lacrimation (11 of 21, 52.4%), and eye dryness (9 of 21, 42.9%) most often. (Frequencies of each symptom are shown in Figure 2). Notably, all patients in this group described their eye discharge as clear and thick mucus secretions. Typical secretions of acute GVHD are shown in Figures 3(a) and 3(b).

3.2.2. Chronic Ocular GVHD Group. Chronic ocular GVHD was diagnosed in 127 patients. Mean latency from transplant to initial ocular symptoms was 10.7 ± 9.1 months (similar to that of acute ocular GVHD, $P = 0.091$). However, mean interval between initial discomfort and first visit was 9.9 ± 14.1 months, and the interval between onset of initial ocular discomfort and first ophthalmologist visit was >2 months for 82 of 127 (64.6%) and >6 months for 59 patients (46.5%).

The symptoms often reported at the first visit were eye dryness (115 of 127, 90.6%), increased eye discharge (68 of 127, 53.5%), photophobia (50 of 127, 39.4%), and alacrimia (45 of 127, 35.4%). Among patients with increased eye discharge, 77.9% (53 of 68) described discharge as white and stringy fibrous secretions, and the other 22.1% (15 of 68) reported mucus secretions. Typical fibrous secretions are shown in Figures 3(g) and 3(h).

TABLE 1: Demographics and transplant characteristic by patient groups.

	Acute GVHD (n = 21, eyes = 42)	Chronic GVHD (n = 127, eyes = 254)
Age (yrs.), mean ± SD	29 ± 12	28 ± 11
P (independent sample T-test)	0.704	
Gender		
Male	13 (61.9%)	79 (62.2%)
Female	8 (38.1%)	48 (37.8%)
P (chi-square test)	0.979	
Primary disease		
Acute lymphoid leukemia	2 (9.5%)	38 (29.9%)
Acute myeloid leukemia	9 (42.9%)	48 (37.8%)
Myelodysplastic syndrome	6 (28.6%)	31 (24.4%)
Chronic myeloid leukemia	1 (4.8%)	5 (3.9%)
Non-Hodgkin's lymphoma	0 (0.0%)	3 (2.4%)
Hodgkin's lymphoma	1 (4.8%)	0 (0.0%)
Aplastic anemia	2 (9.5%)	2 (1.6%)
Donor-recipient gender disparity		
Female donor to male recipient	8 (38.1%)	36 (28.3%)
Male donor to female recipient	4 (19.0%)	33 (26.0%)
Essential time points		
Interval from transplant to initial ocular symptoms (months), mean ± SD	8.0 ± 5.0	10.7 ± 9.1
P (Mann–Whitney U test)	0.091	
Interval between initial symptoms and first visit (months), mean ± SD	0.6 ± 0.7	9.9 ± 14.1
P (Mann–Whitney U test)	<0.001	
Interval between transplant and first visit (months), mean ± SD	8.6 ± 5.4	20.4 ± 17.7
P (Mann–Whitney U test)	<0.001	

GVHD = graft-versus-host disease.

Among initial symptoms recalled at the first visit, increased eye discharge (90 of 127, 70.9%), red eye (76 of 127, 59.8%), eye dryness (69 of 127, 54.3%), and fluctuating vision (32 of 127, 25.2%) were most common. In addition, 44.1% (56 of 127) of patients reported symptoms (mucus ocular secretions, red eye and systemic symptoms) that were similar to typical acute ocular GVHD manifestations in our study, and they could recall definite events related to the occurrence of initial ocular symptoms. The events included increased intensity of conditioning regimens (35 of 52, 67.3%), treatment with interferon (IFN)-a2b (10 of 52, 19.2%),

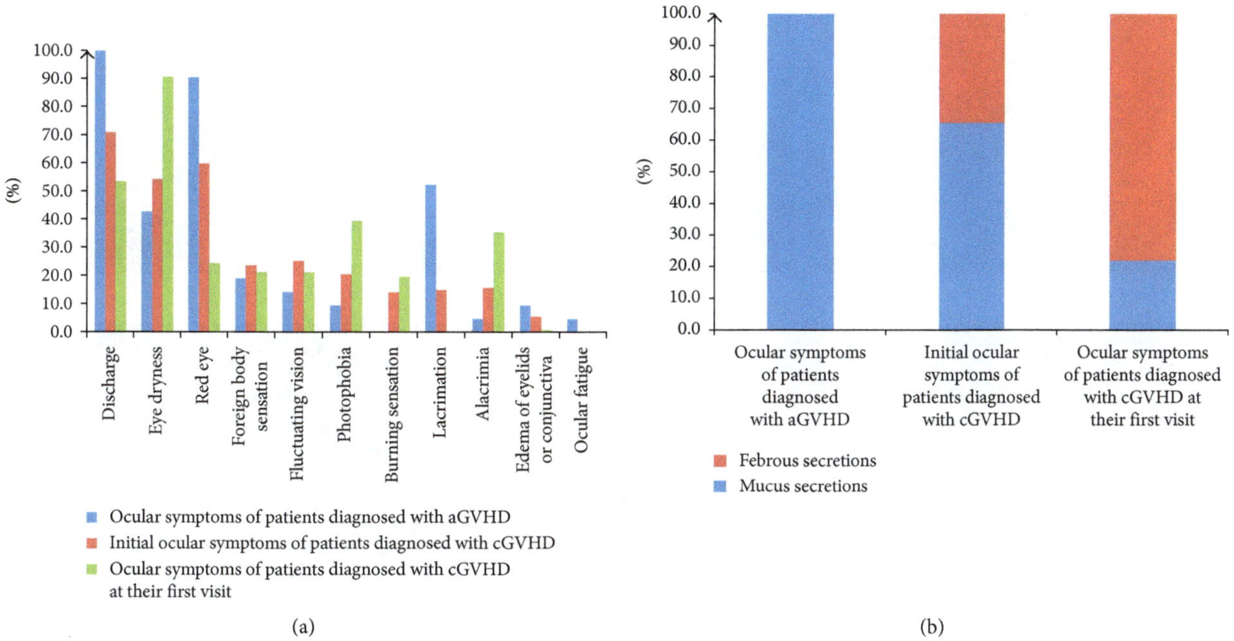

Figure 2: Symptoms of different clinical ocular GVHD categories. (a) Frequencies of different subjective symptoms. (b) Secretion compositions of different ocular disease GVHD categories. cGVHD = chronic graft-versus-host disease; aGVHD = acute graft-versus-host disease.

retransplant or reinfusion of donor lymphocyte (5 of 52, 9.6%), fatigue (1 of 52, 1.9%), and pulmonary infection (1 of 52, 1.9%). Ocular manifestations improved with intensive conditioning immunosuppressant, and these patients were followed in oncology or internal medicine departments until severe ocular complications occurred or symptoms became unbearable.

Frequencies of subjective symptoms of different clinical ocular GVHD categories are shown in Figure 2(a). In Figure 2(b), we analyzed secretion composition differences between GVHD categories. The frequencies of characteristic symptoms (increased mucus secretion, red eye, and lacrimation) in the acute ocular GVHD group differed significantly from those inherent to the chronic ocular GVHD group (eye dryness, increased fibrous secretion, alacrimia, and photophobia) ($P < 0.05$).

3.2.3. Objective Ocular Examinations. Best corrected visual acuities and intraocular pressures were all within normal limits and were similar between the two groups. Patients in the acute GVHD group had different levels of conjunctival involvement but few had keratopathy (corneal fluorescein staining score 2.5 ± 3.8) (Figures 3(c) and 3(d)). 59.5 percent (25 of 42) of eyes were in stage I of conjunctival disease, and 21.4 percent (9 of 42) of eyes (stage III and stage IV) appeared to have severe conjunctival and corneal involvement of pseudomembranous conjunctivitis, corneal epithelial sloughing, and limbus damage. However, the chronic group had severe eye dryness and further corneal lesions: 30 (11.8%) eyes developed filamentary keratitis (Figure 3(i)), 20 (7.9%) eyes developed corneal ulcer, 6 (2.4%) eyes developed spontaneous corneal perforation (Figure 3(j)), and 2 (0.8%) eyes developed corneal vascularization (Figure 3(k)). Corneal fluorescein staining, TBUT, and Schirmer's tear secretion score were also significantly different from the acute GVHD group ($P < 0.05$) (Table 2).

4. Discussion

4.1. Manifestations of Acute Ocular GVHD. According to previous studies, the prevalence of ocular involvement in post-HSCT patients is approximately 30%–40%; acute GVHD only accounts for 1% of this [13, 14]. Studies of acute ocular GVHD are limited. Jabs et al. [12] described distinct-appearing conjunctivitis as an acute GVHD involvement of the conjunctiva and formulated a clinical-staging system from mild conjunctival hyperemia to severe pseudomembranous conjunctivitis with corneal epithelial sloughing (see disease-grading details in *Materials and Methods*). Uchino et al. [15] reported a juvenile case of pseudomembranous conjunctivitis accompanied with corneal ulcer (stage IV) and corneal epithelial defects, which eventually disappeared after pseudomembrane excision. Inflammatory cells, including macrophages, neutrophils, T cells, and natural killer cells that accumulate in the conjunctiva in acute ocular GVHD promote the release of cytokines (tumor necrosis factor (TNF)-α, interleukin (IL)-6, etc.) that resulted in further corneal epithelial defects [8, 15]. Thus, it is our belief that conjunctival involvement is the early and primary manifestation of acute ocular GVHD.

In our study, patients with acute ocular GVHD all demonstrated acute conjunctival inflammation but fewer had lacrimal secretion dysfunction and corneal lesions. The most characteristic acute ocular GVHD manifestation was increased mucus eye secretions. We found corresponding signs in each affected eye. Red eye and lacrimation were also

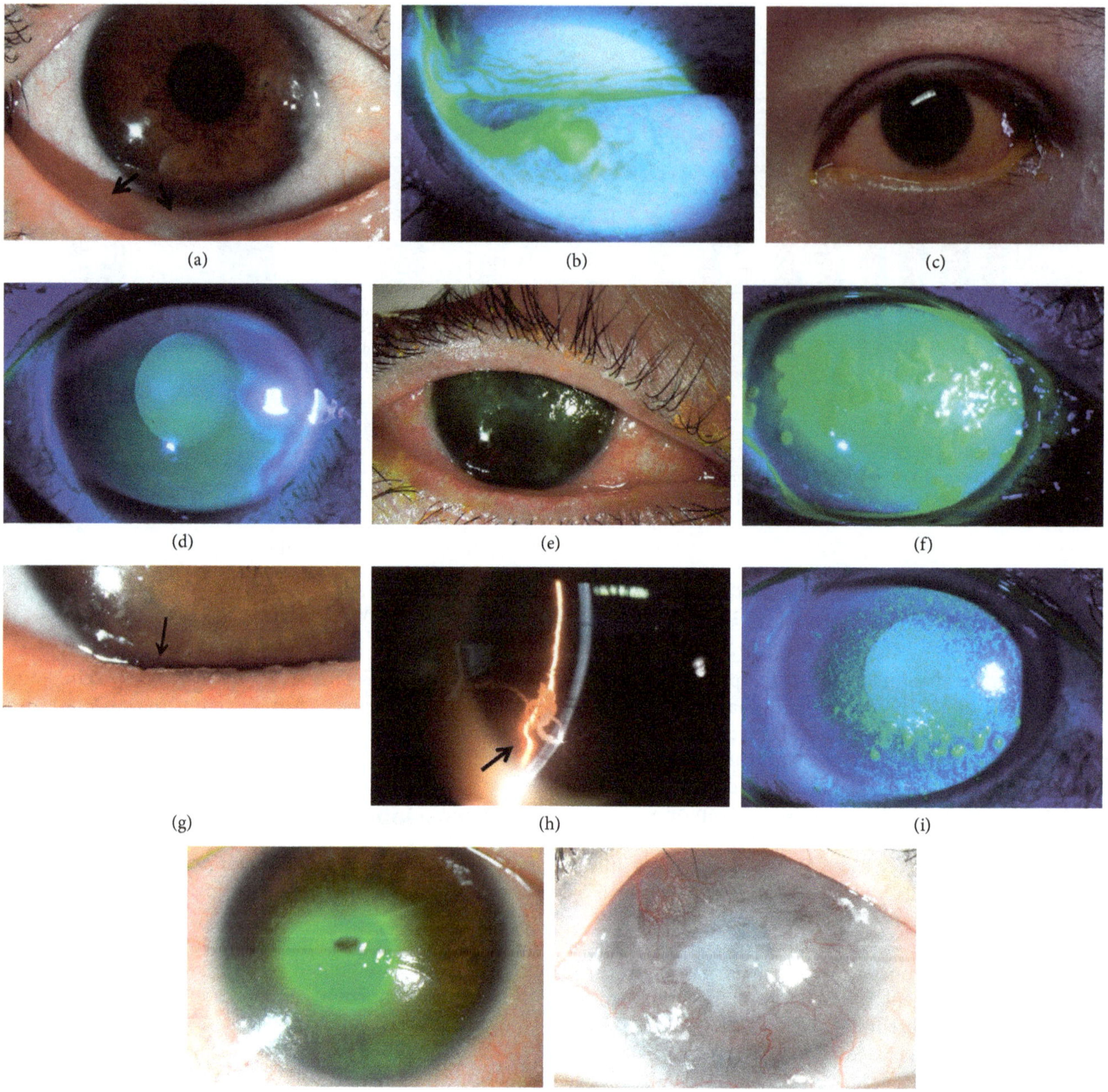

(a) (b) (c) (d) (e) (f) (g) (h) (i) (j) (k)

Figure 3: Typical ocular signs of ocular GVHD. (a)–(f) Signs of acute ocular GVHD and differential diagnosis: (a) mucus secretion (arrow) and conjunctival injection of acute ocular GVHD; (b) mucus secretion using fluorescein dye and visualized under a cobalt blue light; (c) and (d) conjunctiva and cornea signs of mild acute ocular GVHD; (e) and (f) conjunctiva and cornea signs of a post allo-HSCT patient who complained of red eye, lacrimation, and increased eye discharge and was diagnosed with viral corneal dermatitis eventually. (g)–(k) Signs and complications of chronic ocular GVHD: (g) and (h) typical fibrous secretion (arrow) of chronic ocular GVHD; (i) filamentary keratitis; (j) corneal perforation; and (k) corneal vascularization.

frequent in this group. In our study, the majority of patients with acute ocular GVHD had mild-moderate involvement and often could be cured with intensive conditioning immunosuppressant. However, it is advantageous to follow these patients closely because patients developed pseudomembrane formation and/or corneal epithelium loss (stage III-IV) that indicated a severe systemic involvement by GVHD as well as decreased survival rate [4, 12]. Moreover, acute ocular involvement is a predecessor of chronic ocular GVHD [16]. It is also important and necessary to exclude the diagnoses of anterior segment infections, including viral keratitis, viral conjunctivitis, and bacterial conjunctivitis that could occur in post-HSCT patients (Figures 1 and 3).

Although eye dryness was frequently reported, Schirmer's test, TBUT, and corneal fluorescein staining scores were almost always within normal limits. Perhaps, poor reading habits, underlying diseases, and conditioning regimens led to dry eye problems.

TABLE 2: Outcomes of objective ocular examinations of two groups.

Outcomes	Acute GVHD (n = 21, eyes = 42)	Chronic GVHD (n = 127, eyes = 254)
Best corrected visual acuity (logMAR)		
Mean ± SD	0.23 ± 0.24	0.24 ± 0.27
Z	−0.165	
P (Mann–Whitney U test)	0.869	
Intraocular pressure (mmHg)		
Mean ± SD	13.42 ± 2.04	14.11 ± 2.70
Z	−1.566	
P (Mann–Whitney U test)	0.117	
Corneal fluorescein staining		
Mean ± SD	2.5 ± 3.8	5.8 ± 3.9
Z	−5.726	
P (Mann–Whitney U test)	<0.001	
Schirmer tear secretion score (mm)		
Mean ± SD	9.0 ± 3.6	2.8 ± 2.0
Z	−9.623	
P (Mann–Whitney U test)	<0.001	
Fluorescein tear film break-up time (seconds)		
Mean ± SD	5.7 ± 3.6	3.2 ± 2.7
Z	−4.054	
P (Mann–Whitney U test)	<0.001	

GVHD = graft-versus-host disease.

4.2. Manifestations of Chronic Ocular GVHD. Dry eye is the most common manifestation of chronic ocular GVHD. The National Institutes of Health censensus document defines dry eye and corresponding ocular signs as distinctive manifestations of chronic ocular GVHD. An ocular distinctive manifestation with impaired Schirmer's test is sufficient for the diagnosis of the disease [6]. The international chronic ocular consensus group strongly recommended dry eye disease as a diagnostic clinical entity for chronic GVHD [4]. In our study, ocular chronic GVHD severe eye dryness predominated and was accompanied by corresponding serious ocular signs, including corneal fluorescein staining (6.7 ± 4.8), decreased TBUT (2.1 ± 1.8 seconds), and Schirmer's tear secretion (3.1 ± 2.4 mm). Those findings are consistent with previous research and consensus findings. Increased fibrous eye secretions, photophobia, and alacrimia were common complaints in this group. Besides, photophobia, burning sensation, foreign body sensation, and fluctuating vision indicated further corneal lesion, for example, punctate keratopathy fusion, filamentary keratitis, corneal ulcer, and corneal perforation occurred in 10%–40% eyes of this group. In our study, 22.8% of chronic ocular GVHD patients developed severe ocular complications; spontaneous corneal perforation, corneal vascularization, and even endophthalmitis have been reported before [17–19]. Moreover, chronic ocular GVHD greatly impairs patient's vision-related quality of life and affects their educational level, job position, and underlying disease [20, 21].

However, we also found that 44.1% (56 of 127) of chronic ocular GVHD patients had a definite history of acute ocular GVHD episode. Ocular symptoms that were mild initially were ignored or only treated with artificial tears. Over time, manifestations progressed and patients were finally referred to ophthalmologists when severe ocular complications arose or symptoms became unbearable. These patients might have missed the best opportunity for prophylaxis and treatment to restore lacrimal secretion function. Had patients reported mild discomfort, we could have detected the ocular surface changes of chronic ocular GVHD directly and, thus, given comprehensive treatments with early intervention and regular follow-up.

Our primary limitation is the retrospective nature of the study; patients' recall of initial subjective symptoms on the questionnaire may also be inaccurate. Ocular GVHD patients always struggle with visiting an ophthalmological clinic promptly due to burdens of relapses of underlying disease, systemic GVHD, and infections. Ophthalmologists and physicians are challenged to recognize, diagnose, and evaluate ocular GVHD, and even more so to understand progression of the disease. We tried to report accurate results. Few essential records were missing, and we confirmed data from medical records with patients or their families through face-to-face interviews. Certainly, further large, long-term, prospective clinical studies are necessary to better describe this disease accurately.

In summary, acute conjunctivitis with increased mucus eye secretions, red eye, and lacrimation indicates a high probability of acute ocular GVHD if differentiated from infections. Chronic ocular GVHD is characterized by severe dry eye and further corneal lesions, including filamentary keratitis, corneal ulcer, and corneal vascularization. After diagnosis, it is not difficult to determine ocular GVHD subsets like classic acute or chronic GVHD, overlap syndrome, and late-onset acute GVHD. At an early stage, most acute ocular GVHD and chronic GVHD cases are overlooked and therefore do not undergo stepwise evaluation or treatment, which eventually leads to serious ocular complications and poor quality of life. The ultimate goal is to offer better, early prophylaxis and treatment of the discussed complications. Ocular GVHD or dry eye syndrome of chronic GVHD should be referred to ophthalmologists who can then intervene early to evaluate, diagnose, and treat the corresponding conditions.

Conflicts of Interest

The authors declare no conflicts of interest.

Acknowledgments

This work was partly supported by National Natural Science Foundation of China (81650027).

References

[1] X. H. Lin and H. D. Cavanagh, "Ocular manifestations of graft-versus-host disease: 10 years' experience," *Clinical Ophthalmology*, vol. 9, pp. 1209–1213, 2015.

[2] T. B. Abud, F. Amparo, U. S. Saboo et al., "A clinical trial comparing the safety and efficacy of topical tacrolimus versus methylprednisolone in ocular graft-versus-host disease," *Ophthalmology*, vol. 123, no. 7, pp. 1449–1456, 2016.

[3] S. C. Balasubramaniam, H. Raja, C. B. Nau, J. F. Shen, and M. M. Schornack, "Ocular graft-versus-host disease," *Eye and Contact Lens: Science and Clinical Practice*, vol. 41, no. 5, pp. 256–261, 2015.

[4] Y. Ogawa, S. K. Kim, R. Dana et al., "International chronic ocular graft-vs-host-disease (GVHD) consensus group: proposed diagnostic criteria for chronic GVHD (Part I)," *Scientific Reports*, vol. 3, no. 1, pp. 3419–3424, 2013.

[5] J. L. Ferrara, J. E. Levine, P. Reddy, and E. Holler, "Graft-versus-host disease," *The Lancet*, vol. 373, no. 9674, pp. 1550–1561, 2009.

[6] M. H. Jagasia, H. T. Greinix, M. Arora et al., "National Institutes of Health consensus development project on criteria for clinical trials in chronic graft-versus-host disease: I. The 2014 diagnosis and staging working group report," *Biology of Blood and Marrow Transplantation*, vol. 21, no. 3, pp. 389–401, 2015.

[7] N. Mirza, M. Zierhut, A. Korn et al., "Graft versus self against T-cell autoantigens is a mechanism of graft-host interaction," *Proceedings of the National Academy of Sciences of the United States of America*, vol. 113, no. 48, pp. 13827–13832, 2016.

[8] H. Shikari, J. H. Antin, and R. Dana, "Ocular graft-versus-host disease: a review," *Survey of Ophthalmology*, vol. 58, no. 3, pp. 233–251, 2013.

[9] S. Herretes, D. B. Ross, S. Duffort et al., "Recruitment of donor T cells to the eyes during ocular GVHD in recipients of MHC-matched allogeneic haematopoietic stem cell transplants," *Investigative Opthalmology and Visual Science*, vol. 56, no. 4, pp. 2348–2357, 2015.

[10] Y. Ogawa, S. Okamoto, M. Wakui et al., "Dry eye after hematopoietic stem cell transplantation," *British Journal of Ophthalmology*, vol. 83, no. 10, pp. 1125–1130, 1999.

[11] W. Shi, L. Xie, Y. Li et al., "Chinese consensus of corneal transplantation," *Chinese Journal of Ophthalmology*, vol. 51, pp. 888–891, 2015.

[12] D. A. Jabs, J. Wingard, W. R. Green, E. R. Farmer, G. Vogelsang, and R. Saral, "The eye in bone marrow transplantation. III. Conjunctival graft-vs-host disease," *Archives of Ophthalmology*, vol. 107, no. 9, pp. 1343–1348, 1989.

[13] K. S. Na, Y. S. Yoo, J. W. Mok, J. W. Lee, and C. K. Joo, "Incidence and risk factors for ocular GVHD after allogeneic hematopoietic stem cell transplantation," *Bone Marrow Transplantation*, vol. 50, no. 11, pp. 1459–1464, 2015.

[14] R. Jacobs, U. Tran, H. Chen et al., "Prevalence and risk factors associated with development of ocular GVHD defined by NIH consensus criteria," *Bone Marrow Transplantation*, vol. 47, no. 11, pp. 1470–1473, 2012.

[15] M. Uchino, Y. Ogawa, M. Kawai et al., "Ocular complications in a child with acute graft-versus-host disease following cord blood stem cell transplantation: therapeutic challenges," *Acta Ophthalmologica Scandinavica*, vol. 84, no. 4, pp. 545–548, 2006.

[16] A. Z. Munir and J. Aylward, "A review of ocular graft-versus-host disease," *Optometry and Vision Science*, vol. 94, no. 5, pp. 545–555, 2017.

[17] H. Westekemper, S. L. Scholz, H. Thomasen, C. Halfwassen, and K. P. Steuhl, "Ocular graft versus host disease: corneal complications," *Der Ophthalmologe*, vol. 114, no. 8, pp. 697–702, 2017.

[18] S. D. Adrean and J. E. Puklin, "Perforated corneal ulcer with subsequent endophthalmitis in a patient with graft-versus-host disease," *Cornea*, vol. 26, no. 1, pp. 107-108, 2007.

[19] M. Mohammadpour, "Progressive corneal vascularization caused by graft-versus-host disease," *Cornea*, vol. 26, no. 2, pp. 225-226, 2007.

[20] Y. C. Sun, X. Chai, Y. Inamoto et al., "Impact of chronic ocular graft-versus-host disease on quality of life," *Biology of Blood and Marrow Transplantation*, vol. 21, no. 9, pp. 1687–1691, 2015.

[21] U. S. Saboo, F. Amparo, T. B. Abud, D. A. Schaumberg, and R. Dana, "Vision-related quality of life in patients with ocular graft-versus-host disease," *Ophthalmology*, vol. 122, no. 8, pp. 1669–1674, 2015.

20

Screening of Primary School Children for Amblyopia and Amblyogenic Factors in Central Cairo, Egypt

Mohammad A. Rashad,[1] Khaled M. Abd Elaziz,[2] Samah Mahmoud Fawzy,[1] Ahmed Abdel Meguid Abdel latif,[1] and Mahmoud Abdel Meguid Abdel latif[1]

[1]*Ophthalmology Department, Faculty of Medicine, Ain Shams University, Cairo, Egypt*
[2]*Community Department, Environmental and Occupational Medicine, Faculty of Medicine, Ain Shams University, Cairo, Egypt*

Correspondence should be addressed to Samah Mahmoud Fawzy; samfzy2@hotmail.com

Academic Editor: Van C. Lansingh

Objective. To measure the prevalence of amblyopia and amblyogenic factors among primary school children and to evaluate distance visual acuity (VA) as a screening test to detect amblyopia and define its cutoff value. *Subjects and Methods.* A cross-sectional study was conducted on primary school children in two schools in Central Cairo. Children underwent assessment of visual acuity using Landolt broken ring. Comprehensive ophthalmologic examination was performed for amblyopia suspects at the Ophthalmology Department of Ain Shams University Hospitals, including reassessment of best-corrected visual acuity (BCVA) using the same chart. *Results.* A total of 352 children were examined. Reduced screening VA (amblyopia suspect) was detected in 47 subjects (13.35%) proved amblyopia after comprehensive examination was 1.98% (7 cases). Refractive errors (REs) were present in all suspected and proved amblyopia cases (100%) but was only present in 11.6% of nonamblyopic students ($P < 0.05$). The prevalence of hyperopia in the whole sample was 3.6%, and was 27.6% in subjects with RE. Thirty percent of hyperopic eyes were amblyopic. The prevalence of myopia was 9.3% of the whole sample and 70% of students with RE. Only 9% of myopic eyes were amblyopic. Mild to moderate amblyopia (VA better than 0.2log MAR) was 42.9%, while severe amblyopia represented 57.1%. *Conclusion.* This study emphasizes the importance of school-based eye care system targeting the detection of amblyopia by application of a fast screening distance VA test with a cutoff value of high sensitivity at log MAR 0.539 (Snellen's VA equivalent 6/18).

1. Introduction

Amblyopia is a potentially treatable decrease in BCVA with no structural pathology [1]. It can be unilateral if two or more line difference in best-corrected visual acuity (BCVA) is present between the two eyes or bilateral if BCVA is equal or less than 6/12 in both eyes [2, 3]. The basic mechanisms in amblyopia could be interactive anomaly between eyes or dissociative disorder in one or both eyes. It is either anisometropic, strabismic, or visual deprivation in nature [4, 5].

Early detection of amblyopia is important for effective treatment; however, it can be still treated in older age [6]. Recent evidences on successful treatment of amblyopia in children up to 12 years old and more encouraged screening programs for older children [7, 8]. This helps discovering undiagnosed amblyopes who have been missed in earlier screening programs or those living in countries with poor medical services and no screening programs [7, 8]. Although the global international prevalence of amblyopia is 1.6–3.6% [9, 10], the available data concerning the prevalence of amblyopia and RE (refractive error) in different geographical areas is still inadequate.

According to the action plan released by the WHO Global Initiative for the Elimination of Avoidable Blindness in 2006–2011, uncorrected refractive errors are the second cause of global blindness (18%) and the main cause of visual impairment in children between 5 and 15 years of age. There are at least 13 million of them all over the world, of which more than 90% live in developing countries [8]. WHO announced refractive errors as one of the five conditions of

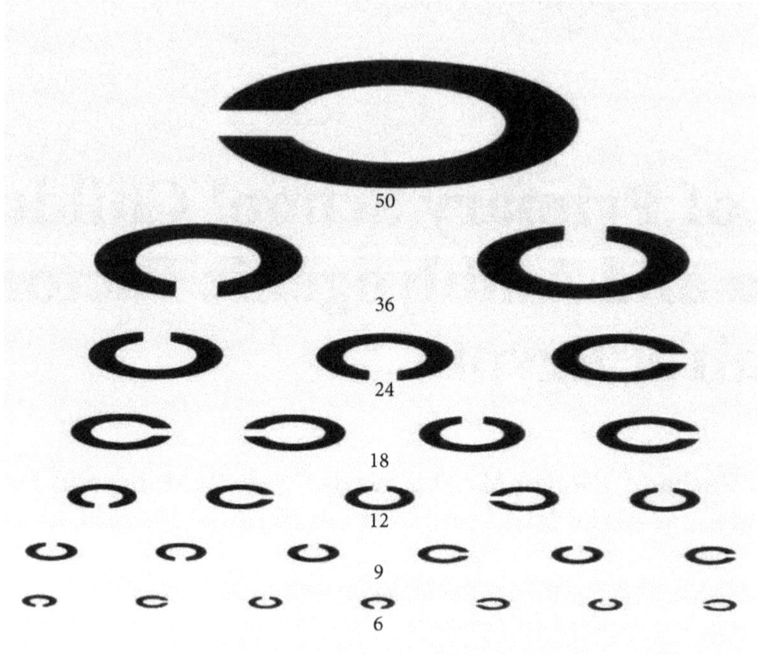

FIGURE 1: Landolt broken ring (C optotype).

immediate management priority and recommended that services for their detection should be integrated in different levels of eye-care provision with special emphasis on primary and secondary school eye-health programs especially in developing countries [8]. However, their plans met some limitations: inadequate population-based prevalence studies, uncertainty of the best cost effective ways to deliver refraction services in those different settings, and lack of awareness among people and the community about proper detection and preventive measures [8].

Following these recommendations, we constructed our study to measure the prevalence of amblyopia and refractive errors as an amblyogenic factor in primary school children in Central Cairo, Egypt, which is a crowded, viable area deficient in such studies. At older age children as our study population, causes of amblyopia other than refractive errors are unlikely, as by this age strabismus and organic causes of visual deprivation should have been discovered and managed. We aimed at identifying the ideal cutoff visual acuity (VA) value for suspecting amblyopia by simply using distance VA chart (Landolt's broken rings), and hence referral to comprehensive examination. A secondary goal of our study is to test the efficacy of Landolt's broken ring chart as a suitable screening tool being simple, low cost, and readily available test at all Egyptian primary schools.

2. Subjects and Methods

Our cross-sectional study was based on multistage sampling. It was carried out in Central Cairo, Egypt. We performed this study in two primary schools, one public and one private school with different socioeconomic standards. Both schools were selected from a list of Central Cairo Educational Directorate, using simple random sampling. Systematic random sampling was also used for children in classes.

The total number of students in both schools was 815 students, 315 in the public school and 500 in the private school. Assuming the prevalence of amblyopia ranges from 1% to 5% [10], with alpha error 5% and power of study 80%, our sample size was calculated to be 378 students. One general ophthalmologist performed the screening and the examination.

The first stage was history taking from children, including name, age, history of wearing glasses, and history of squint or surgery. The second stage was examination using simple pin light for gross media opacity, lid position, and pupillary light reflex. Ocular motility examination and cover uncover test were also performed.

The third stage involved the assessment of monocular uncorrected VA and BCVA with glasses for students who were wearing glasses. Assessment of VA was done at the school premises using Landolt broken ring self-illuminated chart at six meters in a dark room at school (Figure 1). The test was performed monocularly using bracketing technique.

The BCVA of each student was recorded and converted to logarithm minimal angle of resolution (log MAR). Suspected cases were defined as students who had difference in BCVA between both eyes of two lines or more, or those who have BCVA of 6/12 or less in both eyes.

The fourth stage was referring amblyopia suspects to ophthalmic comprehensive examination at Ain Shams University Hospitals. Distant BCVA and pinhole VA were assessed using Landolt broken ring chart. Refraction before and after cycloplegia was performed using both autorefractometer and streak retinoscopy. Cyclopentolate 1% one drop was instilled at 10 minutes interval, repeated for 3 times. Postmydriatic test was performed after one week. Slit lamp and fundus examinations were performed with dilated pupils. Children with reduced BCVA with no organic eye disease are considered proven amblyopia cases to be included in the statistical analysis.

Unilateral amblyopia was defined as ≥2 line difference in BCVA between the two eyes, and bilateral amblyopia as BCVA worse than 6/12 in both eyes. Significant RE was defined as myopia if ≥−0.50 diopter spherical equivalent (D SE), hyperopia if ≥1.0 DSE and astigmatism if ≥1.0 diopter of cylinder (DC).

2.1. Statistical Methods. Data was revised for its completeness and consistency. Double data entry on SPSS program version 16 was done. Quantitative data was summarized by mean standard deviation, qualitative data was summarized by frequencies and percentages, and significance was analysed by chi-square test. A "*P* value" of less than 0.05 was considered statistically significant. Sensitivity, specificity, and positive and negative predictive values were also calculated. Distant visual acuity log MAR and log MAR ROC curve analysis were plotted.

3. Ethical Considerations

The presented study received the official approval of the Central Cairo Educational Directorate of the screened schools, the two administrators of the selected schools, parents of screened children at school, and the Ethical Committee of the Faculty of Medicine, Ain Shams University. Parents (guardians) of children who had the comprehensive examination provided written informed consents allowing their children to be further examined.

4. Results

Our study included initially 378 children between 8 and 12 years of age. Dropouts were 4 children, and absent students were 24. Our actual final sample size was 352 students; 191 public school students (54.3%) and 161private school students (45.7%). The males were 193 (54.8%) and females were 159 students (45.2%). Amblyopia suspects were 47 students (13.4% with 95% CI 9.9–17.3), while7 children were proven amblyopia cases (1.98% with 95% CI 0.8–4.1). Mild to moderate amblyopia (VA better than 0.2 log MAR) was 42.9%, while severe amblyopia represented 57.1%. All proved amblyopia cases were unilateral.

The mean age was 9.5 years among the 345 nonamblyopic children and 9.4 years in the 7 amblyopic cases, with no statistically significant difference. Amblyopia prevalence was higher in the private school and in females. It was also significantly higher in children wearing glasses as shown in Table 1.

The total percentage of RE among all studied students was 13.4%. Refractive errors were present in 100% of suspected and proved amblyopia patients. In nonamblyopic children, only 11.6% (40/345) had RE. The difference was highly significant ($P < 0.01$ chi-square test). The prevalence of hyperopia, myopia, anisometropia, and astigmatism in all students and in cases with RE is illustrated in Table 2.

Table 1: Risk factors affecting amblyopia occurrence.

Risk factors	Amblyopia *n*	Amblyopia Percent	*P*
Gender			
Male (193)	1/193	0.5%	0.02*
Female (159)	6/159	3.8%	
School			
Public (191)	2/191	1%	0.1
Private (161)	5/161	3.1%	
Wearing spectacles			
No (332)	5/332	1.5%	0.008**
Yes (20)	2/20	10%	

n: number; $^{*}P < 0.05$ significant; $^{**}P < 0.01$ highly significant.

Table 2: Distribution of different RE in all students and in RE cases.

RE type	Number of cases	Percent of each RE type in all (352) students	Percent of each RE type in (47) students with RE
Hyperopia (≥+1.0 diopter)	13	3.6%	27.6%
Myopia (≥−0.5 diopter)	33	9.37%	70.2%
Anisometropia (≥1.0 diopter)	29	8.23%	61.7%
Astigmatism (>1.0 diopter)	12	3.4%	25.5%

Table 3: Amblyopia prevalence in different types of RE.

RE type	Amblyopic eyes **n	Amblyopic eyes %	Nonamblyopia n	Nonamblyopia %
Hyperopia ($n = 13$)*	4/13	30.7%	9/13	69.3%
Myopia ($n = 33$)*	3/33	9%	30/33	91%
Anisometropia ($n = 29$)*	7/29	24.1%	22/29	75.8%
Astigmatism ($n = 12$)*	2/12	16.7%	10/12	83.3%

$^{*}P > 0.05$ not significant; $^{**}n$: number.

Amblyopia was more common in hyperopic children 30.7% compared to myopics 9% (*P* value is 0.0867). Amblyopia prevalence in each type of RE is illustrated in Table 3.

Validity of our screening test was evaluated by specificity, sensitivity, positive predictive value (PPV), and positive predictive value (NPV) in different cutoff values for detection of suspected and proved cases of amblyopia as shown in Table 4 and Figures (2) and (3). At low cutoff value (0.539 log MAR), sensitivity was 100% at specificity 96% in detection of proved amblyopia. At high cutoff value (0.238 log MAR), sensitivity was also 100% but with 89% specificity in the detection of proved amblyopia.

Table 4: Sensitivity and specificity of VA in the detection of amblyopia (weaker eye inclusion) among all subjects and amblyopic suspected subjects.

Log MAR	Sensitivity	Specificity	PPV	NPV
All subjects *$n = 352$				
0.238	100%	89%	15.2%	100%
0.389	100%	90%	16.7%	100%
0.539	100%	96%	33.3%	100%
0.690	85%	99%	50%	99.7%
Amblyopia-suspected cases $n = 47$				
0.238	100%	5%	15.6%	100%
0.389	100%	12.5%	16.7%	100%
0.539	100%	65%	33.3%	100%
0.690	85%	85%	50%	97.1%

*n: number.

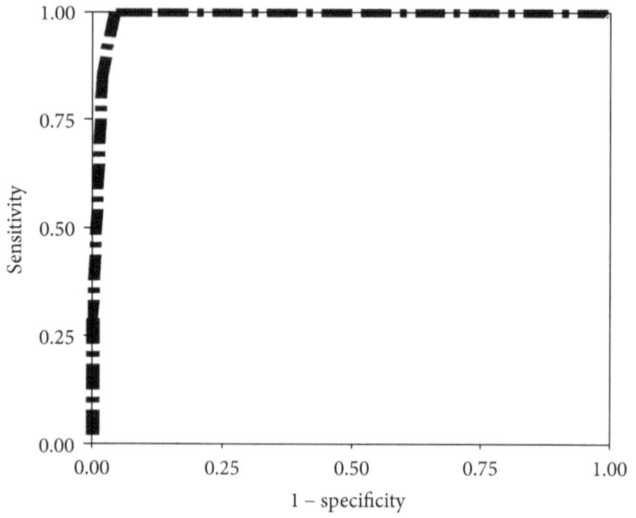

Figure 2: ROC curve sensitivity analysis for VA in detection of amblyopia (all children).

5. Discussion

Vision screening in children is recommended for detection of potentially treatable disorders [8, 11]. In a large population country with moderate resources like Egypt, lack of early eye care services for preschoolers makes the selected age group of our study (8–12 years old); ideal for screening because of their mandatory presence at schools at regular basis, reliable responses, and possible treatment of discovered amblyopia as proven by recent researches [7]. Moreover, in a society like ours, ease of examination with a single, fast, low cost, and readily available test is necessary for successful screening.

In our study, the amblyopia rate in Central Cairo was found to be 1.98%, which is very close to the Menia city in south of Egypt where it was reported to be 1.49% in primary school children [12]. They screened children of narrower age range (7–9 years) and used different screening test, Kay

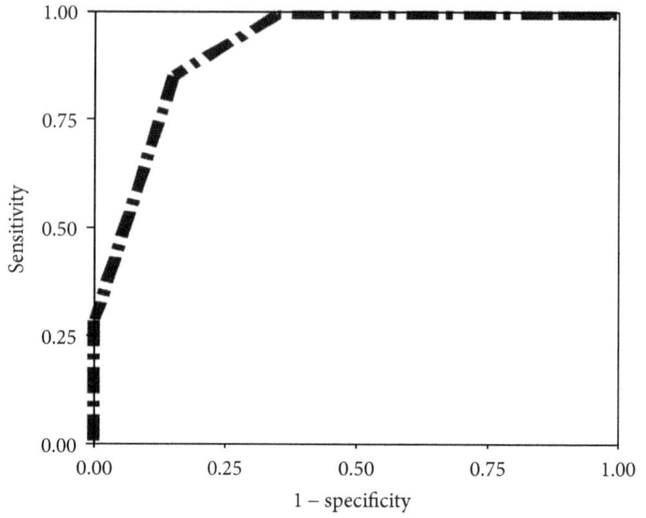

Figure 3: ROC curve sensitivity analysis for VA in detection of amblyopia in suspected subjects.

pictures that is not available in Egyptian primary schools [12]. They also reported a higher rate of amblyopia in rural areas (2%) compared to urban areas (1.04%), although they did not state whether this difference was significant or not.

A much lower prevalence of amblyopia was reported in another Egyptian study conducted in Alexandria in north of Egypt where it was only 0.1% in school children 6–12 years of age [13]. Astonishingly, screen failures in their study were only 6% in comparison to 13.4% (CI 9.9–17.3%) in our study [13]. Underestimation of the actual prevalence is suspected in their study as they used a team of technicians of questionable experience, who used Snellen or Tumbling E optotype VA charts for screening [13].

The prevalence of amblyopia in our study is consistent with international results of 1.6–3.6% [8]. It is very comparable to regional developing countries like Saudi Arabia (1.85% in 6–12 years children) [14] and Central China (2.16% in primary school children) with nearly similar prevalence of severe amblyopia to ours (36% and 42%, resp.) [15]. It is also quite similar to developed countries as Sweden where prevalence of deep amblyopia (VA</=0.3) is 2%, reduced to 0.2% with treatment [16].

In our study the prevalence of refractive errors was 13.4% in general, which is lesser than the 22.5% reported in the El-Bayoumy et al. study who screened older school children in Cairo [17] and found that 85.4% of the reported RE was in children ≥ 12 years. We had almost the same prevalence of hyperopia, although more myopia and astigmatism were found in our study (70.2% versus 55.7% and 25.5% versus 17%) [17]. Setting a definite value for every refractive error in our study might have contributed to better discovery of cases as El-Bayoumy et al. [17] did not define values for the included RE nor screened for amblyopia.

Our results were quite similar to Goh et al. in Malaysia [18] who conducted their study by retinoscopy on children aged 7 years. On the other hand, we had more myopia and less hyperopia than Elsahn [13] in north of Egypt (myopia: 70.2% versus 22.0% and hyperopia: 27.6% versus 52%, resp.), which may be due to the slightly older age range of our study children in addition to his questionable screening team [13]. We also had more astigmatism than Elsahn (25.5% of RE versus 10%) as he included cases with pure astigmatism while we included all astigmatic types [13]. We also reported a much higher anisometropia incidence than him [13] (61.7% of RE versus 3%) as he included only eyes with >4.0 diopter interocular difference, while we included cases with >1.0 diopter interocular difference which is more appropriate for scientific and statistical purposes.

Jing et al. [15] defined their cutoff values before starting the screening and described test failures of 73% with high cutoff value and 31% with low cutoff value in comparison to 13.4% in general in our study. We defined our cutoff values after obtaining the results which allowed us to locate accurately the smallest VA measure that achieved 100% sensitivity and 96% specificity and defined it as the low cutoff value (at log MAR 0.539, equivalent to 6/18 Snellen's fraction), and a high cutoff value with 100% sensitivity and 89% specificity (at log MAR 0.238, equivalent to 6/10 Snellen's fraction).

Our results were better than Jing et al. [15] even when they tried to improve sensitivity of their screening program by doing simultaneous VA and stereo acuity testing [16]. They had lower sensitivity and specificity than us at their most close low cutoff value to ours in both situations (log MAR of 0.17 = 6/9 Snellen's fraction; 92% sensitivity and 68% specificity with distance VA alone and 94% sensitivity and 66% specificity with combined tests). They still had lower specificity than ours when they used a high cutoff value of 0 log MAR = 6/6 Snellen's fraction, which is rather impractical in screening (100% sensitivity, 22.7% specificity with distance VA alone, and 100% sensitivity, 21% specificity with combined tests). The high sensitivity and specificity of our test were also attributed to the selected older age subjects with better performance of distance VA testing [19, 20].

Very close to our results, Gracia et al., [21] found 80% unilateral amblyopia and 100% anisometropia in their amblyopic cases, in comparison to 100% and 75% in our study, respectively. They used the same criteria of our research of ≥1D interocular difference, while Lee et al. [7], who used an interocular difference of ≥2D, reported amblyopia in 52% of anisometropic eyes. In accordance with other studies on similar age groups, we found neither strabismic nor sensory deprivation amblyopia [22, 23], while we had more amblyopic females than males ($p = 0.02$), in contrary to Chinese population who showed no difference between boys and girls ($P = 0.782$) [15].

Based on our results, we do recommend obligatory regular screening of primary school children using simple distance VA chart by well-trained health care providers. Child referral to consultation is mandatory if having VA of 6/18 or worse in one or both eyes or not adequately corrected by his own glasses. We hope that would help over the lack of awareness among parents and community and promote better quality of life for growing children [8, 24].

Conflicts of Interest

The authors declare that they have no conflicts of interest.

References

[1] J. M. Holmes and M. P. Clarke, "Amblyopia," *The Lancet*, vol. 367, no. 9519, pp. 1343–1351, 2006.

[2] G. Ashok, E. P. Marek, A. Rajvardhan et al., *Surgical and Medical Management of Paediatric Ophthalmology*, section 6; Strabismus and amblyopia, sensory adaptation in strabismus, Jaypee Brothers Medical Publisher, New Delhi, India, 1st edition, 2007.

[3] S. Ganekal, V. Jhanji, Y. Liang, and S. Dorairaj, "Prevalence and etiology of amblyopia in Southern India: results from screening of school children aged 5-15 years," *Ophthalmic Epidemiology*, vol. 20, no. 4, pp. 228–231, 2013.

[4] E. Kanonidou, "Amblyopia: a mini review of the literature," *International Ophthalmology*, vol. 31, no. 3, pp. 249–256, 2011.

[5] D. F. Chang, R. S. Feder, S. D. McLeod et al., "Paediatric ophthalmology and strabismus," in *Amblyopia Preferred Practice Pattern Guidelines, Springer Science & Business Media*, pp. 5–30, American Academy of Ophthalmology, San Francisco, 2012.

[6] N. W. Daw, "Critical periods and amblyopia," *Archives of Ophthalmology*, vol. 116, no. 4, pp. 502–505, 1998.

[7] C. E. Lee, Y. C. Lee, and S. Y. Lee, "Factors influencing the prevalence of amblyopia in children with anisometropia," *Korean Journal of Ophthalmology*, vol. 24, no. 4, pp. 225–229, 2010.

[8] K. Simons, "Amblyopia characterization, treatment, and prophylaxis," *Survey of Ophthalmology*, vol. 50, no. 2, pp. 123–166, 2005.

[9] (WHO) Vision 2020 (The Right to Sight), "Global Initiative for the Elimination of Avoidable Blindness: Action Plan 2006-2011," in WHO Press, World Health Organization, Switzerland, 2007.

[10] Committee on Practice and Ambulatory Medicine, Section on Ophthalmology, American association of certified orthoptists, American association for pediatric ophthalmology and strabismus, American academy of pediatrics, and American academy of ophthalmology, "Eye Examination in Infants, Children, and Young Adults by Pediatricians," *Pediatrics*, vol. 111, no. 4, Part 1, pp. 904–907, 2003.

[11] M. M. Scheiman, R. W. Hertle, R. T. Kraker et al., "Patching vs atropine to treat amblyopia in children aged 7 to 12 years: a randomized trial," *Archives of Ophthalmology*, vol. 126, no. 12, pp. 1634–1642, 2008.

[12] S. T. Abdelrazik and M. F. Khalil, "Prevalence of amblyopia among children attending primary schools during the amblyogenic period in Minia county," *Journal of Egyptian Ophthalmological Society*, vol. 107, no. 4, pp. 220–225, 2014.

[13] M. Elsahn, "International vision screening: results from Alexandria, Egypt," *Current Ophthalmology Reports*, vol. 2, no. 4, pp. 137–141, 2014.

[14] M. A. Abolfotouh, I. Badawi, and Y. Faheem, "Prevalence of amblyopia among schoolboys in Abha City, Asir Region, Saudi Arabia," *The Journal of the Egyptian Public Health Association*, vol. 69, no. 1-2, pp. 19–30, 1994.

[15] J. Fu, S. M. Li, J. L. Li et al., "Screening of amblyopia among grade 1 students in primary school with uncorrected vision

and stereopsis test in central China," *Chinese Medical Journal*, vol. 126, no. 5, pp. 903–908, 2013.

[16] G. Kvarnstrom, P. Jakobsson, and G. Lennerstrand, "Visual screening of Swedish children: an ophthalmological evaluation," *Acta Ophthalmologica Scandinavica*, vol. 79, no. 3, pp. 240–244, 2001.

[17] B. M. El-Bayoumy, A. Saad, and A. H. Choudhury, "Prevalence of refractive error and low vision among schoolchildren in Cairo," *Eastern Mediterranean Health Journal*, vol. 13, no. 3, pp. 575–579, 2007.

[18] P. Goh, Y. Abqariyah, G. Pokharel, and L. Ellwein, "Refractive error and visual impairment in school age children in Gombak District, Malaysia," *Ophthalmology*, vol. 112, no. 4, pp. 678–685, 2005.

[19] Y. Pan, K. Tarczy-Hornoch, S. A. Cotter et al., "Visual acuity norms in pre-school children: the multi-ethnic pediatric eye disease study," *Optometry and Vision Science*, vol. 86, no. 6, pp. 607–612, 2009.

[20] D. E. Shaw, A. R. Fielder, C. Minshull, and A. R. Rosenthal, "Amblyopia-factors influencing age of presentation," *The Lancet*, vol. 2, no. 8604, pp. 207–209, 1988.

[21] C. A. de Amorim Garcia, E. de Araújo Dantas, A. B. de Souza, R. A. C. Uchoa, and F. Oréfice, "Epidemiologic study of anisometropia in students of Natal, Brazil," *Arquivos Brasileiros de Oftalmologia*, vol. 68, no. 1, pp. 75–77, 2005.

[22] G. Woodruff, F. Hiscox, J. R. Thompson, and L. K. Smith, "The presentation of children with amblyopia," *Eye*, vol. 8, no. 6, pp. 623–626, 1994.

[23] C. Williams, K. Northstone, R. A. Harrad, J. M. Sparrow, I. Harvey, and ALSPAC Study Team, "Amblyopia treatment outcomes after preschool screening v school entry screening: observational data from a prospective cohort study," *British Journal of Ophthalmology*, vol. 87, no. 8, pp. 988–993, 2003.

[24] B. Chua and P. Mitchell, "Consequences of amblyopia on education, occupation, and long term vision loss," *British Journal of Ophthalmology*, vol. 88, no. 9, pp. 1119–1121, 2004.

21

Comparison of SNP Genotypes Related to Proliferative Vitreoretinopathy (PVR) across Slovenian and European Subpopulations

Xhevat Lumi,[1] Mateja M. Jelen,[2] Daša Jevšinek Skok,[2] Emanuela Boštjančič,[2] Metka Ravnik-Glavač,[2] Marko Hawlina,[1] and Damjan Glavač[2]

[1] *Eye Hospital, University Medical Centre Ljubljana, Ljubljana, Slovenia*
[2] *Department of Molecular Genetics, Institute of Pathology, Faculty of Medicine, University of Ljubljana, Ljubljana, Slovenia*

Correspondence should be addressed to Damjan Glavač; damjan.glavac@mf.uni-lj.si

Academic Editor: Stephen T. Armenti

The present study investigated the distribution of genotypes within single nucleotide polymorphisms (SNPs) in genes, related to PVR pathogenesis across European subpopulations. Genotype distributions of 42 SNPs among 96 Slovenian healthy controls were investigated and compared to genotype frequencies in 503 European individuals (Ensembl database) and their subpopulations. Furthermore, a case-control status was simulated to evaluate effects of allele frequency changes on statistically significant results in gene-association studies investigating functional polymorphisms. In addition, 96 healthy controls were investigated within 4 SNPs: rs17561 (*IL1A*), rs2069763 (*IL2*), rs2229094 (*LTA*), and rs1800629 (*TNF*) in comparison to PVR patients. Significant differences ($P < 0.05$) in distribution of genotypes among 96 Slovenian participants and a European population were found in 10 SNPs: rs3024498 (*IL10*), rs315952 (*IL1RN*), rs2256965 (*LST1*), rs2256974 (*LST1*), rs909253 (*LTA*), rs2857602 (*LTA*), rs3138045 (*NFKB1A*), rs3138056 (*NFKB1A*), rs7656613 (*PDGFRA*), and rs1891467 (*TGFB2*), which additionally showed significant differences in genotype distribution among European subpopulations. This analysis also showed statistically significant differences in genotype distributions between healthy controls and PVR patients in rs17561 of the *IL1A* gene (OR, 3.00; 95% CI, 0.77–11.75; $P = 0.036$) and in rs1800629 of the *TNF* gene (OR, 0.48; 95% CI, 0.27–0.87; $P = 0.014$). Furthermore, we have shown that a small change (0.02) in minor allele frequency (MAF) significantly affects the statistical *p* value in case-control studies. In conclusion, the study showed differences in genotype distributions in healthy populations across different European countries. Differences in distribution of genotypes may have had influenced failed replication results in previous PVR-related SNP-association studies.

1. Introduction

The impact of genome-wide association studies and genetic-association studies has become enormous in the past ten years, providing researchers with extensive data repositories [1]. As genetic factors affect susceptibility to certain diseases, identifying the relevant genes and/or their polymorphisms contribute greatly to the development of novel prevention programs and treatments of disease. Numerous evaluations of genetic association have also led to the remarkable potential for the discovery of novel genetic biomarkers. However, the execution of such analysis in many cases is cumbersome with considerable statistical and computational challenges and also requires reproducibility [2]. The potential for the discovery of false positive findings when results are not properly corrected is high and represents the most conspicuous problem in gene-disease-association studies [3–5].

Proliferative vitreoretinopathy (PVR) represents the growth and contraction of cellular membranes on both retinal surfaces and within the vitreous cavity in patients with rhegmatogenous retinal detachment (RRD) [6–8]. It is the major complication following retinal detachment surgery and a leading cause of failure in the management of RRD [6, 9]. It is estimated to occur in 5–10% of patients with RRD [6]. Technological advances in high-throughput screening have been introduced in gene-association studies, including PVR. These studies revealed numerous inflammatory molecules to be implicated in the PVR development, such as growth factors (PDGF, HGF, VEGF, and EGF), transforming growth factors (TGFA, TGFB), molecules from the SMAD family and interleukins (IL1, IL6, IL8, and IL10), tumor necrosis factors (TNF), and tumor suppressor protein (p53) [10–15]. Studies, published in the past ten years, by the "Retina 4 Project" consortium, have demonstrated that specific single nucleotide polymorphisms (SNPs), located in genes involved in PVR pathways, may represent potential predictive factors for the PVR development [10, 11, 14, 16–20]. Among 200 studied SNPs in more than 30 candidate genes, the "Retina 4 Project" identified 8 SNPs in 7 genes, encoding CCL2, FGF2, IL1RN, LTA, NFKBIA, SMAD7, and TGFB2, as significant individual predictors for PVR [11] and demonstrated associations between PVR and SNPs in *BAX*, *p53*, *PIK3CG*, *MDM2*, *SMAD7*, and *TNFB2* in the TNF locus [10, 16–19]. A more recent genetic-association study, on a Slovenian PVR patient population, demonstrated significant differences in genotype distributions between RRD patients with and without PVR in SNPs within *IL6*, in the vicinity of *IL10*, and the *TGFB1* gene. Interestingly, several associations between SNP genotypes and the PVR phenotype could not be replicated throughout a series of "Retina 4 Project" studies and by a recent study on a Slovenian population. To establish the credibility of an association between a SNP and disease, a replication of SNP effect among different study populations is essential. It is possible that fluctuations between genotype frequencies across studied countries reflect the difference in population ancestry, which could influence the variability in allele frequencies even in unrelated conditions of interest [21]. As success of replication of a genetic-association study depends on many factors, including enrollment of independent population datasets, information on the effect of different allele frequencies in genetic-association studies remains scarce.

The present study is a part of an ongoing gene-association study in Slovenian RRD patients who developed PVR after vitrectomy. In order to expand the current perspective on differences between PVR patients and healthy controls and SNP effects in patients with different geographical background, we further investigated our previously established in-house genomic databases. Firstly, we aimed to assess basic differences in SNP genotype distributions among European subpopulations. For this purpose, we compared distributions of 42 SNP genotypes between a Slovenian healthy population and European subpopulations and among European subpopulations. Additionally, this study designed a simulation of a case-control gene-association study in order to demonstrate that even a minor allele frequency (MAF) change could result in a considerable increase in the power to replicate the previously established SNP effect. In the second part of the study, we examined differences in distribution of SNP genotypes between Slovenian healthy controls and PVR patients.

2. Methods

2.1. Study Population. The genetic-association study conducted on 191 Slovenian patients with primary RRD, who underwent vitrectomy at the Eye Hospital, University Medical Centre Ljubljana, Slovenia. In the study we recruited 153 patients who developed PVR grade C1 or higher within 3 months after the surgery. We also enrolled 96 healthy controls without retinal detachment. The study was approved by the National Medical Ethics Committee of the Republic of Slovenia and followed the tenets of the Helsinki Declaration. All patients provided written informed consent.

Ninety-six healthy Slovenian blood donors (52 men and 44 women), aged between 20 and 55 years, originating from 11 geographic areas, representative for the country of Slovenia, were statistically analyzed in 4 SNPs.

2.2. Blood Collection and DNA Extraction. Six milliliters of peripheral blood were collected from each participant and stored until DNA extraction at −20°C. DNA was extracted using QIAamp DNA Blood Midi Kit (100) (QIAGEN, Hilden, Germany), according to the manufacturer's instructions. Extracted DNA was stored until used for amplification at −20°C.

2.3. Genotype Distribution in Slovenian and European Populations. Genotype distributions of 42 SNPs of 96 Slovenian healthy controls, genotyped using HumanOmniExpress-14 platform (Illumina, San Diego, CA, USA), were compared across 503 European residents, using data on specific SNP genotypes obtained from the Ensembl database (release 83) (Supplemental Table 1). In case a difference among SNP genotype distribution was observed among Slovenian and European populations, the differences between the populations were further examined, as follows: the frequencies of genotypes were subsequently compared between the Slovenian and three European subpopulations, namely, 99 Utah residents with northern and western European ancestry (CEU), 91 residents from Britain in England and Scotland (GBR), and 107 Iberian residents from Spain (IBS).

2.4. Evaluation of Genetic Effects in a Simulated Population Dataset. We hypothesized that some statistically significant differences in SNP genotype distributions could not be replicated due to even small changes in allele frequencies. To test this hypothesis, we designed a simulated case-control status. The genotype frequency of the original case dataset was AA = 1, AG = 39, and GG = 73, and the minor allele frequency (MAF) was 0.18 ($P = 0.13$). The control dataset remained unchanged. Genotypes were added one by one in each homozygote or heterozygote category to evaluate effects of minor allele frequency (MAF) changes on statistically significant results (Table 1).

2.5. Genotyping of 96 Healthy Participants. Ninety-six Slovenian healthy controls were genotyped for 713,014 markers, using HumanOmniExpress-14 platform (Illumina, San Diego, CA, USA). Genotypes were assigned according to the standard Illumina protocol in GenomeStudio Software,

Table 1: Simulation of genotype distribution in a potential population dataset.

Number of simulations	Genotype case dataset (n)			Number of genotypes added to the case dataset (n)			Allele frequency		MAF	P value
	AA	AG	GG	AA	AG	GG	A	G		
1	1	39	73	0	0	0	0.18	0.82	0.18	0.130
2	1	40	73	0	1	0	0.18	0.82	0.18	0.110
3	1	41	73	0	2	0	0.19	0.81	0.19	0.092
4	1	42	73	0	3	0	0.19	0.81	0.19	0.078
5	1	43	73	0	4	0	0.19	0.81	0.19	0.066
6	1	44	73	0	5	0	0.19	0.81	0.19	0.056
7	1	45	73	0	6	0	0.20	0.80	0.20	0.047
8	2	39	73	1	0	0	0.19	0.81	0.19	0.091
9	2	40	73	1	1	0	0.19	0.81	0.19	0.077
10	2	41	73	1	2	0	0.19	0.81	0.19	0.065
11	2	42	73	1	3	0	0.20	0.80	0.20	0.055
12	2	43	73	1	4	0	0.20	0.80	0.20	0.047
13	3	39	73	2	0	0	0.20	0.80	0.20	0.065
14	3	40	73	2	1	0	0.20	0.80	0.20	0.055
15	3	41	73	2	2	0	0.20	0.80	0.20	0.046
16	4	39	73	3	0	0	0.20	0.80	0.20	0.041

Note: original case dataset is shown in the second column. The control dataset is not shown. Added genotypes to the original dataset are represented in the third column. Genotypes were added one by one in each homozygote or heterozygote category. Allele frequency, MAF, and *P* values changed according to the performed simulation.

version V2011.1. Only individuals with a genotyping success rate of >95% were considered as positive for a respective genotype. The HumanOmniExpress-14 platform included only 4 SNPs, investigated previously in RRD and PVR patients. Therefore, our subsequent analysis included comparison of 96 control PVR patients for 4 SNPs: rs17561 (*IL1A*), rs2069763 (*IL2*), rs229094 (*LTA*) and rs1800629 (*TNF*).

2.6. TaqMan Genotyping of PVR Patients. Genotypes of 4 SNPs, located within or in the vicinity of the 4 genes rs17561 (*IL1A*), rs2069763 (*IL2*), rs2229094 (*LTA*), and rs1800629 (*TNF*), were determined using TaqMan assay (Applied Biosystems, Foster City, CA, USA) according to the manufacturer's instructions.

2.7. Statistical Analysis. Differences in genotype distributions among Slovenian healthy controls and European subpopulations were evaluated with the chi-square test, calculated using SAS software version 9.2 (JMP®, SAS Institute Inc., 2010, Cary, North Carolina, USA) and presented as pie charts (Figures 1 and 2).

To assess the differences in SNP genotype distribution among healthy population and PVR patients, odds ratios (ORs) with 95% confidence intervals (95% CIs) were calculated in SNPStats software [22], using the unconditional logistic regression. For inheritance model identification, the Akaike information criteria (AIC) were used, according to the authors' instructions. An α value was set to 0.05 in all calculations.

3. Results

The genotype distribution comparison of 42 SNPs among 96 Slovenian healthy controls (SLO) and a European population (data for 503 individuals were obtained from the Ensembl database) revealed significant differences ($P < 0.05$) in distribution of genotypes in 10 SNPs: rs3024498 (*IL10*), rs315952 (*IL1RN*), rs2256965 (*LST1*), rs2256974 (*LST1*), rs909253 (*LTA*), rs2857602 (*LTA*), rs3138045 (*NFKB1A*), rs3138056 (*NFKB1A*), rs7656613 (*PDGFRA*), and rs1891467 (*TGFB2*) (see Figures 1 and 2).

The frequencies of genotypes rs315952 (*IL1RN*), rs2256965 (*LST1*), and rs2256974 (*LST1*) varied significantly between SLO and CEU, SLO and GBR, and SLO and IBS, while the differences between GBR and IBS were not observed. Similar differences were observed for SNP rs1891467 (*TGFB2*), where we noticed the differences between all comparisons with the Slovenian population, as well as between GBR and IBS. Differences in the frequency of genotypes for the SNP rs3024498 (*IL10*) were observed between SLO and GRB, SLO and IBS, and between GBR and IBS. For the SNP rs3138056 (*NFKB1A*), differences between SLO and CEU and between SLO and IBS were observed. The differences in the frequencies of genotypes for the SNP rs3138045 (*NFKB1A*) were observed between SLO and IBS and GBR and IBS, while the frequencies of genotypes rs7656613 (*PDGFRA*), rs909253 (*LTA*), and rs2857602 (*LTA*) differ between populations of SLO and CEU and SLO and GBR.

Simulation of the potential population dataset of SNP genotypes revealed that adding six heterozygotes (AG) to the

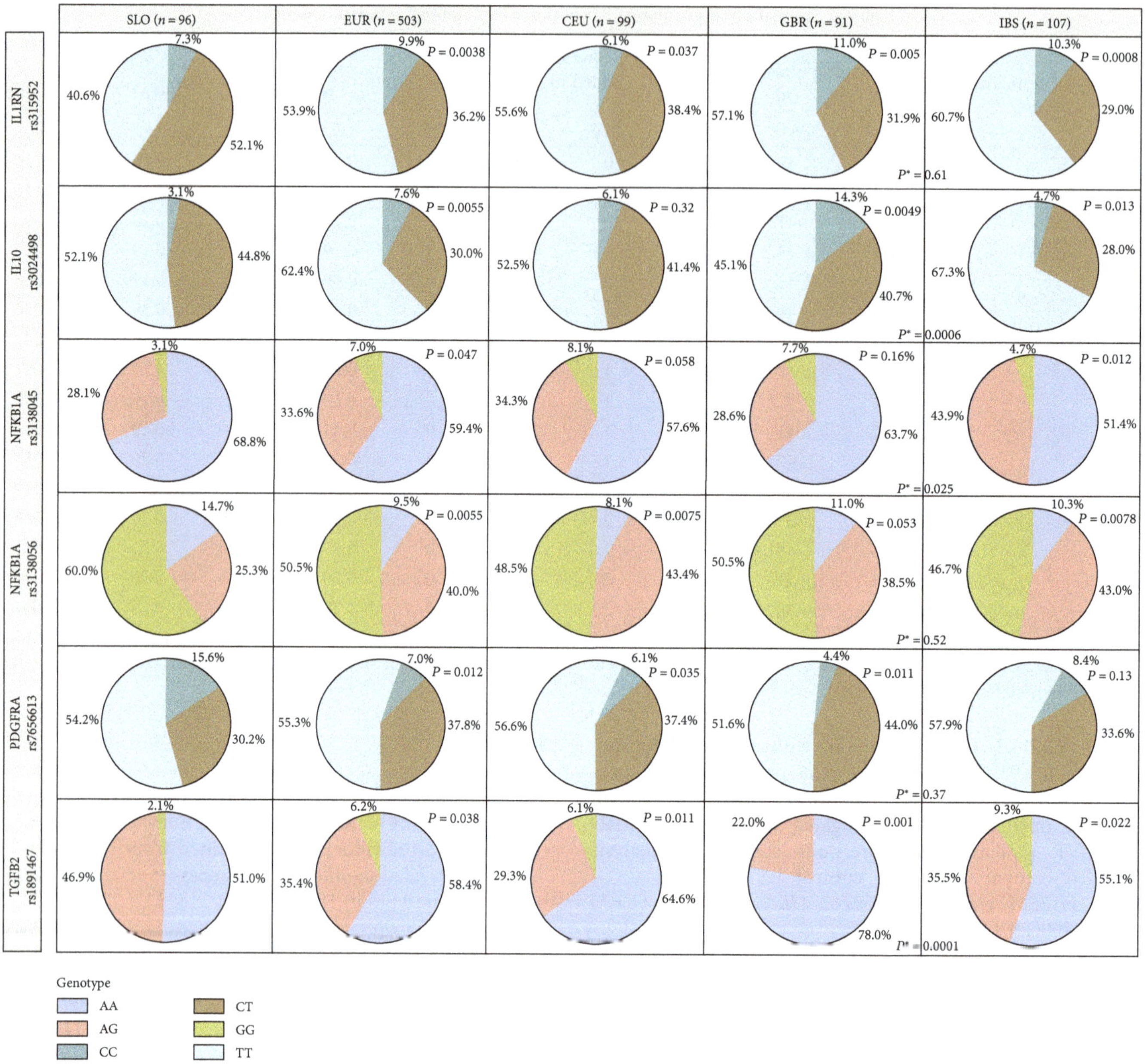

FIGURE 1: The genotype frequencies for 6 SNPs across European subpopulations. P value means difference in genotype distribution between Slovenian population (SLO) and other populations (EUR, CEU, GBR and IBS). P^* value means difference in genotype distribution between Great Britain population (GBR) and Iberian population (IBS) only.

original case dataset showed a statistically significant difference between the two populations ($P = 0.047$) (Table 1). Similarly, statistically significant differences were shown when one homozygote (AA) and four heterozygotes (AG), or two homozygotes (AA) and two heterozygotes (AG), or three homozygotes (AA), were added to the original case dataset. Despite the fact that MAF increased from 0.18 to 0.20 in all described cases of events, the small change (0.02) in MAF showed an important decrease of the P value below 0.05.

In addition, the analysis showed two statistically significant differences in genotype distributions between 96 healthy controls and PVR patients (Table 2). In *IL1A* (rs17561), a statistically significant difference in distribution of genotypes was found between PVR patients and healthy controls (OR, 3.00; 95% CI, 0.77 to 11.75; $P = 0.036$). A significantly different distribution of genotypes was found also in rs1800629 of the *TNF* gene (OR, 0.48; 95% CI, 0.27 to 0.87; $P = 0.014$).

4. Discussion

Numerous inflammatory mediators, growth factors, and cytokines have been implicated in PVR pathogenesis. Statistical results of several genetic-association studies within the "Retina 4 Project" have emphasized the possible potential of those inflammatory mediators as novel biomarkers in the diagnostics and treatment of PVR [7, 8, 20, 23]. Replication

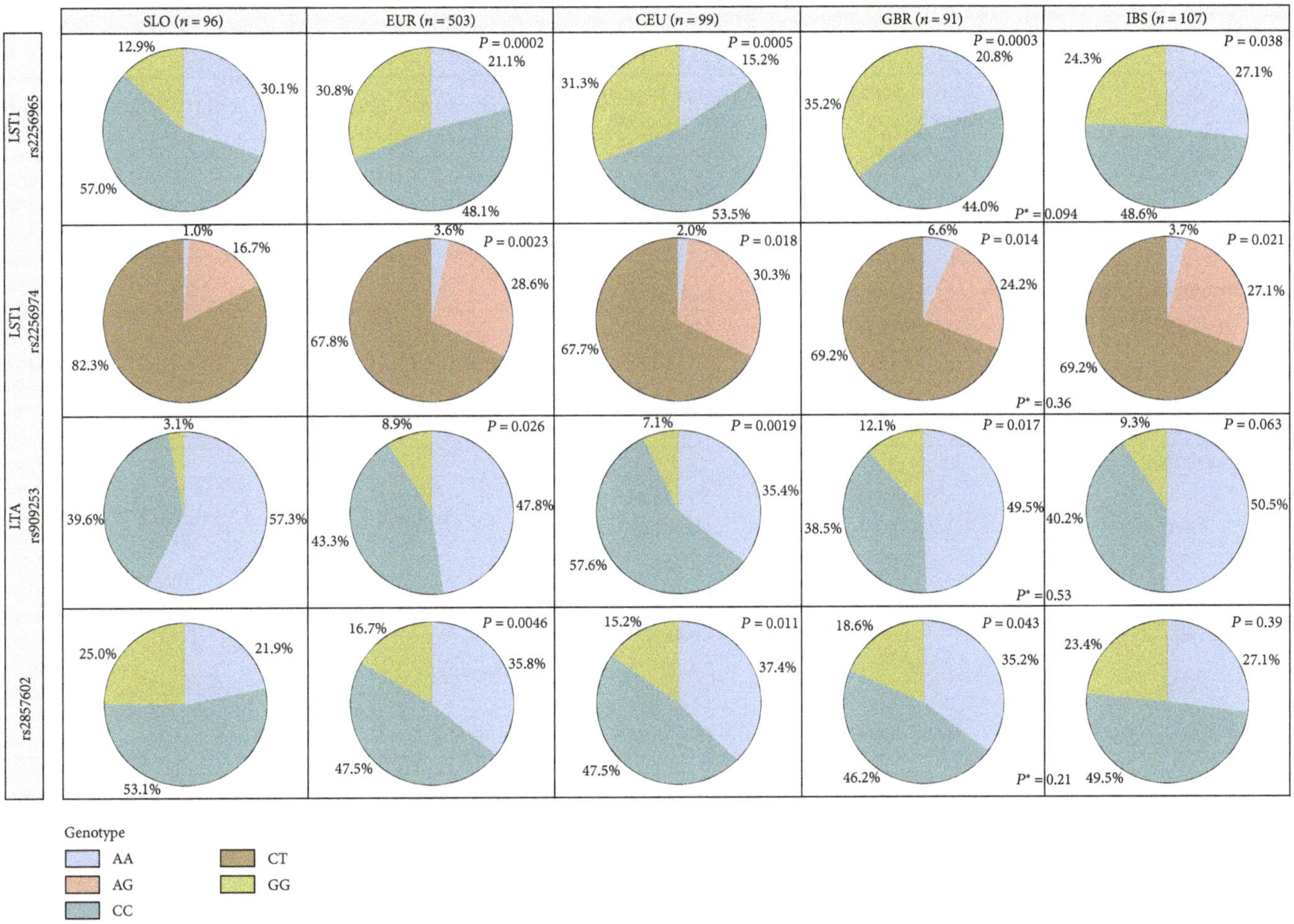

FIGURE 2: The genotype frequencies for 4 SNPs across European subpopulations. P value means difference in genotype distribution between Slovenian population (SLO) and other populations (EUR, CEU, GBR and IBS). P^* value means difference in genotype distribution between Great Britain population (GBR) and Iberian population (IBS) only.

of statistical results in gene-association studies has become the golden standard for assessing the independent effect of SNP and/or its genomic location to a certain disease [3]. Unfortunately, reproducibility is frequently challenging to achieve due to genetic heterogeneity, inadequate population size, or variability in phenotype definitions, environmental interactions, inadequate statistical power, and age-dependent effects [1, 2, 24–26].

Previous gene-association studies investigating SNPs in PVR have demonstrated significant differences between PVR cases, RRD controls, and healthy controls and predicted several genetic associations for PVR development [10, 16–19]. Fundamental studies in PVR research were based on international investigation of SNP genotype associations and included patients from Spain, Portugal, UK, and Netherlands [18, 19]. However, these studies did not include the comparison of genotype distributions in healthy populations across European subpopulations. For this reason, it is possible that failed replications of SNP effects in studies that followed were a consequence of different genetic structures across studied populations *per se*.

The present study compared the distribution of 42 SNP genotypes between Slovenian and European healthy populations and revealed significant differences in 10 SNPs, suggesting a somewhat similar distribution of genotypes among residents of common European ancestry. Our results firstly suggest that genotype polymorphisms more frequently identified in individuals from one European country could probably share a similar genotype pattern in individuals from other European countries as well. Our observations also indicate that different allele frequencies across independent datasets indeed influence the final SNP effect, frequently leading to spurious results in replication studies. The mentioned bias has been confirmed in our study by manipulating a simulated case-control dataset, which revealed that already a small change of 0.02 in MAF indeed causes important differences in statistical significance in genetic-association studies. Similar results were obtained in a simulation study of two interacting SNPs by Greene et al. which showed that the power to replicate the statistically significant independent effect of one SNP can drop dramatically with a change in allele frequency of less than 0.1 at the second interacting polymorphism [3]. On the other hand, it has been proposed that population structure has so far caused less inaccurate associations in genetic-association studies than it was initially predicted. When systematic ethnicity

Table 2: Genotype distributions of 4 SNPs in Slovenian patients with PVR and 96 healthy controls. Inheritance models and odds ratios (ORs) were determined.

Gene	SNP	Genotype	Genotype frequency in healthy controls (%)	Genotype frequency in cases (%)	Inheritance model*	OR (95% CI)	P value
IL1A	rs17561	CC	49 (51)	49 (43.39)	Codominant (CC-CA/AA)	3.00 (0.77–11.75)	**0.036**
	C/A	CA	38 (40)	59 (52.29)			
		AA	9 (9)	3 (2.7)			
		ND	0 (0)	2 (1.8)			
Total number of participants			96 (100)	113 (100)			
IL2	rs2069763	CC	39 (41)	52 (46.0)	Recessive** (CC/CA-AA)	1.51 (0.71–3.18)	0.28
	C/A	CA	39 (41)	46 (40.7)			
		AA	18 (19)	15 (13.3)			
Total number of participants			96 (100)	113 (100)			
LTA	rs2229094	CC	8 (8.3)	15 (9.8)	Additive	1.15 (0.78–1.70)	0.49
	T/C	TC	33 (34.4)	55 (36.0)			
		TT	55 (57.3)	79 (51.6)			
		ND	0 (0)	4 (2.6)			
Total number of participants			96 (100)	153 (100)			
TNF	rs1800629	GG	74 (77)	96 (62.7)	Overdominant (GG-AA/AG)	0.48 0.27–0.87	**0.014**
	G/A	AG	20 (21)	54 (35.3)			
		AA	2 (2)	3 (2.0)			
Total number of participants			96 (100)	153 (100)			

Abbreviations: OR: odds ratio; 95% CI: 95% confidence interval; ND: patients, in which genotype could not be identified. *Inheritance models: additive: each copy of the rare variant modifies the risk; dominant: a single copy of the frequent variant is enough to modify the risk; recessive: two copies of the variant allele are necessary to change the risk; overdominant: heterozygosity modifies the risk. **In case of IL2, the inheritance model could be also additive (OR, 1.23; 95% CI, 0.84–1.80; $P = 0.28$).

matching and application of standard quality control measures are not provided by research executors, population effect can still represent a major bias in these studies [5]. In the second part of our study, we have found a statistically significant difference in distribution of genotypes between healthy controls and PVR patients in rs17561 within the *IL1A* gene and rs1800629 (*TNF*). Similar significance was observed in a previously published study by Sanabria Ruiz-Colmenares et al. for *TGFB1* (rs1800471), when no significant difference in genotype distribution was observed between patients with and without PVR; instead, a statistically significant difference was observed between PVR patients and healthy controls [14].

The impact of different distributions of genotypes in SNPs in TNF locus, which encodes also TNF-α, has been investigated in three subsequent studies by a Spanish group of the Retina 4 Project [10, 11, 16]. Various SNPs in *TNF* have been shown to be associated with increased risk of PVR development, including the rs1800629. However, we have found a statistically significant difference in distributions of genotypes between healthy controls and PVR patients. In conclusion, the ultimate goal in PVR research as well as in other human diseases is to detect genetic associations, which replicate in studies without a significant bias. Our study showed that differences in genotype distributions exist between healthy populations across different European countries and may have had influenced the failed replication results in PVR SNP-association studies. This study confirmed the importance of baseline screening of the healthy population before investigating patients originating from the same dataset. Considering the fact that genotype distributions in patients with PVR and RRD patients without PVR have been compared within a limited number of European countries (Netherlands, Portugal, Slovenia, Spain, and United Kingdom), and that results of different previous PVR studies failed to be replicated, it is crucial to conduct larger multicentric population-based study.

Conflicts of Interest

None of the authors has any conflicting interests to disclose.

Acknowledgments

The authors thank Borut Jerman, PhD, for technical support with PLINK software. This work is a part of the PhD thesis of candidate Xhevat Lumi, MD. This work was supported by the Slovenian Research Agency (ARRS) (Programs P3-054 and P3-0333).

References

[1] T. A. Pearson and T. A. Manolio, "How to interpret a genome-wide association study," *JAMA*, vol. 299, no. 11, pp. 1335–1344, 2008.

[2] J. N. Hirschhorn and M. J. Daly, "Genome-wide association studies for common diseases and complex traits," *Nature Reviews Genetics*, vol. 6, no. 2, pp. 95–108, 2005.

[3] C. S. Greene, N. M. Penrod, S. M. Williams, and J. H. Moore, "Failure to replicate a genetic association may provide important clues about genetic architecture," *PLoS One*, vol. 4, no. 6, article e5639, 2009.

[4] P. Gorroochurn, S. E. Hodge, G. A. Heiman, M. Durner, and D. A. Greenberg, "Non-replication of association studies: "pseudo-failures" to replicate?," *Genetics in Medicine*, vol. 9, no. 6, pp. 325–331, 2007.

[5] J. Nsengimana and D. T. Bishop, "Design considerations for genetic linkage and association studies," *Methods in Molecular Biology*, vol. 850, pp. 237–262, 2012.

[6] J. C. Pastor, "Proliferative vitreoretinopathy: an overview," *Survey of Ophthalmology*, vol. 43, no. 1, pp. 3–18, 1998.

[7] J. C. Pastor, J. Rojas, S. Pastor-Idoate, S. di Lauro, L. Gonzalez-Buendia, and S. Delgado-Tirado, "Proliferative vitreoretinopathy: a new concept of disease pathogenesis and practical consequences," *Progress in Retinal and Eye Research*, vol. 51, pp. 125–155, 2016.

[8] S. Yang, H. Li, M. Li, and F. Wang, "Mechanisms of epithelial-mesenchymal transition in proliferative vitreoretinopathy," *Discovery Medicine*, vol. 20, no. 110, pp. 207–217, 2015.

[9] A. Sadaka and G. P. Giuliari, "Proliferative vitreoretinopathy: current and emerging treatments," *Clinical Ophthalmology*, vol. 6, pp. 1325–1333, 2012.

[10] J. Rojas, I. Fernandez, J. C. Pastor et al., "A genetic case-control study confirms the implication of *SMAD7* and *TNF locus* in the development of proliferative vitreoretinopathy," *Investigative Ophthalmology & Visual Science*, vol. 54, no. 3, pp. 1665–1678, 2013.

[11] J. Rojas, I. Fernandez, J. C. Pastor et al., "Development of predictive models of proliferative vitreoretinopathy based on genetic variables: the Retina 4 Project," *Investigative Ophthalmology & Visual Science*, vol. 50, no. 5, pp. 2384–2390, 2009.

[12] S. Pennock, L. J. Haddock, D. Eliott, S. Mukai, and A. Kazlauskas, "Is neutralizing vitreal growth factors a viable strategy to prevent proliferative vitreoretinopathy?," *Progress in Retinal and Eye Research*, vol. 40, pp. 16–34, 2014.

[13] F. Rouberol and C. Chiquet, "Proliferative vitreoretinopathy: pathophysiology and clinical diagnosis," *Journal Français d'Ophtalmologie*, vol. 37, no. 7, pp. 557–565, 2014.

[14] M. R. Sanabria Ruiz-Colmenares, J. C. Pastor Jimeno, J. A. Garrote Adrados, J. J. Telleria Orriols, and M. I. Yugueros Fernández, "Cytokine gene polymorphisms in retinal detachment patients with and without proliferative vitreoretinopathy: a preliminary study," *Acta Ophthalmologica Scandinavica*, vol. 84, no. 3, pp. 309–313, 2006.

[15] S. Saika, O. Yamanaka, I. Nishikawa-Ishida et al., "Effect of Smad7 gene overexpression on transforming growth factor β-induced retinal pigment fibrosis in a proliferative vitreoretinopathy mouse model," *Archives of Ophthalmology*, vol. 125, no. 5, pp. 647–654, 2007.

[16] J. Rojas, I. Fernandez, J. C. Pastor et al., "A strong genetic association between the tumor necrosis factor locus and proliferative vitreoretinopathy: the Retina 4 Project," *Ophthalmology*, vol. 117, no. 12, pp. 2417–2423.e2, 2010.

[17] S. Pastor-Idoate, I. Rodríguez-Hernández, J. Rojas et al., "BAX and BCL-2 polymorphisms, as predictors of proliferative vitreoretinopathy development in patients suffering retinal detachment: the Retina 4 Project," *Acta Ophthalmologica*, vol. 93, no. 7, pp. e541–e549, 2015.

[18] S. Pastor-Idoate, I. Rodríguez-Hernández, J. Rojas et al., "The T309G MDM2 gene polymorphism is a novel risk factor for proliferative vitreoretinopathy," *PLoS One*, vol. 8, no. 12, article e82283, 2013.

[19] S. Pastor-Idoate, I. Rodriguez-Hernández, J. Rojas et al., "The *p53* codon 72 polymorphism (rs1042522) is associated with proliferative vitreoretinopathy: the Retina 4 Project," *Ophthalmology*, vol. 120, no. 3, pp. 623–628, 2013.

[20] J. Rojas, I. Fernandez, J. C. Pastor et al., "Predicting proliferative vitreoretinopathy: temporal and external validation of models based on genetic and clinical variables," *The British Journal of Ophthalmology*, vol. 99, no. 1, pp. 41–48, 2015.

[21] J. Attia, J. P. A. Ioannidis, A. Thakkinstian et al., "How to use an article about genetic association: B: are the results of the study valid?," *JAMA*, vol. 301, no. 2, pp. 191–197, 2009.

[22] X. Sole, E. Guino, J. Valls, R. Iniesta, and V. Moreno, "SNPStats: a web tool for the analysis of association studies," *Bioinformatics*, vol. 22, no. 15, pp. 1928-1929, 2006.

[23] K. Nassar, S. Grisanti, A. Tura et al., "A TGF-β receptor 1 inhibitor for prevention of proliferative vitreoretinopathy," *Experimental Eye Research*, vol. 123, pp. 72–86, 2014.

[24] J. Ott, "Association of genetic loci: replication or not, that is the question," *Neurology*, vol. 63, no. 6, pp. 955–958, 2004.

[25] J. P. A. Ioannidis, "Non-replication and inconsistency in the genome-wide association setting," *Human Heredity*, vol. 64, no. 4, pp. 203–213, 2007.

[26] J. Lasky-Su, H. N. Lyon, V. Emilsson et al., "On the replication of genetic associations: timing can be everything!," *The American Journal of Human Genetics*, vol. 82, no. 4, pp. 849–858, 2008.

22

Decorin, Tenascin C, Total Antioxidant, and Total Oxidant Level Changes in Patients with Pseudoexfoliation Syndrome

Yavuz Oruc,[1] Sinem Keser,[1] Elif Yusufoglu,[1] Fatih Celik,[1] İbrahim Sahin,[2,3] Meltem Yardim,[2] and Suleyman Aydin[2]

[1]*Department of Ophthalmology, Elazig Research and Education Hospital, Health Science University, 23119 Elazig, Turkey*
[2]*Department of Medical Biochemistry and Clinical Biochemistry, Firat Hormones Research Group, Medical School, Firat University, 23119 Elazig, Turkey*
[3]*Department of Medical Biology, Medical School, Erzincan Binali Yildirim University, 24100 Erzincan, Turkey*

Correspondence should be addressed to Suleyman Aydin; saydin1@hotmail.com

Academic Editor: Maurizio Uva

Purpose. Pseudoexfoliation syndrome (PEX) is an eye disease that develops under the influence of regional population differences, genetic factors, age, and environmental factors and is characterized by visualization of a gray-white fibrogranular substance in the lens anterior capsule and/or pupil margin during anterior segment examination. The underlying biochemical mechanisms of the disease have not yet been fully elucidated. Therefore, this study was designed to show the changes in aqueous humor and blood serum levels of matrix metalloproteinases (decorin and tenascin C), total antioxidants (TAS), and total oxidants (TOS) in both cataract patients who have unilateral PEX material and cataract patients who do not have unilateral PEX material. *Methods.* Biological samples were simultaneously collected from 22 cataract patients who had unilateral pseudoexfoliation (PEX patients) and 22 cataract patients who did not have unilateral pseudoexfoliation (control patients). From the collected biological samples, decorin (DEC) and tenascin C (TN-C) were measured with the enzyme-linked immunosorbent assay (ELISA) method, and TAS and TOS were measured with an autoanalyzer. *Results.* When decorin, tenascin C, and TOS values of PEX patients were compared with those of control patients, there was a statistically significant increase in all three parameters. Conversely, TAS values showed a statistically significant decrease in PEX patients compared to controls. DEC, TN-C, TAS values, and TOS values were significantly higher in aqueous fluid than in blood in both the PEX patient and control groups. *Conclusions.* We suggest that parameters such as DEC, TN-C, TAS, and TOS play a role in the etiopathology of pseudoexfoliation syndrome. Thus, bringing these increased levels of extracellular proteins and TOS and decreased levels of TAS back to within physiological limits can mediate the reorganization of the blood-aqueous fluid barrier and slow the progression of pseudoexfoliation syndrome.

1. Introduction

Pseudoexfoliation syndrome (PEX) is a systemic disease with a 5–25% prevalence in all societies worldwide (genetically linked and influenced by race, age, and environmental factors). PEX is characterized by a grayish-white, bran-like fibrillar extracellular material in the intraocular and extraocular structures such as the pupillary flank, lens anterior capsule, iridocorneal angle, ciliary body and zonules, anterior hyaloid face, trabecular meshwork, corneal endothelium, and lid conjunctiva [1–3].

However, although the abovementioned features of PEX are known, the definitive etiopathology has not been fully elucidated. Studies to date have reported that this condition is associated with extreme accumulation of abnormally structured extracellular material in intraocular and ectodermal tissues [4]. Therefore, associations between molecules such as elastin, fibronectin, amyloid, fibrilin-1, and PEX were investigated, and their relationship was revealed. In addition, other studies have reported increased growth factors in the aqueous humor of patients with PEX. Another study group (Schlotzer-shrehud et al.) reported that the concentrations of matrix metalloproteinases and their inhibitors in the aqueous humor of PEX patients were increased [5].

Two of the most important members of the matrix metalloproteinase family are decorin (DEC) and tenascin C

(TN-C). DEC is a proteoglycan that is rich in leucine amino acids. This protein is associated with collagen fibrils from all connective tissues, and the average molecular weight ranges from 90 to 140 kilodaltons (kDa). The main function of DEC is to regulate cellular proliferation and differentiation in newly formed bone [6]. DEC also mediates the stabilization of the collagen skeleton, supporting ligaments and tendons. Histochemical and immunochemical studies have reported that glycoprotein/proteoglycan molecules play a role in the etiopathology of PEX [7–14]. Thus, we believe that it is scientifically worthwhile to show whether decorin, a proteoglycan-structured molecule as described above, is involved in the etiopathogenesis of PEX. According to an extensive literature review, there is no scientific study investigating this linkage.

Similarly, TN-C is one of the glycoprotein/proteoglycan-forming matrix metalloproteinases, and a study investigating its association with PEX has not yet been performed. TN-C induces smooth muscle cell proliferation in collaboration with growth factors. The molecular weight of TN-C ranges from 250 to 300 kilodaltons (kDa). Glycoproteins and proteoglycans encircle the retinal cells. TN-C, a proteoglycan, is a key molecule in the immune system and neuroinflammatory processes. TN-C also plays a role in the etiopathogenesis of macular degeneration, diabetic retinopathy, glaucoma, and retinal vascular occlusion [15]. It has been studied in many biological fluids, cartilage extracts, synovial fluid, and blood. TN-C has not yet been studied in the aqueous humor [16, 17].

Pseudoexfoliation is a syndrome associated with cataracts. Thirty-five percent of cataract formation is caused by genetic factors, and the other 65 percent is caused by environmental factors such as nutrition, age, alcohol, cigarette consumption, diabetes, and excessive daylight exposure [18]. Antioxidants protect cells from free radicals. There is evidence that abundant intake of antioxidant vitamin C reduces the risk of cataracts, slows down cataract progression, and reduces the need for cataract surgery [19, 20]. This means that the coexistence of PEX and cataracts is one of the oxidative stress states in which antioxidant mechanisms are inhibited.

Oxidative damage has been demonstrated to play a major role in ocular diseases including cataracts and macular degeneration [21, 22]. Increasing evidence indicates that oxidative stress plays a key role in the pathogenesis of PEX syndrome [23–27]. Oxidative stress causes the production of free radicals, which are reactive chemical species generated during normal metabolic processes that can damage lipids and proteins when present in excess [28].

Therefore, it is also within the objectives of this work to establish whether total antioxidant capacity (TAS) and total oxidant capacity (TOS) have links to PEX. The diagnosis of PEX is usually made with a biomicroscope. However, this does not provide clues into the etiopathogenesis of the disease. It is important to examine aqueous humor and blood materials to reveal the biological mechanisms underlying PEX. Therefore, this study was designed in order to show whether there is a relationship between TAS or TOS and PEX and determine the changes in the levels of matrix metalloproteinases (DEC and TN-C), TAS, and TOS in aqueous humor and serum in cataract patients with unilateral PEX material and in cataract patients who do not have unilateral PEX material.

2. Material and Method

This study was approved by the Noninterventional Ethics Committee of Firat University on 5 January 2018 with decision number 10; informed consent forms were obtained from the subjects. The study was originally planned to be performed with 30 patients who had unilateral PEX and cataracts together (PEX group) and 30 patients with cataracts who did not have unilateral PEX (control group). However, 8 patients from each group left the study; therefore, 22 subjects for each group remained in the analysis. Patients were evaluated before surgery, and age, sex, and cataract types were recorded. The type of surgery performed (phacoemulsification, extracapsular lens extraction, intracapsular lens extraction, and insertion of the intraocular lens), approach (into the lens capsule, sulcus, anterior chamber, and fixation to sclera or aphakia), and occurrence of any complications during surgery (posterior capsule opening, zonular dialysis, drop of lens parts in the vitra, and vitreous loss) were assessed as described previously. Participants with diabetes, systemic arterial hypertension, systemic vasculopathies, retinal diseases (macular degeneration, etc.), ocular surgery, ocular trauma, or ocular inflammation were excluded from the study. In patients with PEX, the material was observed and detected on the biomicroscope at the edge of the pupil and on the anterior capsule of the lens. All of the patients included in this study were operated on using the phaco method.

A blood sample and 0.1 mL aqueous humor sample taken from the anterior chamber during cataract surgery were simultaneously collected into biochemistry centrifuge tubes and delivered to the biochemical laboratory within an ice basket. After samples were centrifuged at 4000 rpm, they were stored at −80°C. TN-C levels (Human TN-C) in the blood and aqueous humor (anterior chamber fluid) of PEX patients and control group were studied with the ELISA method (catalog number 201-12-1415 Sunred Biological Technology Co., Ltd., Shanghai, China) in accordance with the operating procedures specified in the kit instructions. The assay range for the Human TN-C ELISA kit was 200–60000 pg/mL; intraassay CV value was <10%, interassay CV value was <12%, and sensitivity was 180.556 pg/mL. As aqueous humor samples were diluted with a 1/2 ratio of pH 7.4 phosphate buffer, values for anterior chamber fluid results were entered by multiplying by a dilution factor of 2. Plate washes were performed with an automatic washer Bio-Tek ELX50 (BioTek Instruments, USA) and absorbance readings were made with ChroMate Microplate Reader P4300 instruments (Awareness Technology Instruments, USA). Test results were reported in pg/mL.

DEC levels (human decorin) in the blood and aqueous humor (anterior chamber fluid) of PEX patients and control patients were studied with the ELISA method in accordance with the operating procedures specified in the kit instructions (catalog number 201-12-3612 Sunred Biological Technology Co., Ltd., Shanghai, China). The assay range for the Human DEC ELISA kit was 0.2–40 ng/mL; intraassay

Table 1: Demographic and cataract characteristics of patients.

Group	Age	BMI	Sex		Location		Type of cataract
			Male	Female	Right eye	Left eye	
Control (cataract)	71.64 ± 6.43	25.46 ± 2.59	4	2	2	4	Posterior subcapsular cataract
			3	2	—	5	Mature cataract
			11	13	11[a]	13[a]	Nuclear cataract
			5	4	6	3	Cortical cataract
			23	**21**	**19**	**25**	*Total* (*n*: 44)
PEX + cataract	70.93 ± 5.63	25.66 ± 2.46	5	2	2	5	Posterior subcapsular cataract
			2	4	2	4	Mature cataract
			12	19	17[a]	14[a]	Nuclear cataract
			—	—	—	—	Cortical cataract
			19	**25**	**21**	**23**	*Total* (*n*: 44)

PEX: pseudoexfoliation syndrome; BMI: body mass index. [a]$p < 0.05$.

CV value was <10%, interassay CV value was <12%, and sensitivity was 144 ng/mL. As aqueous humor samples were diluted with a 1/2 ratio of pH 7.4 phosphate buffer, values for anterior chamber fluid results were entered after multiplying by a dilution factor of 2. Plate washes were performed with an automatic washer Bio-Tek ELX50 (BioTek Instruments, USA) and absorbance readings were made with ChroMate Microplate Reader P4300 instruments (Awareness Technology Instruments, USA). Test results were reported in ng/mL.

TN-C measurements were initially given in pg/mL, per the manufacturing company, but were converted to ng/mL for easy comparison with DEC values. In this study, TAS and TOS values were measured according to the previously mentioned method. As TAS and TOS kits were produced in order to measure blood TAS and TOS levels, a validity test was carried out in order to see whether these kits could measure TAS and TOS levels from the aqueous humor.

TAS was measured using a fully automatic method that detects the TAS and produces a Fenton-type reaction with oxygen peroxide and Fe^{+2} o-dianisidine, resulting in OH radicals [29]. This strongly reactive oxygen species is reduced and reacts with the o-dianisidine molecule at acidic pH to form yellow-brown dianisidine radicals. These radicals produce color formations by participating in oxidation reactions. However, antioxidants present in these samples suppress these oxidation reactions and stop color formation. These reaction results are obtained automatically with an autoanalyzer measurement.

TOS is a fully automated system that oxidizes the ferrozine o-dianisidine complex to the ferric ion, showing the TOS with the uptake of the oxidants present in the material; ferric ions form a colored complex with xylenol orange at an acidic pH [30]. The intensity of the color, which is associated with the level of oxidants present in the samples, is measured spectrophotometrically. The mmol value of the TAS test was converted to μmol units as in the TOS test, and the oxidative stress index (OSI) was calculated according to the following formula: OSI (arbitrary unit) = TOS (μmol H_2O_2 Eq/L)/TAS (μmol Trolox Eq/L) [31].

The intraassay CV value of TAS was <10%, while the intraassay CV value of TOS was <12%. Interassay CV values of TAS and TOS were detected as <15%. The intraassay CV value of decorin was <10% and the interassay CV value was detected as <15%. The recovery results of the kits were ranged between 98 and 114%. It was recorded that there was linearity in the measurements across dilutions. According to all the validity tests, the kits used in this study were determined to have the same sensitivity in the measurements of eye liquid as those of the blood.

2.1. Statistical Analysis. Differences in the preoperative distribution of age, sex, cataract type, type of operation, and complication rate during surgery were examined between groups. Statistical analyses were performed using the SPSS 22.00 package program. The Mann–Whitney *U* test was used for comparison between groups. The difference between the groups was considered significant when p was < 0.05.

3. Results

The demographic characteristics of the subjects are summarized in Table 1. There was no statistically significant difference between the PEX and control groups with regard to body mass index and age. Within the PEX group, 19 (43.2%) were male, and 25 (56.8%) were female. Within the control group, 23 (52.3%) were male and 21 (47.7%) were female. When the groups were examined according to preoperative cataract types, it was found that nuclear cataracts were seen most frequently in both groups. According to the eye symmetry, 11 (45.8%) of the cataracts were in the right eye, and 13 (542%) were in the left eye in the group without PEX ($n = 24$, 54.55%). However, in PEX group ($n = 31$, 70.45%), 17 of the cataracts were in the right eye (54.8%), and 14 of them were in the left eye (45.2%) according to eye symmetry. There was a significant difference in the distribution of cataract type according to the groups ($p = 0.02$) (Table 1).

The values of decorin in the aqueous humor and in the blood were significantly higher in the PEX group than in the control group (Figure 1). When we compared the aqueous humor values of decorin with the blood values, we observed statistically significantly higher levels in both the patient group and the control group (Figure 1). Similarly, when compared with the control group (patients with cataracts

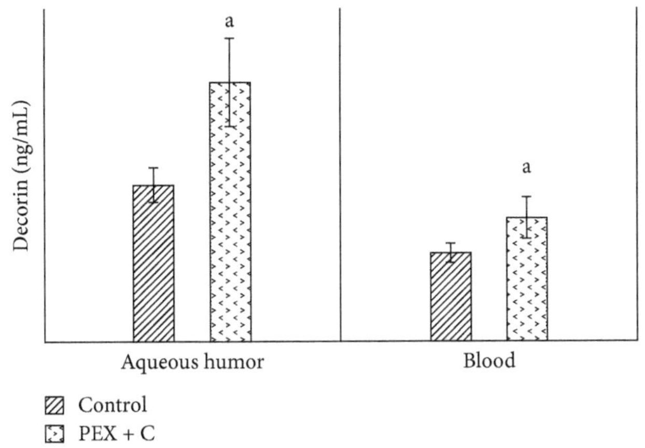

Figure 1: Comparison of decorin levels in intraocular fluid and blood between patients with and without pseudoexfoliation syndrome. C: cataract; PEX: unilateral pseudoexfoliation syndrome. (a) $p < 0.05$.

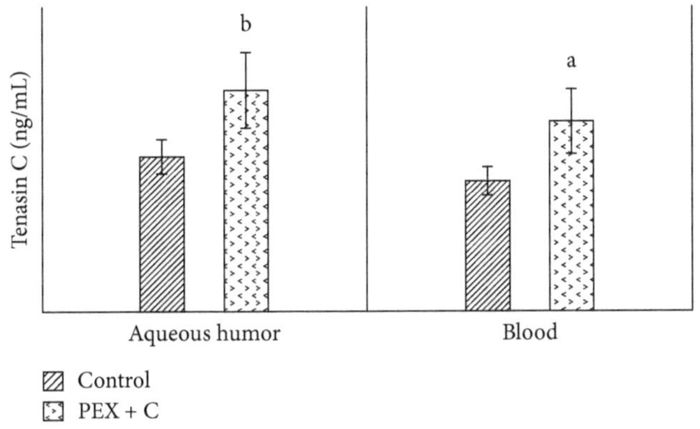

Figure 2: Comparison of tenascin C levels in aqueous humor and blood between cataract patients with and without pseudoexfoliation syndrome. C: cataract; PEX: unilateral pseudoexfoliation syndrome. (a) $p < 0.05$. (b) $p < 0.01$.

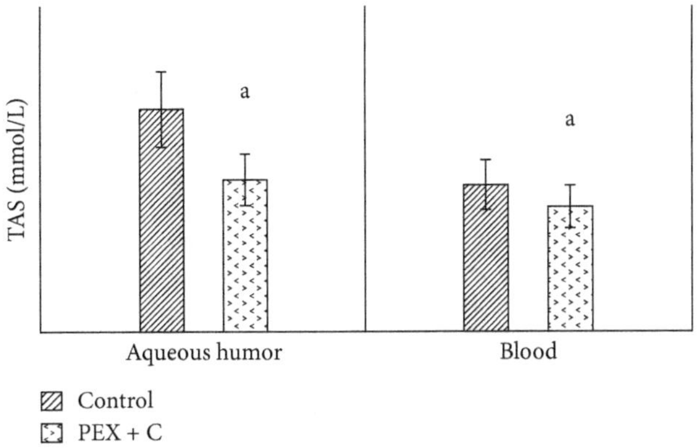

Figure 3: Comparison of TAS levels in aqueous humor and blood between cataract patients with and without pseudoexfoliation syndrome. C: cataract; PEX: unilateral pseudoexfoliation syndrome; TAS: total antioxidant. (a) $p < 0.05$.

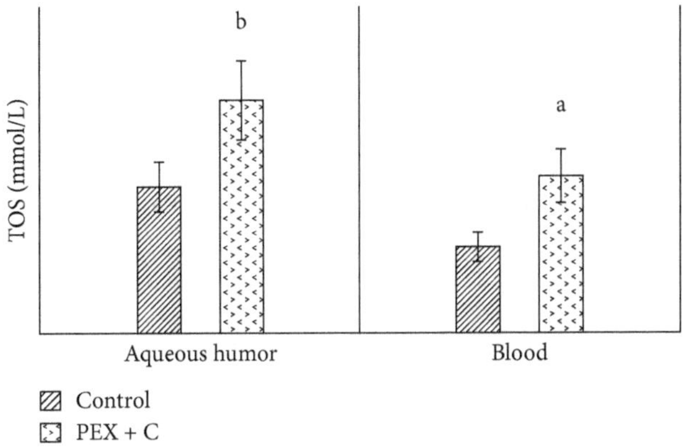

Figure 4: Comparison of TOS levels in aqueous humor and blood between patients with and without pseudoexfoliation syndrome. C: cataract; PEX: unilateral pseudoexfoliation syndrome; TOS: total oxidant. (a) $p < 0.05$. (b) $p < 0.01$.

who did not have pseudoexfoliation), tenascin C values in both the aqueous humor and blood were significantly high in the PEX group (Figure 2). When we compared the aqueous humor values of tenascin C with the blood values, we observed that they were significantly higher in both the patient and control groups (Figure 2). Compared with the control group, the TAS values in both the aqueous humor and blood were detected to be significantly lower in the PEX group (Figure 3). When we compared the aqueous humor values of TAS with the blood values, it was observed that they were significantly higher in both the PEX and control groups (Figure 3). The values of TOS in the aqueous humor and blood were significantly higher in the PEX group than in the control group (Figure 4). When we compared the aqueous humor values of TOS with the blood values, we observed that they were significantly higher in both the PEX group and the control group (Figure 4). There was local tissue reduction of TAS activity in PEX. Compared with the control group, we found the OSI values of the PEX group to be increased in both the aqueous humor and blood, and these increases were found to be significant (Figure 5).

4. Discussion

Pseudoexfoliation syndrome is an eye disease in which an extracellular matrix disorder is observed. PEX is often associated with cataracts, which causes ocular involvement and systemic involvement [1]. The worldwide incidence of PEX varies according to regional population differences and genetic variations, and etiopathology maintains its place on the agenda as an important eye health problem that needs to be fully addressed [3, 32, 33]. In recent years, matrix metalloproteinases have moved to the top of the list of the most frequently studied molecules with regard to the etiopathology of this disease [7]. DEC and TN-C are glycoprotein/proteoglycan-structured matrix metalloproteinases, and a study investigating their association with PEX has not been performed yet. Oxidative stress also plays a role in the etiopathology of many diseases. Therefore, the relationship between DEC, TN-C, TAS values, TOS values, and PEX was shown for the first time in this study. However, before the possible roles of these parameters in patients with PEX are discussed individually, we must first discuss the observed demographic characteristics, since the

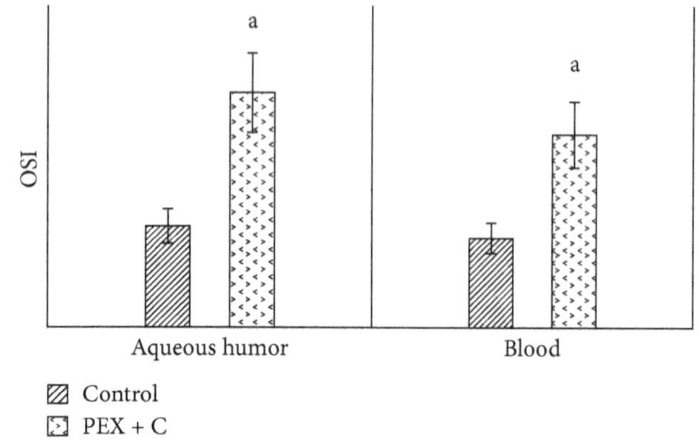

Figure 5: Comparison of OSI in aqueous humor and blood between patients with and without pseudoexfoliation syndrome. C: cataract; OSI: oxidative stress index; PEX: unilateral pseudoexfoliation syndrome. (a) $p < 0.05$.

association of both age and sex with cataracts has been revealed by many researchers in academic studies.

For example, many studies have shown that there is a significant positive correlation between age and the incidence of PEX. Moreover, the incidence after 50 years of age increases by a factor of two in each decade. Although PEX is often unilateral, it has also been shown that PEX appears in both eyes with advancing age in 13% of patients. In our study, we reported that the age averages of PEX and PEX-free cases were close to each other (no statistically significant difference) and that PEX was generally seen in only one eye.

Increased cataract prevalence is observed in patients with PEX. Both conditions occur with advanced age, and their co-occurrence is also frequent. This co-occurrence was reported with different ratios by different researchers as follows: Lumme 31%, Elibol 13.7%, Yalaz 17.7%, Drolsum 16%, Naumann 3%, Schönberr 5%, and Freyler 0.98% [34–40].

In addition, the complication rate in the PEX group was higher in this study than in the control group, but this was not statistically significant. Similarly, the complication rates in the PEX group were found to be high in many studies, but this was not statistically significant [41]. These complications, which are not statistically significant, are predicted to be due to differences in cataract morphology and the ages of the patients.

The incidence of PEX among sexes is debatable. Some studies reported that PEX can be seen more frequently in men, while other studies reported that PEX can be more frequent in women [42, 43]. However, many studies have shown that there is no significant relationship between sex and PEX [44]. There was no significant relationship between sex and PEX frequency in this present study. Therefore, TAS, TOS, TN-C, and DEC levels in this study were evaluated without sex distinction.

In this study, when levels of TAS in the aqueous humor and blood of patients with PEX were compared with those of the control group, TAS levels were significantly lower; however, TOS levels were reported to be significantly higher. We suggest that the observed decrease in TAS level and increase in TOS level in PEX syndrome increases oxidative stress, which makes cell membranes brittle, and extracellular matrix disorders may occur after increased cell destruction. This is further supported by our observed oxidative stress index values. In addition, oxidative damage is related to many pathological problems of the eye [45–47]. Several investigators have suggested that the reduction in antioxidant enzyme activities in ocular degenerative diseases may be a cause of oxidative stress in ocular degenerative diseases. Ferreira et al. conducted a study including patients with primary open-angle glaucoma. According to this study, TAS values in the aqueous humor of patients were significantly lower than those in the control group. The results of Ferreira et al. are consistent with our results, which were observed in patients with PEX syndrome [48].

A unilateral PEX group and control group (cataract patients without pseudoexfoliation) were compared in this study. DEC and TN-C values, in both aqueous humor and blood, were detected to be significantly higher in the unilateral PEX group.

DEC and TN-C are two important members of the matrix metalloproteinase class. Matrix metalloproteinases (MMPs) are involved in many physiological processes including embryogenesis and wound healing [49]. In addition, MMPs mediate cell penetration, leading proteins to pass the extracellular matrix (ECM) [50]. Presumably, MMP-2 also plays a major role in epithelial cell migration in the human eye lens. The increased levels of DEC and TN-C in PEX may be due to increased synthesis by the residual lens epithelial cells. Increased levels of these two molecules in aqueous humor in this study, when compared with blood, indicates that these two molecules are also synthesized in these tissues. In another study, TN-C expression has been reported to be upregulated in human lens epithelial cells during posterior capsule opacification (PCO) [51]. Therefore, it is considered that the levels of DEC and TN-C are increased in order to establish the tissue structure in PEX and the adaptation of individuals to PEX.

To determine whether the kits used in this study (DEC, TN-C, TAS, and TOS) can measure the values of interest in both aqueous humor and blood with the same sensitivity, the kits were tested with Aydin's previously specified assay validation experiment [52]. The kits were confirmed to measure with the same sensitivity in aqueous humor as in blood. Although kits are generally produced by manufacturers to detect biological molecules in blood, it has been reported by researchers that similar kits can be used with the same precision for many biological samples, including breast milk. The manufacturers of the kits specifically used in this study have indicated in their catalog that they can measure other biological fluids aside from blood.

As a result, PEX is a common condition in societies given the prevalence of general cataracts. When the patient and control groups were compared in this study, DEC and TN-C showed a statistically significant increase in the PEX group. In addition, the TAS level in the PEX group was statistically decreased, while the TOS level was statistically increased. In relation to the ways that these parameters may play a role in the etiopathology of PEX, we suggest that bringing these extracellular proteins, TOS levels and TAS levels back to within physiological limits can mediate the reorganization of the blood-aqueous fluid barrier and slow the progression of PEX. Additionally, these outcomes might be interrelated with a gradual deposition of fibrillary residue from the lens, ciliary body, iris, zonules, and corneal endothelium.

Conflicts of Interest

The authors declare that there are no conflicts of interest.

References

[1] H. Forsius, E. Forsman, J. Fellman, and A. W. Eriksson, "Exfoliation syndrome: frequency, gender distribution and association with climatically induced alterations of the cornea and conjunctiva," *Acta Ophthalmologica Scandinavica*, vol. 80, no. 5, pp. 478–484, 2002.

[2] H. Aasved, "Prevalence of fibrillopathia epitheliocapsularis (pseudoexfoliation) and capsular glaucoma," *Transactions of the ophthalmological societies of the United Kingdom*, vol. 99, no. 2, pp. 293–295, 1979.

[3] N. Yildirim, E. Yasar, H. Gursoy, and E. Colak, "Prevalence of pseudoexfoliation syndrome and its association with ocular and systemic diseases in Eskisehir, Turkey," *International Journal of Ophthalmology*, vol. 10, no. 1, pp. 128–134, 2017.

[4] M. Zenkel, "Extracellular matrix regulation and dysregulation in exfoliation syndrome," *Journal of Glaucoma*, vol. 10, pp. S24–S28, 2018.

[5] U. Schlötzer-Schrehardt, J. Lommatzsch, M. Küchle, A. G. Konstas, and G. O. Naumann, "Matrix metalloproteinases and their inhibitors in aqueous humor of patients with pseudoexfoliation syndrome/glaucoma and primary open-angle glaucoma," *Investigative Ophthalmology and Visual Science*, vol. 44, no. 3, pp. 1117–1125, 2003.

[6] D. J. Kirby and M. F. Young, "Isolation, production, and analysis of small leucine-rich proteoglycans in bone," *Methods in Cell Biology*, vol. 143, pp. 281–296, 2018.

[7] P. Sahay, A. Rao, D. Padhy et al., "Functional activity of matrix metalloproteinases 2 and 9 in tears of patients with glaucoma," *Investigative Ophthalmology and Visual Science*, vol. 58, no. 6, pp. BIO106–BIO113, 2017.

[8] S. Kara, N. Yildirim, A. Ozer, O. Colak, and A. Sahin, "Matrix metalloproteinase-2, tissue inhibitor of matrix metalloproteinase-2, and transforming growth factor beta 1 in the aqueous humor and serum of patients with pseudoexfoliationsyndrome," *Clinical Ophthalmology*, vol. 8, pp. 305–309, 2014.

[9] N. Fountoulakis, G. Labiris, A. Aristeidou et al., "Tissue inhibitor of metalloproteinase 4 in aqueous humor of patients with primary open angle glaucoma, pseudoexfoliation syndrome and pseudoexfoliative glaucoma and its role in proteolysis imbalance," *BMC Ophthalmology*, vol. 13, no. 1, p. 69, 2013.

[10] N. Zimmermann and C. Erb, "Immunoassay for matrix metalloproteinase-9 in the tear film of patients with pseudoexfoliationsyndrome-a pilot study," *Klinische Monatsblätter für Augenheilkunde*, vol. 230, no. 8, pp. 804–807, 2013.

[11] E. Elhawy, G. Kamthan, C. Q. Dong, and J. Danias, "Pseudoexfoliation syndrome, a systemic disorder with ocular manifestations," *Human Genomics*, vol. 6, no. 1, p. 22, 2012.

[12] U. Schlötzer-Schrehardt, "New pathogenetic insights into pseudoexfoliation syndrome/glaucoma. Therapeutically relevant?," *Ophthalmologe*, vol. 109, no. 10, pp. 944–951, 2012.

[13] J. Djordjević-Jocić, G. Zlatanović, D. Veselinović et al., "Transforming growth factor beta1, matrix-metalloproteinase-2 and its tissue inhibitor in patients with pseudoexfoliation glaucoma/syndrome," *Vojnosanitetski Pregled*, vol. 69, no. 3, pp. 231–236, 2012.

[14] S. L. Ho, G. F. Dogar, J. Wang et al., "Elevated aqueous humour tissue inhibitor of matrix metalloproteinase-1 and connective tissue growth factor in pseudoexfoliation syndrome," *British Journal of Ophthalmology*, vol. 89, no. 2, pp. 169–173, 2005.

[15] J. Reinhard, L. Roll, and A. Faissner, "Tenascins in retinal and optic nerve neurodegeneration," *Frontiers in Integrative Neuroscience*, vol. 11, pp. 30, 2017.

[16] L. Patel, W. Sun, S. S. Glasson, E. A. Morris, C. R. Flannery, and P. S. Chockalingam, "Tenascin-C induces inflammatory mediators and matrix degradation in osteoarthritic cartilage," *BMC Musculoskeletal Disorders*, vol. 12, no. 1, p. 164, 2011.

[17] R. G. Mansour, L. Stamper, F. Jaeger et al., "The presence and anti-HIV-1 function of tenascin C in breast milk and genital fluids," *PLoS One*, vol. 11, no. 5, Article ID e0155261, 2016.

[18] E. Yonova-Doing, Z. A. Forkin, P. G. Hysi et al., "Genetic and dietary factors influencing the progression of nuclear cataract," *Ophthalmology*, vol. 123, no. 6, pp. 1237–1244, 2016.

[19] K. A. Weikel, C. Garber, A. Baburins, and A. Taylor, "Nutritional modulation of cataract," *Nutrition Reviews*, vol. 72, no. 1, pp. 30–47, 2014.

[20] M. Pastor-Valero, "Fruit and vegetable intake and vitamins C and E are associated with a reduced prevalence of cataract in a Spanish Mediterranean population," *BMC Ophthalmology*, vol. 13, no. 1, pp. 52, 2013.

[21] J. Kruk, K. Kubasik-Kladna, and H. Y. Aboul-Enein, "The role oxidative stress in the pathogenesis of eye diseases: current status and a dual role of physical activity," *Mini-Reviews in Medicinal Chemistry*, vol. 16, no. 3, pp. 241–257, 2015.

[22] V. Agte and K. Tarwadi, "The importance of nutrition in the prevention of ocular disease with special reference to cataract," *Ophthalmic Research*, vol. 44, no. 3, pp. 166–172, 2010.

[23] M. Tetikoğlu, H. M. Sağdik, S. Aktas, F. Uçar, and F. Özcura, "Serum prolidase activity and oxidative stress in patients with pseudoexfoliation syndrome," *Graefe's Archive for Clinical and Experimental Ophthalmology*, vol. 254, no. 7, pp. 1339–1343, 2016.

[24] E. Ergan, F. Ozturk, E. Beyazyildiz et al., "Oxidant/antioxidant balance in the aqueous humor of patients with glaucoma," *International Journal of Ophthalmology*, vol. 9, no. 2, pp. 249–252, 2016.

[25] F. Dursun, A. Vural Ozec, and H. Aydin, "Total oxidative stress, paraoxonase and arylesterase levels at patients with pseudoexfoliation syndrome and pseudoexfoliative glaucoma," *International Journal of Ophthalmology*, vol. 8, no. 5, pp. 985–990, 2015.

[26] M. Tanito, S. Kaidzu, Y. Takai, and A. Ohira, "Status of systemic oxidative stresses in patients with primary open-angle glaucoma and pseudoexfoliation syndrome," *PLoS One*, vol. 7, no. 11, Article ID e49680, 2012.

[27] T. Cumurcu, A. Gunduz, H. Ozyurt, H. Nurcin, O. Atis, and M. Egri, "Increased oxidative stress in patients with pseudoexfoliation syndrome," *Ophthalmic Research*, vol. 43, no. 4, pp. 169–172, 2010.

[28] L. M. Pujol-Lereis, N. Schäfer, L. B. Kuhn, B. Rohrer, and D. Pauly, "Interrelation between oxidative stress and

complement activation in models of age-related macular degeneration," *Advances in Experimental Medicine and Biology*, vol. 854, pp. 87–93, 2016.
[29] O. Erel, "A novel automated direct measurement method for total antioxidant capacity using a new generation, more stable ABTS radical cation," *Clinical Biochemistry*, vol. 37, no. 4, pp. 277–285, 2004.
[30] O. Erel, "A new automated colorimetric method for measuring total oxidant status," *Clinical Biochemistry*, vol. 38, no. 12, pp. 1103–1111, 2005.
[31] S. Aydin, M. Ogeturk, T. Kuloglu, A. Kavakli, and S. Aydin, "Effect of carnosine supplementation on apoptosis and irisin, total oxidant and antioxidants levels in the serum, liver and lung tissues in rats exposed to formaldehyde inhalation," *Peptides*, vol. 64, pp. 14–23, 2015.
[32] S. Y. Lee, S. Kim, J. H. Kim et al., "Prevalence of pseudoexfoliation syndrome in an isolated island population of Korea: the Woodo study," *Journal of Glaucoma*, vol. 26, no. 8, pp. 730–734, 2017.
[33] H. Hashemi, M. Khabazkhoob, M. H. Emamian, A. Jafari, S. Mohazeb-Torabi, and A. Fotouhi, "The prevalence of exfoliation syndrome in an Iranian population aged 45-69 years," *Ophthalmic Epidemiology*, vol. 23, no. 5, pp. 303–308, 2016.
[34] P. Lumme and L. Laatikainen, "Exfoliation syndrome and cataract extraction," *American Journal of Ophthalmology*, vol. 116, no. 1, pp. 51–55, 1993.
[35] M. Yalaz, I. Otman, K. Nas et al., "The frequency of pseudoexfoliation syndrome in the eastern Mediterranean area of Turkey," *Acta Ophthalmologica*, vol. 70, no. 2, pp. 209–213, 1992.
[36] O. Elibol, C. Güler, T. Alçelik, and T. Erdoğan, "Eksfoliasyon sendromunun PEKKE ve arka kamara göz içi lens implantasyonuna etkisi," *Medical Network Oftalmoloji*, vol. 2, no. 4, pp. 342–345, 1995.
[37] G. O. H. Naumann, M. Küchle, and U. Schönherr, "Pseudoexfoliation syndrome as a risk factor for vitreus loss in ECCE," *Fortschritte Der Ophthalmologie*, vol. 86, pp. 543–545, 1989.
[38] L. Drolsum, E. Haaskjold, and M. Davanger, "Results and complications after extracapsular cataract extraction in eyes with pseudoexfoliation syndrome," *Acta Ophthalmologica*, vol. 71, no. 6, pp. 771–776, 1993.
[39] H. Freyler and U. Radax, "Pseudoexfoliation syndrome–a risk factor in modern cataract surgery?," *Klinische Monatsblätter für Augenheilkunde*, vol. 205, no. 5, pp. 275–279, 1994.
[40] U. Schönherr, M. Küchle, A. Händel, G. K. Lang, and G. O. Naumann, "Pseudoexfoliation syndrome with and without glaucoma as a major risk factor in extracapsular cataract extraction. A prospective clinical study," *Fortschritte Der Ophthalmologie*, vol. 87, no. 6, pp. 588–590, 1990.
[41] N. R. Dwivedi, A. K. Dubey, and P. R. Shankar, "Intraoperative and immediate postoperative outcomes of cataract surgery using phacoemulsification in eyes with and without pseudoexfoliation syndrome," *Journal of Clinical and Diagnostic Research*, vol. 8, no. 12, pp. VC01–VC05, 2014.
[42] A. Arnarsson, H. Sasaki, and F. Z. Jonasson, "Twelve-year incidence of exfoliation syndrome in the reykjavik eye study," *Acta Ophthalmologica*, vol. 91, no. 2, pp. 157–162, 2013.
[43] S. Åström and C. Lindén, "Incidence and prevalence of pseudoexfoliation and open-angle glaucoma in northern Sweden: I. Baseline report," *Acta Ophthalmologica Scandinavica*, vol. 85, no. 8, pp. 828–831, 2007.
[44] G. E. Erkayhan and S. Dogan, "Cataract surgery and possible complications in patients with pseudoexfoliation syndrome," *Eurasian Journal of Medicine*, vol. 49, no. 1, pp. 22–25, 2017.
[45] R. Shetty, A. Sharma, N. Pahuja et al., "Oxidative stress induces dysregulated autophagy in corneal epithelium of keratoconus patients," *PLoS One*, vol. 12, no. 9, Article ID e0184628, 2017.
[46] R. A. Kowluru and Y. Shan, "Role of oxidative stress in epigenetic modification of MMP-9 promoter in the development of diabetic retinopathy," *Graefe's Archive for Clinical and Experimental Ophthalmology*, vol. 255, no. 5, pp. 955–962, 2017.
[47] O. Awodele, I. A. Oreagba, S. O. Olayemi et al., "Evaluation and comparison of the indices of systemic oxidative stress among black-africans with age-related cataracts or primary glaucoma," *Middle East African Journal of Ophthalmology*, vol. 22, no. 4, pp. 489–494, 2015.
[48] S. M. Ferreira, S. F. Lerner, R. Brunzini, P. A. Evelson, and S. F. Llesuy, "Oxidative stress markers in aqueous humor of glaucoma patients," *American Journal of Ophthalmology*, vol. 137, no. 1, pp. 62–69, 2004.
[49] B. J. Rose and D. L. Kooyman, "A tale of two joints: the role of matrix metalloproteases in cartilage biology," *Disease Markers*, vol. 2016, Article ID 4895050, 7 pages, 2016.
[50] S. Kumar, A. Das, A. Barai, and S. Sen, "MMP secretion rate and inter-invadopodia spacing collectively govern cancer invasiveness," *Biophysical Journal*, vol. 114, no. 3, pp. 650–662, 2018.
[51] F. A. Mamuya, Y. Wang, V. H. Roop, D. A. Scheiblin, J. C. Zajac, and M. K. Duncan, "The roles of αV integrins in lens EMT and posterior capsular opacification," *Journal of Cellular and Molecular Medicine*, vol. 18, no. 4, pp. 656–670, 2014.
[52] S. Aydin, "A short history, principles, and types of ELISA, and our laboratory experience with peptide/protein analyses using ELISA," *Peptides*, vol. 72, pp. 4–15, 2015.

23

Vision-Threatening Behcet's Disease: Severity of Ocular Involvement Predictors

Mohammed A. Hussein,[1] Iman M. Eissa,[2] and Ahmed A. Dahab[2]

[1]*Internal Medicine Department, Rheumatology and Clinical Immunology Division, Cairo University, Cairo, Egypt*
[2]*Ophthalmology Department, Cairo University, Cairo, Egypt*

Correspondence should be addressed to Iman M. Eissa; iman_eissa@yahoo.com

Academic Editor: Anna Nowinska

Purpose. To examine and spot systemic findings commonly associated with a serious form of ocular Behcet's disease. This could potentially help ophthalmologists categorize their patients based on future risk and plan treatment accordingly. *Subjects and Methods.* The data of 249 patients with Behcet's disease were examined thoroughly. Correlations between systemic and ocular findings were recorded. Patients were further subgrouped by the authors as having a vision-threatening form of the disease or not. Regression analysis was done to spot predictors for a vision-threatening form of the disease. *Results.* The presence of systemic vasculitis and oral and genital ulcers in a patient with Behcet's disease was found to be associated with a milder form of ocular affection or none at all and vice versa. Certain correlations between findings were also found. *Conclusion.* Certain findings in Behcet's disease may act as predictors for the severity of ocular affection. Directing our attention to these factors by the internist and ophthalmologist can help plan the frequency of follow-up as well as the aggressiveness of treatment in patients with Behcet's disease.

1. Introduction

Behcet's disease (BD) is a chronic, relapsing, inflammatory vascular disease of unknown etiology that commonly affects the eye with unpredictable exacerbations and remissions. Various visual complications may occur and are potentially sight threatening [1]. Male sex and a younger age of disease onset (younger than 40 years) were found to be associated with a higher frequency of ocular affection as well as of more severe form of the disease [1]. To date however, there are no gold standard criteria for the diagnosis/classification of Behcet's disease, with more than 15 available sets of criteria used around the world [2]. Two of the most commonly used classification criteria are the ICBD (International Criteria for Behcet's Disease) which was used in this study and the ISG (International Study Group) criteria. Egypt is one of the countries with a high incidence of Behcet's disease. A 4-year follow-up study done on Egyptian patients with Behcet's disease demonstrated a higher male-to-female ratio and a higher incidence of neurological (34.9%) and vascular (57.1%) lesions than other countries. This study also demonstrated a 47.6% ocular affection of varying degrees among its 63 studied patients [3]. Another study done in Cairo University, Egypt, found that the ICBD criteria perform better on Egyptian patients more than other available classifications [4]. Performance of the ISG, ICBD 2006, revised Japanese criteria, and the revised ICBD 2010 was evaluated in terms of sensitivity, specificity, negative likelihood ratio (NLR), negative predictive value (NPV), positive predictive value (PPV), positive likelihood ratio (PLR), diagnostic odds ratio (DOR), and Youden's index (YI), and it was found that the ICBD 2010 carried the highest sensitivity (98.83%), NPV (98.48%), DOR (1645), and YI (0.94) and the lowest NLR (0.01) [4].

The common ocular manifestations of Behcet's disease which potentially threaten vision include anterior and posterior uveitis, vitritis, panuveitis, retinal vasculitis, papillitis, and chorioretinitis. Complications like retinal detachment, secondary glaucoma, and optic atrophy often cause irreversible visual loss. It is thus very important for an ophthalmologist to be able to predict which case of Behcet's disease will pursue a vision-threatening course and which case will not. To date, no enough data exists regarding the presence of general predictors for vision-threatening disease. If vision-threatening disease has certain predictors (clinical as well as demographic), detecting these predictors early in the course of the disease may help alter the course of the disease in these high-risk patients. A patient with a potentially vision-threatening form of the disease can be given special ophthalmological care, closer follow-up appointments, more aggressive treatment, and/or earlier intervention.

The authors further pursued this point of research in an attempt to look for clinical predictors for the potentially vision-threatening form of Behcet's disease. In the hope that this can allow ophthalmologists and internists to take appropriate measures in a timely fashion, it was for this purpose that this work was done.

2. Subjects and Methods

The study was done in accordance with the ethical standards of the national research committee and the 1964 Helsinki Declaration and its later amendments [5].

This retrospective analytical database study targeted patients attending the outpatient clinic of Internal Medicine, Rheumatology and Clinical Immunology Division of Kasr Al Ainy Medical School, Cairo University. The data of this historical cohort were collected from the available fully completed and revised files of 249 Egyptian patients with Behcet's disease recorded from the end of 2012 to the end of 2017.

The revised International Criteria for Behcet's Disease (ICBD) 2010 [6] was chosen to confirm patients to have the disease according to a recent work by Hussein et al. [4]. These criteria include the following:

(i) Recurrent oral ulcers (OU) of at least 3 times/year

(ii) Recurrent genital ulcers (GU)

(iii) Cutaneous manifestations including papulopustular rash and erythema nodosum

(iv) Ocular manifestations consistent with the disease as uveitis (anterior, posterior, or panuveitis) and retinal vasculitis, chorioretinitis, or papillitis

(v) Vascular manifestations including venous thromboembolism, superficial thrombophlebitis, arterial thrombosis, and aneurysms, especially aortic and pulmonary aneurysms

(vi) Central nervous system (CNS) lesions consistent with the disease, namely, parenchymal CNS involvement and/or venous sinus thrombosis

(vii) Pathergy test as an extra criterion to be used if conducted and positive

A weighted point value system was given: two points for oral ulcers (OU), genital ulcers (GU), and ocular manifestations and only one point for the others, and at least four points are required for diagnosing the patient as having the disease. Patients who had other autoimmune and/or autoinflammatory diseases were excluded from the study. All patients had a duration of illness of at least 4 years and were treated by corticosteroids and methotrexate.

Ophthalmologically, patients' data was thoroughly examined and the cohort was divided by the authors into two groups: a group with a "vision-threatening form of Behcet's disease" and another group with "non-vision-threatening Behcet's disease." The full ophthalmological examination done at the ophthalmology department outpatient clinics included anterior segment examination by slit lamp biomicroscopy, posterior segment examination by 90-diopter lens, and indirect ophthalmoscopy. Fundus fluorescein angiography was done if needed to confirm posterior segment findings like retinal vasculitis. Visual acuity was measured as well as intraocular pressure by applanation tonometry for each patient. Patients with a best-corrected visual acuity (BCVA) of 6/60 or less due to an irreversible cause, as well as those with documented panuveitis, retinal vasculitis, chorioretinitis, and/or papillitis or a combination of these findings, were classified by the authors as having a vision-threatening form of the disease (VTD), while patients whose BCVA was 6/36 or better, those who had a reversible cause of visual loss, or those who were found to have mild-to-moderate anterior uveitis, vitritis (diffuse vitreous cells and/or mild-to-moderate vitreous haze), complicated cataract (which can be surgically removed), episcleritis, and/or a combination of these were classified as having a non-vision-threatening form of the disease (NVTD).

Each ocular finding (like the presence of anterior or posterior uveitis, panuveitis, vitritis, retinal vasculitis, chorioretinitis, papillitis, and ocular complications like cataract, glaucoma, macular edema, and retinal detachment) was recorded if present for each included patient. Each systemic finding (like the presence of oral ulcers, genital ulcers, cutaneous manifestations, a positive pathergy test, systemic vasculitis, CNS manifestations, arthralgia, arthritis, and/or gastrointestinal tract (GIT) symptoms) was also recorded if present for each participating patient. Age, sex, laterality of ocular disease, and any family history for the disease were also recorded for each patient.

Data were statistically described in terms of mean ± standard deviation (SD), range, or frequencies (number of cases) and percentages when appropriate. Comparison between the study groups was done using the chi-square (χ^2) test. An exact test was used instead when the expected frequency was less than 5. Correlation between various variables was done using Spearman's rank correlation equation. Multivariate logistic regression analysis was used to test for the preferential effect of all important variables on the occurrence of vision-threatening affection. A p value of less than 0.05 was considered statistically significant. All statistical calculations were done using the computer program IBM SPSS (Statistical Package for the Social Science; IBM Corp., Armonk, NY, USA) release 22 for Microsoft Windows.

3. Results

3.1. Descriptive Statistics. The records of 249 patients were included in our study. The mean age in our study was 32.3

± 8.47 years (mean ± SD). 85.1% of our patients were males (212 patients), and 14.9% (37 patients) were female (yielding a male-to-female ratio of 5.7 : 1). Of these, 38.2% (95 patients) had bilateral ocular affection. A positive family history was only found in 3.2% of patients (8 patients).

As for overall ocular affection, a total of 51% (127 patients) of all patients were found to have some form of ocular involvement by the disease.

Of these, 59% suffered from anterior uveitis, 74.8% from posterior uveitis, and 33.8% from panuveitis. 54.3% of these patients had retinitis, 46.4% had vitritis, 66.9% had chorioretinitis, 31.4% had retinal vasculitis, 7.8% had papillitis, 9.4% had macular edema, and 7.8% had secondary retinal detachment. Patients frequently suffered from more than one ocular finding.

According to the authors' suggested classification previously described, 74.01% of these patients (94 patients) were found to fall within the category of having vision-threatening disease (decreased vision due to an irreversible cause), while 25.98% (33 patients) fell in the category of having non-vision-threatening disease.

Systemically, 98.8% of all patients suffered from oral ulceration, 90% had genital ulceration, 36.5% had different skin manifestations of Behcet's disease, 34.5% suffered from arthralgia, 31.3% had systemic vasculitis, 17.7% manifested a positive pathergy test, 12% had CNS manifestations, 10% had arthritis, and 2.8% had different GIT manifestations of Behcet's disease, with most patients displaying more than one systemic finding.

3.1.1. Correlation between Individual Ocular and Systemic Variables. Upon correlating all variables with each other, many correlations were found. Some were statistically significant, and some showed only a trend towards being significant. Table 1 displays these correlations and their correlation coefficient (r) and p value. It was generally noted that genitourinary ulcers as well as peripheral vasculitis almost always had a significant negative correlation with all forms of ocular affection whether uveitis, vitritis, chorioretinitis, or retinal vasculitis. Oral ulcers were also inversely correlated with the presence of retinal vasculitis, as well as with overall ocular involvement. However, this correlation was only close to being statistically significant (Table 1).

Secondary glaucoma and complicated cataract were both significantly positively correlated with the presence of GIT symptoms, and secondary retinal detachment was significantly positively correlated with the presence of a positive pathergy test.

3.1.2. Correlation between Different Variables and the Occurrence of Vision-Threatening Disease (VTD). Upon correlating systemic variables with the development of the vision-threatening form of ocular affection (as previously described), it was found that 65.2% of participants with genitourinary ulcerations did not develop vision-threatening disease, whereas 34.8% with genitourinary symptoms had vision-threatening disease. 64% of patients with no genitourinary affection developed VTD. This relationship was statistically highly significant ($p = 0.008$).

Table 1: Correlation between individual variables.

Correlated variables	Correlation coefficient (r)	p value
Bilaterality & GU	−0.15	0.018*
Bilaterality & systemic vasculitis	−0.21	0.001*
Bilaterality & arthralgia	0.108	0.09
Anterior uveitis & systemic vasculitis	−0.198	0.002*
Anterior uveitis & CNS	−0.109	0.08
Anterior uveitis & arthralgia	0.112	0.07
Anterior uveitis & male gender	−0.119	0.06
Posterior uveitis & GU	−0.178	0.005*
Posterior uveitis & systemic vasculitis	−0.245	0.001*
Retinitis & systemic vasculitis	−0.186	0.003*
Vitritis & GU	−0.191	0.002*
Vitritis & pathergy	0.113	0.07
Vitritis & systemic vasculitis	−0.193	0.002*
Vitritis & CNS	−0.14	0.019*
Chorioretinitis & GU	−0.12	0.047*
Chorioretinitis & systemic vasculitis	−0.26	0.001*
Chorioretinitis & CNS	−0.13	0.031*
Retinal vasculitis & OU	−0.15	0.016*
Retinal vasculitis & GU	−0.109	0.08
Retinal vasculitis & pathergy	0.11	0.07
Retinal vasculitis & systemic vasculitis	−0.13	0.04*
Retinal vasculitis & age	0.11	0.06
Panuveitis & systemic vasculitis	−0.19	0.002*
Panuveitis & male gender	−0.138	0.03*
Ocular involvement & OU	−0.1	0.08
Ocular involvement & GU	−0.22	0.001*
Ocular involvement & systemic vasculitis	−0.27	0.001*
Ocular involvement & CNS	−0.13	0.03*
Glaucoma & GIT	0.227	0.001*
Cataract & GIT	0.149	0.019*
Synechia & male gender	−0.13	0.03*
Retinal detachment & pathergy	0.17	0.006*

*Statistically significant.

Patients with systemic vasculitis largely developed non-vision-threatening disease, as 79.5% of them exhibited a mild form of ocular affection as opposed to 20.5% of patients with systemic vasculitis who exhibited VTD. This again was statistically highly significant ($p = 0.001$).

More than 50% of patients with oral ulcers developed non-vision-threatening disease. Meanwhile, 66.7% of patients without oral ulceration (2 out of 3 patients) developed VTD. The difference was however statistically nonsignificant ($p = 0.55$) and of limited clinical significance due to the small number of patients having no oral ulcers (3 patients).

The rest of systemic variables, as well as family history ($p = 0.26$), had no significant effect on the development of VTD. It seems that the presence of genital ulcers and systemic vasculitis may have a significant protective role against the development of the vision-threatening form of the disease.

3.1.3. Logistic Regression and Predictive Factors. Upon logistic regression analysis, taking into consideration each variable alone (Table 2), the authors found a significant predictive value for both the presence of genital ulcers ($p = 0.004$) and that of systemic vasculitis ($p = 0.001$) on the development of NVTD.

Upon logistic regression analysis with all variables taken into consideration (Table 3), the authors found that three factors have a predictive value on the development of the non-vision-threatening form of the disease. Namely, these are the presence of genital ulcers ($p = 0.003$) and systemic vasculitis ($p = 0.001$) which both showed a highly significant predictive value on the development of non-vision-threatening disease. The presence of oral ulcers with a p value close to being significant ($p = 0.07$) may have a predictive value as to the development of NVTD, yet still it is statistically nonsignificant. In other words, absence of these systemic criteria (GU, systemic vasculitis, and maybe OU as well) may put the eye at higher risk for the development of vision-threatening disease (VTD).

Table 2: Univariate regression analysis and significance of each variable.

Variables	Score	df	p value
OU	1.080	1	0.299
GU	8.148	1	0.004*
Cutaneous	0.516	1	0.472
Pathergy	0.671	1	0.413
Systemic vasculitis	14.362	1	0.001*
CNS	1.783	1	0.182
Arthralgia	0.944	1	0.331
Arthritis	0.391	1	0.532
GIT	1.153	1	0.283
Family history	2.243	1	0.134
Age	0.157	1	0.692
Male gender	0.000	1	0.991

*Statistically significant.

Table 3: Multivariate regression analysis with all variables in the equation.

Variables	B	SE	df	p value
OU	−2.29	1.29	1	0.077*
GU	−1.45	0.48	1	0.003*
Cutaneous	0.32	0.30	1	0.294
Pathergy	0.38	0.37	1	0.311
Systemic vasculitis	−1.37	0.35	1	0.001*
CNS	−0.46	0.47	1	0.328
Arthralgia	0.18	0.30	1	0.543
Arthritis	−0.28	0.50	1	0.574
GIT	1.25	0.86	1	0.146
Family history	−1.40	1.11	1	0.208
Age	−0.01	0.01	1	0.452
Male gender	0.23	0.40	1	0.561

*Statistically significant.

4. Discussion

Behcet's disease (BD) is named after Turkish dermatologist Hulusi Behçet who reported three cases with recurrent oral and genital ulceration together with hypopyon anterior uveitis [7]. It is a chronic relapsing multisystem disease of yet nonconclusive etiology. A complex causality involving infectious agent exposure as well as genetic and environmental factors may play a role [8]. A previous study done on 63 Egyptian patients with BD studying their demographics found that a very high male-to-female ratio was exhibited (30.5 : 1) as well as a mean age of 32.8 ± 8.3 years [3]. The commonest manifestation of BD in this study was oral ulcers (100%), followed by genital ulcers (96.8%), vascular lesions (57.1%), cutaneous manifestations (55.5%), ocular affection (47.6%), joint affection (36.5%), CNS (34.9%), gastrointestinal manifestations (19%), and lastly cardiac manifestations (6.3%) [3]. Despite the difference in sample size (249 versus 63 subjects), the reported percentages were comparable to ours except for CNS, GIT, and cardiac manifestations. We also reported a different male-to-female ratio (5.7 : 1) which was lower than the ratio of this study but higher than the ratio of most studies done in the Mediterranean region.

Another study on the demographics of BD in the North African Mediterranean region (Tunisia) implementing a closer sample size to ours (260) showed a male-to-female ratio of 2.6 : 1, oral ulcers in 100% of patients, genital ulcers in 83%, ocular involvement in 51% (the same percentage as ours), arthritis in 38.8%, vasculitic and thrombotic lesions in 33%, neurological lesions in 24.2%, and GIT symptoms in 1.5%. These results are almost identical to what we found in our study. This study also reported a high overall incidence of DVT and a low incidence of GIT symptoms which were similar to our results [9].

We found that different correlations exist between different variables. Genital ulcers were almost always negatively correlated with all sorts of ocular inflammation, and so was systemic vasculitis. A significant negative correlation existed between these two variables and the development of anterior or posterior uveitis, vitritis, retinitis, chorioretinitis, panuveitis, and overall ocular involvement. This finding was similar to that of the previous study where the authors reported less frequent occurrence of deep vein thrombosis as well as GU in patients with ocular involvement [9].

We found a predictive potential for the presence of GU, systemic vasculitis, and OU on the development of what we classified as non-vision-threatening disease, where we reported a milder form of eye affection in the presence of one or more of these three systemic criteria. Interestingly, a previous study by Hazirolan et al. found that GU were significantly lower among BD patients with ocular (71.4%) compared to those without ocular affection ($p = 0.04$), but the authors did not propose any explanation for this in their study [10]. To date, no studies have proposed evidence-based explanation for this phenomenon of what we call "immunological targeting" and why severe inflammation of ocular structures is usually associated with a milder peripheral inflammatory process and vice versa "reverse immunological targeting." A lot of research can be started to fully explain this phenomenon. However, we postulate that retinal pericytes, which may play a role in intravascular immunity, are derived from the same embryologic origin as CNS pericytes and thus may behave differently from peripheral vascular pericytes [11]. The eye as an embryologic outgrowth from the brain may be immunologically protected, so that in the setting of a florid form of peripheral vasculitis, orogenital ulcers, and mucocutaneous manifestations, the eye may still be relatively protected. It is however still not understood why absence of these peripheral findings is usually associated with the vision-threatening form of ocular inflammation. Further investigation is thus needed to investigate this finding shedding more light on the possibility of having two immunological variants of Behcet's disease, one with a central impact (more severe ocular affection) and the other with a peripheral one (more severe systemic vasculitis). HLA subtypes of the disease may also contribute to the type of systemic involvement, a point which needs further study and is somehow a limitation to our study.

Besides, the immune privilege (IP) manifested by ocular and brain tissue in particular and described as a suppressed or extremely extinguished immune response to foreign antigens, particularly alloantigens, functions normally as a homeostatic mechanism preserving function in highly specialized tissues with a limited capacity for renewal such as those of the brain and eye [12]. However, IP (in the form of blood-ocular barriers, induction of T regulatory cells, intraocular immune modulators, lack of lymphatics, and other properties) is relatively easily bypassed when facing a sufficiently strong immunological response. Under these circumstances, these privileged tissues (those of the eye and brain) may be at greater risk of collateral damage because the natural defence mechanisms of these privileged tissues are more easily breached than those of a fully immunocompetent tissue which quickly rejects foreign antigens and restores integrity [13]. This acts like a double-edged knife to an organ like the eye. Under most circumstances, immune privilege (IP) mechanisms maintain tissue integrity; however, when these mechanisms are breached, various degrees of tissue damage occur from severe tissue destruction in retinal viral infections and other forms of uveoretinal inflammation. Immune privilege does not appear to offer much protection against the damaging effects of uveitis possibly because IP serves mainly to maintain homeostasis, mainly keeping healthy tissue free of random antigens which may provoke inflammation. However, when facing a serious challenge, IP drearily fails to prevent severe inflammation. In uncontrolled vision-threatening uveitis, both infection and the immune response to it can cause permanent structural damage. Therapies such as anti-TNFα are claimed to impair the destructive effects of inflammation while permitting monocytes to traverse tissues without causing damage [14]. This whole IP mechanism may partially explain the exaggerated ocular immune response to Behcet's disease in certain cases that the authors postulate. However, it does not fully explain the opposite scenario where in the presence of marked ocular inflammation, a quiet systemic (peripheral) pattern of disease usually coexists. This is a limitation to our study that needs further research.

In our study, we noted a positive correlation between bilaterality of ocular affection and the presence of arthralgia, the presence of vitritis and positive pathergy, anterior uveitis and arthralgia, retinal vasculitis and positive pathergy, retinal vasculitis and increasing age, GIT symptoms and the development of glaucoma and cataract (this specific correlation may be attributed to complications of prolonged use of corticosteroids), and finally retinal detachment and positive pathergy. All these correlations—except the last three—were close to being statistically significant. Whether immunologic variants or HLA subtypes of the disease exist that could be responsible for this "symptom pairing" needs to be further investigated. HLA subtypes of the disease may also contribute to the type of systemic involvement, a point which needs further study and is somehow a limitation to our study.

Most vision-threatening conditions were of posterior segment origin and were largely inversely correlated with the presence of genital ulcers and systemic vasculitis. This agrees with what another study reported, in which posterior segment lesions in Behcet's disease are of a persistent nature and lead to significant visual loss [15]. However, this study did not shed any light on the strong negative correlation we reported between the severity of posterior segment affection and certain systemic features.

Behcet's disease remains an immunologic mystery, a clinical and a therapeutic challenge to internists, immunologists, and ophthalmologists alike. The importance of long-term follow-up remains crucial in the prognosis of the disease. Potential benefits of long-term colchicine treatment were previously discussed and showed some promising results [16]. With further collaborative research and understanding of the disease and its patterns of organ affection and/or avoidance, we may reach new classifications which will help us better plan our treatment and follow-up regimens and even develop prophylactic options. We recommend that predictors for severity of ocular diseases mentioned in this study be implemented in the initial assessment for disease and its diagnostic criteria and eventually be taken into consideration when designing the treatment plan.

Conflicts of Interest

The authors report no conflicts of interest.

References

[1] E. Alpsoy, L. Donmez, M. Onder et al., "Clinical features and natural course of Behçet's disease in 661 cases: a

multicentre study," *British Journal of Dermatology*, vol. 157, no. 5, pp. 901–906, 2007.

[2] F. Davatchi, B. SadeqhiAbdollahi, C. Chams-Davatchi et al., "The saga of diagnostic/classification criteria in Behcet's disease," *International Journal of Rheumatic Diseases*, vol. 18, no. 6, pp. 594–605, 2015.

[3] M. M. El Menyawi, H. M. Raslan, and A. Edrees, "Clinical features of Behcet's disease in Egypt," *Rheumatology International*, vol. 29, no. 6, pp. 641–646, 2009.

[4] M. A. Hussein, M. I. Ellawindi, and G. Ragab, "Performance of classification criteria for Behcet's disease in an Egyptian cohort," *Indian Journal of Rheumatology*, vol. 12, no. 3, pp. 152–155, 2017.

[5] World Medical Association, "World Medical Association Declaration of Helsinki: ethical principles for medical research involving human subjects," *JAMA*, vol. 310, no. 20, pp. 2191–2194, 2013.

[6] International Team for the Revision of the International Criteria for Behçet's Disease (ITR-ICBD), F. Davatchi, S. Assaad-Khalil et al., "The International Criteria for Behçet's Disease (ICBD): a collaborative study of 27 countries on the sensitivity and specificity of the new criteria," *Journal of the European Academy of Dermatology and Venereology*, vol. 28, no. 3, pp. 338–347, 2013.

[7] H. Behçet, "Überrezidivierendeaphthöse, durchein Virus verursachte Geschwüre am Mund, am Auge und an den Genitalien," *Dermatologische Wochenschrift*, vol. 36, pp. 1152–1157, 1937.

[8] R. Rokutanda, M. Kishimoto, and M. Okada, "Update on the diagnosis and management of Behçet's disease," *Open Access Rheumatology: Research and Reviews*, vol. 7, pp. 1–8, 2015.

[9] M. H. Houman, H. Neffati, A. Braham et al., "Behçet's disease in Tunisia. Demographic, clinical and genetic aspects in 260 patients," *Clinical and Experimental Rheumatolology*, vol. 25, no. 4, Supplement 45, pp. S58–S64, 2007.

[10] D. Hazirolan, G. Sungur, and S. Duman, "Demographic, clinical, and ocular features in patients with late-onset Behçet disease," *Ocular Immunology and Inflammation*, vol. 20, no. 2, pp. 119–124, 2012.

[11] A. Trost, S. Lange, F. Schroedl et al., "Brain and retinal pericytes: origin, function and role," *Frontiers in Cellular Neuroscience*, vol. 10, article 20, 2016.

[12] J. V. Forrester and H. Xu, "Good news–bad news: the yin and yang of immune privilege in the eye," *Frontiers in Immunology*, vol. 3, p. 338, 2012.

[13] H. Wekerle, "Breaking ignorance: the case of the brain," *Current Topics in Microbiology and Immunology*, vol. 305, pp. 25–50, 2006.

[14] T. K. Khera, A. D. Dick, and L. B. Nicholson, "Mechanisms of TNFα regulation in uveitis: focus on RNA-binding proteins," *Progress in Retinal and Eye Research*, vol. 29, no. 6, pp. 610–621, 2010.

[15] I. Tugal-Tutkun, S. Onal, R. Altan-Yaycioglu, H. Huseyin Altunbas, and M. Urgancioglu, "Uveitis in Behçet disease: an analysis of 880 patients," *American Journal of Ophthalmology*, vol. 138, no. 3, pp. 373–380, 2004.

[16] B. Wechsler, "Colchicine et maladie de Behçet : une efficacité enfin reconnue!," *La Revue de Médecine Interne*, vol. 23, no. 4, pp. 355-356, 2002.

24

Ocular Manifestations of Alzheimer's and Other Neurodegenerative Diseases: The Prospect of the Eye as a Tool for the Early Diagnosis of Alzheimer's Disease

Pade Colligris,[1,2] Maria Jesus Perez de Lara,[2,3] Basilio Colligris,[2,3] and Jesus Pintor[2,3]

[1]*Universidad Alfonso X, Madrid, Spain*
[2]*Ocupharm Diagnostics SL, Madrid, Spain*
[3]*Universidad Complutense de Madrid, Madrid, Spain*

Correspondence should be addressed to Jesus Pintor; jpintor@ucm.es

Academic Editor: László Módis

Dementia, including Alzheimer's disease (AD), is a major disorder, leading to several ocular manifestations amongst the elderly population. These visual disorders may be due to retinal nerve degenerative changes, including nerve fibre layer thinning, degeneration of retinal ganglion cells, and changes to vascular parameters. There is no cure for Alzheimer's, but medicines can slow down the development of many of the classic symptoms, such as loss of memory and communication skills, mood swings, and depression. The disease diagnosis is difficult, and it is only possible through PET scans of the brain, detecting evidence of the accumulation of amyloid and tau. PET is expensive and invasive, requiring the injection of radioactive tracers, which bind with these proteins and glow during scanning. Recently, scientists developed promising eye-scan techniques that may detect Alzheimer's disease at its earliest stage, before major symptoms appear, leading to improved management of the disease symptoms. In this review, we are discussing the visual abnormalities of Alzheimer's and other neurodegenerative diseases, focused on ocular functional-visual-structural biomarkers, retinal pathology, and potential novel diagnostic tools.

1. Introduction

AD is a degenerative disorder of the nervous system, eventually affecting over 10% of individuals aged 65 or over. It is the fifth-leading cause of death among people older than 65 years and a major cause of disability and poor health [1–4]. According to the World Alzheimer Report of 2016, it is estimated that 47 million people suffer from dementia worldwide, and this number could increase to more than 131 million by 2050, as populations age [5]. Life expectancy has increased dramatically over the past century across the globe and consequently has been detected an increase in the observed prevalence of chronic diseases among the elderly people.

While the optical examination sector appears extremely interesting for the development of a novel noninvasive diagnostic tool [6], genome-wide association studies have identified more than 20 AD risk genes [7–10], but the exact mechanism through which these genes are associated with AD remains unknown [11–13]. More promising are the studies on amyloid precursor protein (APP), presenilin 1 (PSEN1), and presenilin 2 (PSEN2) mutations, identifying them as important factors of autosomal-dominant early-onset AD and FAD [14].

As of 2018, there is no modifying therapy for AD [15], and only two families of medications are approved as palliatives for AD symptoms: the cholinesterase inhibitors and the N-methyl-D-aspartate receptor (NMDAR) antagonists, while various new drugs are under clinical trials evaluations, among them the promising new family of secretase inhibitors [16–18].

Even though many preclinical and clinical trials on AD drugs are underway, it is becoming obvious that the concept of the simplistic therapy of one compound against one target is failing, due to the complex pathophysiology of the disease, and future treatment will be based on drug combinations to intensify the results [19]. In any case, the onset of Alzheimer's disease cannot yet be stopped or reversed but might be manageable.

Diagnosis of the disease is difficult and frequently is subjective. There is no single diagnostic test and specialists are using various methods, including physical examination and brain scans, such as computed tomography (CT), magnetic resonance imaging (MRI), or positron emission tomography (PET), to rule out other probable causes for the symptoms [20]. For the moment, early diagnosis is based on the early recognition of the various signs and symptoms, as the most common sign of the disease is memory loss, especially forgetting recently learned information.

Generally, a timely and accurate diagnosis is considered to be important, as treatment of Alzheimer's and other dementia-causing diseases is typically most effective when started early in the disease process [21, 22]. Additionally, accurate diagnosis could transform the design and execution of clinical trials to test new AD treatments [23–27].

Current diagnosis methods mainly rely either on subjective tests or invasive methods with a limited accuracy. Definite AD diagnosis is possible only through postmortem observation of the aberrant accumulation of β-amyloid peptides (Aβ) extracellular aggregates, β-amyloid plaques, and protein tau intracellular twisted strands (neurofibrillary tangles, NFTs) [26–31]. The inaccuracy of the existing diagnostic methods, limits the general applicability for vast population screening and underlines the need for the identification of easily accessible tools for the identification of high-risk subjects. To better serve the population at risk of developing AD, new methods of definitive, noninvasive and lower cost diagnosis are needed.

AD could be categorized in familial Alzheimer's disease (FAD, also known as early-onset Alzheimer's disease) and sporadic type (also known as late onset Alzheimer's disease; LOAD) [32]. The eye offers a natural window to the brain as the retina, the light-sensitive layer lining the interior of the eye is considered part of the central nervous system (CNS) and the only optically accessible nervous tissue [33]. Neurodegenerative changes in the brain produced by AD are accompanied by structural and possible functional changes in the neuroretina and the ocular vasculature.

Numerous recent studies reported the presence of β-amyloid plaques in the retina of patients, opening the possibility of detecting AD though simple noninvasive eye scans [34–38]. In a parallel way, other studies revealed degenerative changes and retinal neuron damage in the retina/eye of AD animal models [39–43]. Consequently, various laboratories are trying to explore this approach, developing optical retinal imaging platforms capable to detect β-amyloid plaques in the retina of AD subjects [38, 44–48]. These novel imaging platforms are expected to early detect the presence of AD hallmarks and assist in monitoring the efficacy of probable future therapeutic agents which target relevant molecular pathways.

Nevertheless, Alzheimer's disease shares common features, mode-of-action, and targets with other neurodegenerative diseases such as, Parkinson's disease, Huntington's disease, amyotrophic lateral sclerosis, frontotemporal dementia, and even glaucoma and macular degeneration [49–52]. Therefore, in the following text, we will analyse the relation between AD and some of these neurodegenerative disorders, focusing on their ocular manifestations on the accessible retina, and the possibility of using these hallmark signs as structural-functional biomarkers for risk assessment-monitoring of disease progression, and evaluation for the drug therapeutic efficacy. In any case, the establishment of a link between neurodegenerative diseases and ocular manifestations is an interesting emerging field of study.

2. Detection and Pathophysiological Processes Involved in Alzheimer's Diseases and Other Neurodegenerative Diseases

Several studies have focused upon the relationship between neurodegenerative diseases and their possible ocular manifestation. There is compelling evidence to suggest that specific ocular biomarkers related to neurodegenerative disorders play a pivotal role in the development of retinal impairment or loss of visual function [53, 54].

The abnormal protein aggregation characterizes numerous neurodegenerative diseases, where insoluble proteins are accumulated in the brain such as AD, the Prion Encephalopathies, Parkinson's disease, Huntington disease, and other polyglutamine disorders [55]. Protein misfolding diseases are not exclusive to the CNS, including disorders implicating amyloidogenic proteins like type 2 diabetes, inherited cataracts, vascular inflammation, atherosclerosis, and haemodialysis-related disorders, among many others [56]. Goldstein et al. reported the detection of nanoaggregates of β-amyloid in the human AD lens [57], a non-CNS structure considering another relevant ocular hallmark in this pathology. Deposits of β-amyloid are a distinct characteristic found in neurodegenerative diseases AD [58–60], Parkinson's disease [60–65], as well as being detected in age-related macular degeneration [66], and glaucoma [67–70].

In fact, there are numerous recent studies connecting glaucoma and AD, and some, bearing in mind the multiple common features to both diseases, including risk factors and pathophysiological mechanisms, are suggesting that Alzheimer's Disease and glaucoma should be considered age-related neurodegenerative diseases, coexisting in the elderly population [71–74]. Adding to the connection link theories between glaucoma and AD is the recent unifying hypothesis of the "glymphatic system." This hypothesis is incorporating various aspects of the vascular, biomechanical, and biochemical theories, based on a few studies suggesting the existence of a paravascular transport system in the eye and optic nerve. However, for the moment, there are not sufficient available research data to totally support this idea [75–78].

On the other hand, recent studies are suggesting that AD and age-related macular degeneration (AMD) share common, pathological signalling defects and disease mechanisms at the molecular genetic level [79, 80]. There is growing evidence that β-amyloid, the main component of senile plaques, the hallmark of AD, is also a vital component of drusen, the hallmark of AMD [81–83]. While AMD is a retinal disease, AD is damaging the brain cells as well as the retina. These two age-related diseases are primarily affecting distinct parts of the central nervous system but are generally similar, concerning the abnormal extracellular deposits, metabolic and oxidative stress, neuroinflammation, and microvascular abnormalities [81, 84].

AD is characterized by visual disturbances at early stages which are correlated to neuronal damage in the inner retina, loss of RGCs, and optic nerve degeneration at postmortem histology, as suggested by several authors [37, 38, 85–91] and is also correlated to Parkinson's disease, as suggested by Bayer et al. [92]. Further studies reported that these inner retinal alterations were correlated with an abnormal pattern electroretinography (pERG) response [93]. From the earliest stages of the disease, amyloid plaque is deposited in retina tissue (including the RGC, retinal nerve fibre layer-RNFL, and inner plexiform layer) which can produce a fluorescence effect by using curcumin as a contrast [94].

An important characteristic of many systemic processes related to AD is the contribution of the energy metabolism, albeit the role of altered metabolic processes implicated in Alzheimer's disease pathogenesis is still unclear [95]. Recent studies discovered that in several CNS disorders, there is evidence of circulating metabolites signatures, suggesting that retinal oxygen metabolism in AD is slightly different from the normal, even though the results are not conclusive (ClinicalTrials.gov Identifier: NCT02253732; ClinicalTrials.gov Identifier: NCT00001972) [96, 97]. Following this discovery, the University of Iceland, Reykjavík, Iceland, is developing a biomarker for AD albeit further studies are necessary, using larger groups, to verify the results and further metabolomic studies and are imperative to demonstrate the correlation between systemic abnormalities and the brain impairment in AD [60].

The Spanish Hospital *Universitari Vall d'Hebron Research Institute* is investigating the association between type 2 diabetes (T2D) and Alzheimer's disease (AD) [98, 99] and in September 2014, started a clinical trial (ClinicalTrials.gov Identifier: NCT02360527) to explore whether diabetic patients are at risk of developing AD based on the assessment of retinal neurodegeneration and if these retina irregularities are related to the severity of AD. The results suggest that retinal sensitivity, assessed by microperimetry, is related to brain neurodegeneration and could be a useful biomarker for the detection of the disease [100].

In *the University Hospital of Bordeaux*, scientists are studying how the reduced thickness of RNFL relates to AD and other degenerative diseases and if RNFL thickness is associated with the development of cognitive impairment. They suggest that this parameter could be used as a biomarker for cerebral axonal degeneration, as RNFL deficits could be an early sign of AD, even before damages occur in the hippocampal region (ClinicalTrials.gov Identifier: NCT01621841- ClinicalTrials.gov Identifier: NCT01555827) [101–104]. The results confirm that the RNFL thickness is associated with changes in patients' memory and could be used as an indicator for the future development of AD [104].

In another instance, in the Department of Neurosurgery and Maxine Dunitz Neurosurgical Research Institute, Cedars-Sinai Medical Centre, Los Angeles, trials have begun to administrate intravenous therapy of curcumin, a fluorophore with high affinity to Aβ, to an AD-Tg mice ($n = 24$) mouse model and performed fluorescent retinal examination in vivo [34]. After systemic administration of curcumin using this method, noninvasive optical imaging of retinal β-amyloid plaques in vivo with high resolution and specificity was allowed [105]. Curcumin is used as an early diagnostic probe due to its inherited fluorescence and high binding affinity to amyloid-β, but it could also be the basis of new drugs for the prevention and treatment of AD [106].

In 2011, Koronyo-Hamaoui and colleagues described the presence of β-amyloid in human retinal whole mount of AD. Posterior studies showed the predominant superior hemiretina damage involving mainly the inner retinal layers and histological analysis provided evidence of increased AβPP in AD retinas [5, 34, 49, 107]. In addition, specific retinal ganglion cells (RGC) and melanopsin retinal ganglion cells (mRGC) are affected by amyloid pathology in AD in and around cells [37].

Numerous studies of transgenic rodent models of AD have identified retinal Aβ depositions in the inner retina (inner plexiform layer, RGC layer, and nerve fibre layers) and the outer nuclear layer. These findings correlate with the burden of amyloid plaques in the brain [34, 38, 107–109]. Furthermore, the pathological mechanisms that involve β-amyloid in neuronal death are similar between RGC loss and neuronal degeneration in hippocampus in different models of AD [66, 85–90, 110]. RGC apoptosis was accompanied by and localized with Aβ deposits in retinas from rodent models, and signalling pathways are similar in retinal and hippocampal neurons death [107, 111]. Based on the observation on the retina of β-amyloid plaques, various companies and research centres started the development of specific biomarkers for the AD early diagnosis. In December 4, 2017 the Canadian company Optina Diagnostics Inc. started the ClinicalTrials.gov Identifier: NCT03420807 for the evaluation of a device called metabolic hyperspectral retinal camera (MHRC) for the detection of β-amyloid plaques. A hyperspectral mydriatic camera is used, producing multiple images of the retina, collecting and processing the light intensity for a large number (225) of contiguous spectral bands at high speeds allowing the noninvasive localization of structures and biomolecules in the retina evaluating their specific spectral signatures [112–114]. This method is based on the β-amyloid plaques hypothesis of AD pathophysiology, even though it generally remains unproven by clinical interventions [115].

Other studies support the hyperspectral imaging microscopy (HSI) method, to examine Aβ presence without the need for exogenous fluorophore. More and colleagues demonstrated the spectral signature of aggregated Aβ in AD mice model retinas and in vivo detection [116, 117].

While the optical examination sector appears extremely interesting for the development of a novel noninvasive diagnostic tool, for the moment, research has barely surpassed the animal model level, and there is limited proof yet that it is possible to detect β-amyloid plaques in the retina by visual means.

In addition to growing reports of retinal Aβ accumulation, other established hallmark of AD is pTau protein aggregates. Alterations in tau protein and gene expression were found in a triple transgenic mouse model revealing neuronal dysfunction that precedes cell death in the AD retina. In addition, these results were correlated to the presence of tau accumulation in the RGC soma and dendrites [38, 41, 118, 119]. Hyperphosphorylated tau was detected in postmortem human retinas and in AD animal models, which led us to the hypothesis that this could be observed at a presymptomatic stage of the disease as tau aggregation was not detected [118, 120, 121].

AD is a progressive brain disorder, with strong genetic determinants and aggregated protein, responsible for dementia. For many decades, the main environmental factors that influence the risk of AD development have been thoroughly studied. The primary risk factors involve hypertension, diabetes, hyperlipidaemia, metabolic syndrome, unhealthy diet, smoking, and physical inactivity among others [1, 122, 123]. It is considered that all these factors may contribute to the dilapidated physiopathological mechanisms in AD development.

Detection of specific biomarkers or advanced AD diagnosis approaches in the preclinical stage would be a potential breakthrough in the management of AD. Recent studies suggest that the retinal alterations occur early, thereby suggesting the necessity of earlier diagnosis and subsequent treatment of AD. Retinal imaging could, therefore, serve as an alternative approach to assessing brain degeneration in AD. Over the last 15 years, a noninvasive optical imaging technique of the retina and OHN has been used as a valuable tool to assess the optic nerve pathology in AD. In vivo detection of amyloid deposits in AD retinas were reported using OCT, and findings included perimacular and perivascular spots in the outer plexiform layer (OPL), ganglion cell layer (GCL), and the nerve fibre layer (NFL) thinning in AD [124–127].

In the Commonwealth Scientific and Industrial Research Organisation (CSIRO), Perth, WA, Australia, scientists began a study of AD patients, to discover whether the vascular analysis of retinal photographs could identify any retinal vascular parameters (RVPs) and when these retinal changes occur. The study demonstrated that retinal vascular biomarker is a potential method for the early detection of AD [128]. Likewise, researchers in Duke University of London developed a diagnostic method based on retinal imaging. In July 2017, a clinical trial with reference ClinicalTrials.gov Identifier: NCT03233646 was undertaken to evaluate a noninvasive OCTA-based retinal microvascular biomarker, as an effective screening tool in cognitive aging. The investigators hypothesize that microvascular network alterations in the retina mirror and possibly precede changes in the cerebral microcirculation seen in AD. Using advanced image analysis, the investigators aim to evaluate markers of reduced capillary blood flow and nonperfusion in the superficial and deep retinal vascular plexuses and choriocapillaris imaging using OCTA that would complement already established retinal-structural markers and increase their sensitivity and specificity in the early detection of AD. Various studies found that patients with AD have less density of retinal microvascular networks than the normal, considering retinal vessel reaction to flicker stimulation as a promising noninvasive, widely available, and easy-to-administer future biomarker for the diagnosis and monitoring of AD [129, 130]. In another study, the OCTA technique was tested on patients with AD, demonstrating its efficacy as a biomarker in the early diagnosis of the disease [131]. Additionally, the Medical University of Vienna is investigating whether more functional changes can be detected in the retina of AD patients, in conjunction with the already identified aberrations. For this purpose, in September 2016, they began a clinical trial (ClinicalTrials.gov Identifier: NCT02663531) evaluating the relationship between neural activity and blood flow, in induced flicker light hyperaemia in the retina, as a possible biomarker for AD. Furthermore, they assessed structural parameters such as retinal nerve fibre layer thickness and function parameters such as ocular blood flow and retinal oxygenation [132, 133]. According to the results, neuritic plaques were detected in representative cortical regions, suggesting OCTA as a useful tool for three-dimensional imaging of retinal Aβ accumulation [134, 135].

In general, advances in the image processing and software have improved the interpreting of anterior segment OCT images. In any case, the technique must advance towards the refinement of assessing vascular networks for the anterior segment and improvement of the histology detail, to become more accurate and to facilitate its use.

Studying the retinal visual changes of patients with neurodegeneration is an emerging field that requires more investigation. Intraocular and systemic therapeutic biomarkers/agents and visualizing techniques may be developed, serving the dual purposes of establishing novel pharmacological targets and new technological sources.

The mentioned areas of research have come a long way with many and important results, allowing us to have a better understanding of the disease [47]. More efforts are still needed, however, to fully understand the aetiology of the disease, to establish reliable individual predictive models, and place us closer to the development of a definitive diagnostic method and a possible personalized treatment.

3. Ophthalmological and Ocular Clinical Symptoms

The ocular alterations in AD involve different structures in the anterior and posterior pole (Table 1). In the anterior pole, tear fluid is considered to be a potential biomarker source. Kallo et al. discovered 100% increase of flow rate and 100% increase in protein levels in AD patients, with respect to the age-matched controls. The combination of four tear proteins lipocalin-1, dermicidin, lysozyme C and lactritin, had 81% sensitivity and 77% specificity for AD [136]. Furthermore, abnormal tear functions and reduced corneal sensibility were described in previous studies of neurodegenerative

TABLE 1: Visual system pathological and functional alterations in Alzheimer's disease.

Ocular structures and clinical facts	Pathological changes
Retina	Deposition of proteins tau, Aβ, and pTAu [35, 38, 39, 118]; accumulation of phosphorylated tau protein [138, 139] Impairment of amyloid β precursor protein (APP) metabolism [140, 141, 142] Reduction in retinal ganglion cells (RGCs) [85–87,143] Reduction of retinal thickness [85, 93, 144] Reduction to the retinal nerve fibre layer (RNFL) thickness [89, 145] Retrograde degeneration from loss of cortical neurons [146, 147] Inflammation [148, 149, 150]
Retinal and choroidal vasculature	Retinal and choroidal vascular β-amyloid deposits in transgenic mouse model of AD lead to retinal degeneration [107] Reduction of vascularization [151]
Retinal vascular blood flow	Blood flow abnormalities may cause neurodegeneration [152]
Optic nerve	Axonal degeneration in the axonal segments [85, 140] Loss of optic nerve thickness [153, 154] Papillary paleness due to axonal loss and perfusion alterations [155]
Lens	Correlation between AD and supranuclear cataract [156, 157] Presence of abnormal protein deposits [124, 157]
Tears Cornea	Changes in the chemical barrier composition of tears [136] Reduced corneal sensitivity [137]
Pupil Choroid	Pupillary responses possible biomarker [158, 159] Attenuation of choroidal thickness [160, 161]
Aqueous humour	Detection of Alzheimer connected, β-amyloid peptides, and chemokines in the aqueous humour [162, 163]
Visual field Visual acuity	Dysfunction in different tasks of basic vision and visual cognition [164] Decreased visual acuity [165]
Sensory perception Visual processing	Clinically important symptoms of visuospatial disorientation [166, 167] Deficits of visual motion perception [168]
Contrast sensitivity Colour vision	Contrast sensitivity disturbances and motion perception [169, 170] Incomplete achromatopsia [171]
Stereopsis	Reduced stereoscopic depth perception [172, 173]
Circadian rhythm	Alterations in the circadian rhythm and β-amyloid deposits inside and surrounding degenerating mRGCs [174–176]

diseases [137]. In 2017, the French company Amoneta Diagnostics SAS started a clinical trial (ClinicalTrials.gov Identifier: NCT03030586) to validate the performance of a noninvasive peripheral blood diagnostic kit for AD, collecting samples from peripheral body fluids, tears being among them.

Pupillary responses are associated with brain impairment in different studies where light reflex amplitude is reduced in AD [177]. Granholm et al. suggest that task-evoked pupillary responses may be a psychophysiological biomarker of early risk for AD [158]. The Massachusetts General Hospital started a clinical trial (ClinicalTrials.gov Identifier: NCT03330353) in 2017 to investigate rod, cone, and melanopsin-driven pupillary light response in individuals, as a possible AD and other neurodegenerative diseases diagnostic method. Furthermore, the Centre Hospitalier Universitaire de Besancon France recently began a clinical trial (ClinicalTrials.gov Identifier: NCT01434940) to validate eye movement recording as an early differential diagnostic tool for AD. Tracking eye movements is becoming an interesting diagnostic technique and could be beneficial in recognizing individuals who will progress to AD, but for the moment, there remain many critical points which require additional investigation.

As previously commented, β-amyloid was detected in the human lens of AD patients, and in a Framingham Offspring Eye Study cohort, a correlation between cortical cataract and AD degeneration was observed [124, 156, 178, 179]. These findings establish the β-amyloid protein as a key pathogenic biomarker between lens and AD. In 2017, the American company Cognoptix, Inc. started a clinical trial to detect β-amyloid in the lens of the eye in patients with mild cognitive impairment (MCI), and mild AD after the instillation of Aftobetin Hydrochloride. Aftobetin, also known as ANCA11 and NCE-11, is an amyloid-binding compound applied topically in the form of an ophthalmic ointment and may be useful as an aid in the diagnosis of AD (ClinicalTrials.gov Identifier: NCT02928211).

Finally, in another ocular fluid, the aqueous humour; higher levels of proteins involved in AD pathology such as β-amyloid peptides; and a series of chemokines, including eotaxin, eotaxin 3, and interleukin [IL]-8 (160) were detected in cataract surgery patients. Additionally, Inoue et al. suggest that open-angle glaucoma patients presented elevated levels of various biomarkers of AD in the aqueous humour, including apolipoprotein (Apo) AI, ApoCIII, ApoE, transthyretin (TTR), complement factor H, complement C3, and α2-macroglobulin (α2M) [162].

In the posterior pole, retinal thickness is correlated to cortical atrophy and choroid and NFL is thinning in AD patients [85, 93, 144, 145, 153, 155, 160]. Several reports in AD patients, showed RGC loss [85, 86, 143]. Additionally, studies in patients and on AD animal models displayed Aβ and tau proteins accumulation in inner retinal layers [138, 143, 180]. Furthermore, Rusu et al. detected APP metabolism impairment in transgenic drosophila [140] and Paris et al. detected a reduction of angiogenesis processes in transgenic mice [151]. In addition, studies on patients and animal models reveal that activated microglia and proinflammatory molecules are contributing to the development of the pathology, and they are degenerating neurons, decreasing retinal activity [111, 148, 149, 181].

All these morphological and/or biochemical changes are leading to decreased visual acuity, deficits in visual perception, anomalies of colour vision, visual cognition impairment, and visuospatial disorientation. In summary, all these findings are creating the certainty that visual abnormalities of the visual axis, from RGC to visual cortex, are common ocular characteristic features of AD [164–166, 168].

4. Conclusions

AD diagnosis is based on the interpretation of the signs and symptoms of the disease in cerebrospinal fluid (CSF) tests and neuroimaging of the brain. Recent major advances in brain imaging are providing opportunities for a more accurate diagnosis, but unfortunately, this technique has limited availability, and its costs are high, making population-wide screening challenging. Consequently, there is a global need for novel early diagnostic methods, more specific, more economic, and with the added ability to distinguish AD among the diverse types of neurodegenerative disorders, bearing in mind that AD diagnosis must identify the disease before the cognitive deficits have reached the threshold of dementia.

The eye shares many neural and vascular similarities with the brain, directing many researchers towards the discovery and development of novel ocular biomarkers, which could have a profound influence on early diagnosis and the discovery of new treatments for the disease.

Numerous recent studies reported the presence of β-amyloid plaques, the hallmark of the disease, in the retina of AD mice models and humans, opening the possibility of detecting AD through a simple noninvasive eye scan. Various laboratories are exploring this approach with the development of optical retinal imaging platforms to detect β-amyloid plaques in the retina of AD subjects. These novel imaging platforms are expected to help aid the early detection of AD and assist in monitoring the efficacy of probable future therapeutic agents which target relevant molecular pathways.

Another imminent change concerning the diagnosis of the neurodegenerative diseases through the eye would be the greater role of the primary eye care practitioners in a sector that previously had little implication.

While a considerable number of clinical trials are currently underway to evaluate novel diagnostic methods, through the eye, and the results are promising, for the moment, the biomarkers for the diagnosis of Alzheimer's disease (AD) are not yet validated for use in clinical settings, and their widespread implementation remains a challenge. Among the reasons for this, we could underline the lack of experience of the researchers to interpret the huge data obtained from these eye images, ethnic variation causing further complications, the overlap with other diseases, and the lack of specificity of these biomarkers. In general, there is a need for a greater number of validation studies involving wider cohorts of various ethnicities and origins. Another question arising in the use of eye biomarkers is that perhaps they are too late as by the time β-amiloide plaques are discovered in the retina, the disease has already progressed.

Finally, the cascade of events resulting in retinal cell death in ocular neurodegenerative pathologies is leading scientists to a new common descriptive term of diseases of the retina. Even though the aetiology of AMD, glaucoma, and AD is still uncertain, studying the common features between them may provide further knowledge about their pathogenesis and could lead to accelerated development of therapies for both diseases. Additionally, studying AD-related retinal degeneration is a promising way forward in the investigation of AD pathologies and therapies, which could eventually benefit the brain and cellular mechanisms in other retinal degenerations.

Conflicts of Interest

There are no existing conflicts for this publication.

Authors' Contributions

Pade Colligris and Maria Jesus Perez de Lara contributed equally to the manuscript.

Acknowledgments

This review was supported by the research grants of SAF2016-77084-R and RETICS RD16/0008/0001.

References

[1] Alzheimer's Association, "2013 Alzheimer's disease facts and figures," *Alzheimer's and Dementia*, vol. 9, no. 2, pp. 208–245, 2013.

[2] H. W. Querfurth and F. M. LaFerla, "Alzheimer's disease," *New England Journal of Medicine*, vol. 362, no. 4, pp. 329–344, 2010.

[3] M. Kivipelto, E. L. Helkala, M. P. Laakso et al., "Midlife vascular risk factors and Alzheimer's disease in later life: longitudinal, population based study," *BMJ*, vol. 322, no. 7300, pp. 1447–1451, 2001.

[4] J. A. Luchsinger and D. R. Gustafson, "Adiposity, type 2 diabetes, and Alzheimer's disease," *Journal of Alzheimers Disease*, vol. 16, no. 4, pp. 693–704, 2009.

[5] S. Ahtiluoto, T. Polvikoski, M. Peltonen et al., "Diabetes, Alzheimer's disease, and vascular dementia a population-based neuropathologic study," *Neurology*, vol. 75, no. 13, pp. 1195–1202, 2010.

[6] I. Moonga, F. Niccolini, H. Wilson, G. Pagano, and M. Politis, "Neuroimaging AsD. Hypertension is associated with worse cognitive function and hippocampal hypometabolism in Alzheimer's disease," *European Journal of Neurology*, vol. 24, no. 9, pp. 1173–1182, 2017.
[7] F. F. Oliveira, G. V. Almeida, S. S. Almeida, E. S. Chen, M. A. C. Smith, and P. H. F. Bertolucci, "Pharmacogenetics of angiotensin receptor blockers in patients with dementia due to Alzheimer's disease," *European Journal of Neurology*, vol. 24, p. 613, 2017.
[8] J. J. Pruzin, J. A. Schneider, A. W. Capuano et al., "Diabetes, hemoglobin A1C, and regional Alzheimer disease and infarct pathology," *Alzheimer Disease and Associated Disorders*, vol. 31, no. 1, pp. 41–47, 2017.
[9] E. Rojas-Gutierrez, G. Munoz-Arenas, S. Trevino et al., "Alzheimer's disease and metabolic syndrome: a link from oxidative stress and inflammation to neurodegeneration," *Synapse*, vol. 71, no. 10, article e21990, 2017.
[10] R. E. Tanzi, "The genetics of Alzheimer's disease," *Cold Spring Harbor Perspectives in Medicine*, vol. 2, no. 10, article a006296, 2012.
[11] C. Iadecola, "The pathobiology of vascular dementia," *Neuron*, vol. 80, no. 4, pp. 844–866, 2013.
[12] A. Kapasi and J. A. Schneider, "Vascular contributions to cognitive impairment, clinical Alzheimer's disease, and dementia in older persons," *Biochimica et Biophysica Acta*, vol. 1862, no. 5, pp. 878–886, 2016.
[13] L. G. Apostolova, S. L. Risacher, T. Duran et al., "Associations of the top 20 Alzheimer disease risk variants with brain amyloidosis," *JAMA Neurology*, vol. 75, no. 3, p. 328, 2018.
[14] H. M. Lanoiselee, G. Nicolas, D. Wallon et al., "APP, PSEN1, and PSEN2 mutations in early-onset Alzheimer's disease: a genetic screening study of familial and sporadic cases," *PLoS Medicine*, vol. 14, no. 3, article e1002270, 2017.
[15] J. L. Cummings, T. Morstorf, and K. Zhong, "Alzheimer's disease drug-development pipeline: few candidates, frequent failures," *Alzheimer's Research and Therapy*, vol. 6, no. 4, p. 37, 2014.
[16] E. J. Mufson, S. E. Counts, S. E. Perez, and S. D. Ginsberg, "Cholinergic system during the progression of Alzheimer's disease: therapeutic implications," *Expert Review of Neurotherapeutics*, vol. 8, no. 11, pp. 1703–1718, 2008.
[17] A. Kumar, C. M. Nisha, C. Silakari et al., "Current and novel therapeutic molecules and targets in Alzheimer's disease," *Journal of the Formosan Medical Association*, vol. 115, no. 1, pp. 3–10, 2016.
[18] D. Kumar, A. Ganeshpurkar, D. Kumar, G. Modi, S. K. Gupta, and S. K. Singh, "Secretase inhibitors for the treatment of Alzheimer's disease: long road ahead," *European Journal of Medicinal Chemistry*, vol. 148, pp. 436–452, 2018.
[19] A. K. Sahoo, J. Dandapat, U. C. Dash, and S. Kanhar, "Features and outcomes of drugs for combination therapy as multi-targets strategy to combat Alzheimer's disease," *Journal of Ethnopharmacology*, vol. 215, pp. 42–73, 2018.
[20] M. W. Weiner, D. P. Veitch, P. S. Aisen et al., "The Alzheimer's disease neuroimaging initiative: a review of papers published since its inception," *Alzheimer's and Dementia: The Journal of the Alzheimer's Association*, vol. 8, no. 1, pp. S1–S68, 2012.
[21] M. E. de Vugt and F. R. Verhey, "The impact of early dementia diagnosis and intervention on informal caregivers," *Progress in Neurobiology*, vol. 110, pp. 54–62, 2013.
[22] L. Robinson, E. Tang, and J. P. Taylor, "Dementia: timely diagnosis and early intervention," *BMJ*, vol. 350, article h3029, 2015.
[23] G. M. McKhann, D. S. Knopman, H. Chertkow et al., "The diagnosis of dementia due to Alzheimer's disease: recommendations from the National Institute on Aging-Alzheimer's Association workgroups on diagnostic guidelines for Alzheimer's disease," *Alzheimer's and Dementia: The Journal of the Alzheimer's Association*, vol. 7, no. 3, pp. 263–269, 2011.
[24] W. M. van der Flier, Y. A. Pijnenburg, N. C. Fox, and P. Scheltens, "Early-onset versus late-onset Alzheimer's disease: the case of the missing APOE varepsilon4 allele," *Lancet Neurology*, vol. 10, no. 3, pp. 280–288, 2011.
[25] P. Scheltens, K. Blennow, M. M. Breteler et al., "Alzheimer's disease," *The Lancet*, vol. 388, no. 10043, pp. 505–517, 2016.
[26] R. D. Terry, E. Masliah, and L. A. Hansen, "Structural basis of the cognitive alterations in Alzheimer disease," in *Alzheimer Disease*, R. D. Terry, R. Katzman, and K. L. Bick, Eds., Raven Press, New York, NY, USA, 1994.
[27] E. M. Mandelkow and E. Mandelkow, "Tau in Alzheimer's disease," *Trends in Cell Biology*, vol. 8, no. 11, pp. 425–427, 1998.
[28] J. Q. Trojanowski and V. M. Lee, ""Fatal attractions" of proteins: a comprehensive hypothetical mechanism underlying Alzheimer's disease and other neurodegenerative disorders," *Annals of the New York Academy of Sciences*, vol. 924, no. 1, pp. 62–67, 2000.
[29] K. Iqbal and I. Grundke-Iqbal, "Neurofibrillary pathology leads to synaptic loss and not the other way around in Alzheimer disease," *Journal of Alzheimer's Disease*, vol. 4, no. 3, pp. 235–238, 2002.
[30] B. Liu, S. Rasool, Z. Yang et al., "Amyloid-peptide vaccinations reduce {beta}-amyloid plaques but exacerbate vascular deposition and inflammation in the retina of Alzheimer's transgenic mice," *American Journal of Pathology*, vol. 175, no. 5, pp. 2099–2110, 2009.
[31] L. Crews and E. Masliah, "Molecular mechanisms of neurodegeneration in Alzheimer's disease," *Human Molecular Genetics*, vol. 19, no. R1, pp. R12–R20, 2010.
[32] M. Saadat, "Distributions of susceptibility loci to late onset Alzheimer's disease on human chromosomes," *EXCLI Journal*, vol. 15, pp. 403–405, 2016.
[33] B. A. Wandell, *Foundations of Vision*, Stanford University, Stanford, CA, USA, 2013.
[34] M. Koronyo-Hamaoui, Y. Koronyo, A. V. Ljubimov et al., "Identification of amyloid plaques in retinas from Alzheimer's patients and noninvasive in vivo optical imaging of retinal plaques in a mouse model," *Neuroimage*, vol. 54, no. 1, pp. S204–S217, 2011.
[35] Y. Koronyo, B. C. Salumbides, K. L. Black, and M. Koronyo-Hamaoui, "Alzheimer's disease in the retina: imaging retinal abeta plaques for early diagnosis and therapy assessment," *Neuro-Degenerative Diseases*, vol. 10, no. 1–4, pp. 285–293, 2012.
[36] J. Jiang, H. Wang, W. Li, X. Cao, and C. Li, "Amyloid plaques in retina for diagnosis in Alzheimer's patients: a meta-analysis," *Frontiers in Aging Neuroscience*, vol. 8, p. 267, 2016.
[37] C. La Morgia, F. N. Ross-Cisneros, Y. Koronyo et al., "Melanopsin retinal ganglion cell loss in Alzheimer disease," *Annals of Neurology*, vol. 79, no. 1, pp. 90–109, 2016.
[38] Y. Koronyo, D. Biggs, E. Barron et al., "Retinal amyloid pathology and proof-of-concept imaging trial in Alzheimer's disease," *JCI Insight*, vol. 2, no. 16, 2017.
[39] P. N. Alexandrov, A. Pogue, S. Bhattacharjee, and W. J. Lukiw, "Retinal amyloid peptides and complement factor H in transgenic models of Alzheimer's disease," *Neuroreport*, vol. 22, no. 12, pp. 623–627, 2011.

[40] Y. Tsai, B. Lu, A. V. Ljubimov et al., "Ocular changes in TgF344-AD rat model of Alzheimer's disease," *Investigative Ophthalmology and Visual Science*, vol. 55, no. 1, pp. 523-534, 2014.

[41] M. Chiasseu, L. Alarcon-Martinez, N. Belforte et al., "Tau accumulation in the retina promotes early neuronal dysfunction and precedes brain pathology in a mouse model of Alzheimer's disease," *Molecular Neurodegeneration*, vol. 12, no. 1, p. 58, 2017.

[42] L. Buccarello, A. Sclip, M. Sacchi et al., "The c-jun N-terminal kinase plays a key role in ocular degenerative changes in a mouse model of Alzheimer disease suggesting a correlation between ocular and brain pathologies," *Oncotarget*, vol. 8, no. 47, pp. 83038–83051, 2017.

[43] C. Criscuolo, E. Cerri, C. Fabiani, S. Capsoni, A. Cattaneo, and L. Domenici, "The retina as a window to early dysfunctions of Alzheimer's disease following studies with a 5xFAD mouse model," *Neurobiology of Aging*, vol. 67, pp. 181–188, 2018.

[44] U. Kayabasi, R. C. Sergott, and M. Rispoli, "Retinal examination for the diagnosis of Alzheimer's disease," *International Journal of Ophthalmic and Pathology*, vol. 1, no. 1, pp. 3-4, 2014.

[45] N. J. Hart, Y. Koronyo, K. L. Black, and M. Koronyo-Hamaoui, "Ocular indicators of Alzheimer's: exploring disease in the retina," *Acta Neuropathologica*, vol. 132, no. 6, pp. 767–787, 2016.

[46] J. Doustar, T. Torbati, K. L. Black, Y. Koronyo, and M. Koronyo-Hamaoui, "Optical coherence tomography in Alzheimer's disease and other neurodegenerative diseases," *Frontiers in Neurology*, vol. 8, p. 701, 2017.

[47] H. Hampel, N. Toschi, C. Babiloni et al., "Revolution of Alzheimer precision neurology passageway of systems biology and neurophysiology," *Journal of Alzheimer's Disease*, vol. 64, no. S1, pp. S47–S105, 2018.

[48] K. Ukalovic, S. Cao, S. Lee et al., "Drusen in the peripheral retina of the Alzheimer's eye," *Current Alzheimer Research*, vol. 15, no. 8, pp. 743–750, 2018.

[49] V. K. Ramanan and A. J. Saykin, "Pathways to neurodegeneration: mechanistic insights from GWAS in Alzheimer's disease, Parkinson's disease, and related disorders," *American Journal of Neurodegenerative Disease*, vol. 2, no. 3, pp. 145–175, 2013.

[50] S. L. Budd Haeberlein and T. J. Harris, "Promising targets for the treatment of neurodegenerative diseases," *Clinical Pharmacology and Therapeutics*, vol. 98, no. 5, pp. 492–501, 2015.

[51] J. Peedicayil, "Epigenetic targets for the treatment of neurodegenerative diseases," *Clinical Pharmacology and Therapeutics*, vol. 99, no. 5, p. 481, 2016.

[52] J. A. Santiago, V. Bottero, and J. A. Potashkin, "Dissecting the molecular mechanisms of neurodegenerative diseases through network biology," *Frontiers in Aging Neuroscience*, vol. 9, p. 166, 2017.

[53] C. Reitz and R. Mayeux, "Alzheimer disease: epidemiology, diagnostic criteria, risk factors and biomarkers," *Biochemical Pharmacology*, vol. 88, no. 4, pp. 640–651, 2014.

[54] P. van Wijngaarden, X. Hadoux, M. Alwan, S. Keel, and M. Dirani, "Emerging ocular biomarkers of Alzheimer disease," *Clinical and Experimental Ophthalmology*, vol. 45, no. 1, pp. 54–61, 2017.

[55] F. Chiti and C. M. Dobson, "Protein misfolding, amyloid formation, and human disease: a summary of progress over the last decade," *Annual Review of Biochemistry*, vol. 86, pp. 27–68, 2017.

[56] E. Herczenik and M. F. B. G. Gebbink, "Molecular and cellular aspects of protein misfolding and disease," *FASEB Journal*, vol. 22, no. 7, pp. 2115–2133, 2008.

[57] L. E. Goldstein, J. A. Muffat, R. A. Cherny et al., "Cytosolic beta-amyloid deposition and supranuclear cataracts in lenses from people with Alzheimer's disease," *The Lancet*, vol. 361, no. 9365, pp. 1258–1265, 2003.

[58] M. B. Pepys, "Amyloidosis," *Annual Review of Medicine*, vol. 57, no. 1, pp. 223–241, 2006.

[59] V. K. Gupta, N. Chitranshi, V. B. Gupta et al., "Amyloid beta accumulation and inner retinal degenerative changes in Alzheimer's disease transgenic mouse," *Neuroscience Letters*, vol. 623, pp. 52–56, 2016.

[60] E. Stefansson, O. B. Olafsdottir, A. B. Einarsdottir et al., "Retinal oximetry discovers novel biomarkers in retinal and brain diseases," *Investigative Ophthalmology and Visual Science*, vol. 58, no. 6, pp. 227–233, 2017.

[61] J. Attems and K. A. Jellinger, "Tau and alpha-synuclein brainstem pathology in Alzheimer disease," *Neuropathology and Applied Neurobiology*, vol. 32, no. 2, pp. 222-223, 2006.

[62] N. A. Verwey, A. Schuitemaker, W. M. van der Flier et al., "Serum amyloid P component as a biomarker in mild cognitive impairment and Alzheimer's disease," *Dementia and Geriatric Cognitive Disorders*, vol. 26, no. 6, pp. 522–527, 2008.

[63] V. L. Villemagne, K. E. Pike, D. Darby et al., "A beta deposits in older non-demented individuals with cognitive decline are indicative of preclinical Alzheimer's disease," *Neuropsychologia*, vol. 46, no. 6, pp. 1688–1697, 2008.

[64] N. K. Archibald, M. P. Clarke, U. P. Mosimann, and D. J. Burn, "The retina in Parkinson's disease," *Brain*, vol. 132, no. 5, pp. 1128–1145, 2009.

[65] I. Bodis-Wollner, P. B. Kozlowski, S. Glazman, and S. Miri, "α-synuclein in the inner retina in Parkinson disease," *Annals of Neurology*, vol. 75, no. 6, pp. 964–966, 2014.

[66] L. V. Johnson, W. P. Leitner, A. J. Rivest, M. K. Staples, M. J. Radeke, and D. H. Anderson, "The Alzheimer's a beta-peptide is deposited at sites of complement activation in pathologic deposits associated with aging and age-related macular degeneration," *Proceedings of the National Academy of Sciences of the United States of America*, vol. 99, no. 18, pp. 11830–11835, 2002.

[67] S. J. McKinnon, N. L. Ransom, N. G. Tahzih, D. M. Lehmann, and H. A. Reitsamer, "A monoclonal antibody to amyloid precursor protein induces apoptosis in rat retinal ganglion cells," *Investigative Ophthalmology and Visual Science*, vol. 43, article U1158-U, 2002.

[68] S. Yoneda, H. Hara, A. Hirata, M. Fukushima, Y. Inomata, and H. Tanihara, "Vitreous fluid levels of beta-amyloid((1-42)) and tau in patients with retinal diseases," *Japanese Journal of Ophthalmology*, vol. 49, no. 2, pp. 106–108, 2005.

[69] D. Goldblum, A. Kipfer-Kauer, G. M. Sarra, S. Wolf, and B. E. Frueh, "Distribution of amyloid precursor protein and amyloid-beta immunoreactivity in DBA/2J glaucomatous mouse retinas," *Investigative Ophthalmology and Visual Science*, vol. 48, no. 11, pp. 5085–5090, 2007.

[70] L. Guo, T. E. Salt, V. Luong et al., "Targeting amyloid-beta in glaucoma treatment," *Proceedings of the National Academy of Sciences*, vol. 104, no. 33, pp. 13444–13449, 2007.

[71] R. Mancino, A. Martucci, M. Cesareo et al., "Glaucoma and Alzheimer disease: a single age-related neurodegenerative disease of the brain," *Current Neuropharmacology*, vol. 16, no. 7, pp. 971–977, 2017.

[72] M. Mirzaei, V. B. Gupta, J. M. Chick et al., "Age-related neurodegenerative disease associated pathways identified in retinal and vitreous proteome from human glaucoma eyes," *Scientific Reports*, vol. 7, no. 1, article 12685, 2017.

[73] E. Cerri, C. Fabiani, C. Criscuolo, and L. Domenici, "Visual Evoked Potentials in Glaucoma and Alzheimer's Disease," *Methods in Molecular Biology*, vol. 1695, pp. 69–80, 2018.

[74] A. Giorgio, J. Zhang, F. Costantino, N. De Stefano, and P. Frezzotti, "Diffuse brain damage in normal tension glaucoma," *Human Brain Mapping*, vol. 39, no. 1, pp. 532-541, 2018.

[75] P. Wostyn, D. Van Dam, K. Audenaert, H. E. Killer, P. P. De Deyn, and V. De Groot, "A new glaucoma hypothesis: a role of glymphatic system dysfunction," *Fluids and Barriers of the CNS*, vol. 12, p. 16, 2015.

[76] N. A. Jessen, A. S. Munk, I. Lundgaard, and M. Nedergaard, "The glymphatic system: a beginner's guide," *Neurochemical Research*, vol. 40, no. 12, pp. 2583–2599, 2015.

[77] P. Wostyn, V. De Groot, D. Van Dam, K. Audenaert, H. E. Killer, and P. P. De Deyn, "The Glymphatic Hypothesis of Glaucoma: A Unifying Concept Incorporating Vascular, Biomechanical, and Biochemical Aspects of the Disease," *BioMed Research International*, vol. 2017, Article ID 5123148, 7 pages, 2017.

[78] P. Wostyn, H. E. Killer, and P. P. De Deyn, "Glymphatic stasis at the site of the lamina cribrosa as a potential mechanism underlying open-angle glaucoma," *Clinical and Experimental Ophthalmology*, vol. 45, no. 5, pp. 539–547, 2017.

[79] L. Biscetti, E. Luchetti, A. Vergaro, P. Menduno, C. Cagini, and L. Parnetti, "Associations of Alzheimer's disease with macular degeneration," *Frontiers in Bioscience*, vol. 9, no. 1, pp. 174–191, 2017.

[80] A. I. Pogue and W. J. Lukiw, "Up-regulated pro-inflammatory microRNAs (miRNAs) in Alzheimer's disease (AD) and age-related macular degeneration (AMD)," *Cellular and Molecular Neurobiology*, vol. 38, no. 5, pp. 1021–1031, 2018.

[81] S. Frost, R. Guymer, K. Z. Aung et al., "Alzheimer's disease and the early signs of age-related macular degeneration," *Current Alzheimer Research*, vol. 13, no. 11, pp. 1259–1266, 2016.

[82] D. Seden, G. Alime, D. Kadir, D. Serpil, T. Levent, and T. Ozlem, "Is Alzheimer disease related to age-related macular degeneration?," *Turkish Journal of Medical Sciences*, vol. 45, no. 5, pp. 1115–1121, 2015.

[83] M. A. Williams, G. J. McKay, R. Carson, D. Craig, G. Silvestri, and P. Passmore, "Age-related macular degeneration-associated genes in Alzheimer disease," *American Journal of Geriatric Psychiatry*, vol. 23, no. 12, pp. 1290–1296, 2015.

[84] R. Sant'Anna, S. Navarro, S. Ventura, L. Paraoan, and D. Foguel, "Amyloid properties of the leader peptide of variant B cystatin C: implications for Alzheimer and macular degeneration," *FEBS Letters*, vol. 590, no. 5, pp. 644–654, 2016.

[85] D. R. Hinton, A. A. Sadun, J. C. Blanks, and C. A. Miller, "Optic-nerve degeneration in Alzheimer's disease," *New England Journal of Medicine*, vol. 315, no. 8, pp. 485–487, 1986.

[86] J. C. Blanks, D. R. Hinton, A. A. Sadun, and C. A. Miller, "Retinal ganglion cell degeneration in Alzheimer's disease," *Brain Research*, vol. 501, no. 2, pp. 364–372, 1989.

[87] A. A. Sadun and C. J. Bassi, "Optic-nerve damage in Alzheimer's disease," *Ophthalmology*, vol. 97, no. 1, pp. 9–17, 1990.

[88] J. C. Blanks, S. Y. Schmidt, Y. Torigoe, K. V. Porrello, D. R. Hinton, and R. H. I. Blanks, "Retinal pathology in Alzheimer's disease. 2. Regional neuron loss and glial changes in GCL," *Neurobiology of Aging*, vol. 17, no. 3, pp. 385–395, 1996.

[89] T. R. Hedges, R. Perez Galves, D. Speigelman, N. R. Barbas, E. Peli, and C. J. Yardley, "Retinal nerve fiber layer abnormalities in Alzheimer's disease," *Acta Ophthalmologica Scandinavica*, vol. 74, no. 3, pp. 271–275, 1996.

[90] J. C. Blanks, Y. Torigoe, D. R. Hinton, and R. H. I. Blanks, "Retinal pathology in Alzheimer's disease. 1. Ganglion cell loss in foveal/parafoveal retina," *Neurobiology of Aging*, vol. 17, no. 3, pp. 377–384, 1996.

[91] P. K. Iseri, O. Altinas, T. Tokay, and N. Yuksel, "Relationship between cognitive impairment and retinal morphological and visual functional abnormalities in Alzheimer disease," *Journal of Neuro-Ophthalmology*, vol. 26, no. 1, pp. 18–24, 2006.

[92] A. U. Bayer, O. N. Keller, F. Ferrari, and K. P. Maag, "Association of glaucoma with neurodegenerative diseases with apoptotic cell death: Alzheimer's disease and Parkinson's disease," *American Journal of Ophthalmology*, vol. 133, no. 1, pp. 135–137, 2002.

[93] V. Parisi, R. Restuccia, F. Fattapposta, C. Mina, M. G. Bucci, and F. Pierelli, "Morphological and functional retinal impairment in Alzheimer's disease patients," *Clinical Neurophysiology*, vol. 112, no. 10, pp. 1860–1867, 2001.

[94] R. Patil, Y. Koronyo, A. V. Ljubimov et al., "Advances in Imaging: brain tumors to Alzheimer's disease," *Bangkok Medical Journal*, vol. 10, no. 1, pp. 83–97, 2015.

[95] J. K. Morris, R. A. Honea, E. D. Vidoni, R. H. Swerdlow, and J. M. Burns, "Is Alzheimer's disease a systemic disease?," *Biochimica et Biophysica Acta*, vol. 1842, no. 9, pp. 1340-1349, 2014.

[96] M. Oresic, G. Anderson, I. Mattila et al., "Targeted serum metabolite profiling identifies metabolic signatures in patients with Alzheimer's disease, normal pressure hydrocephalus and brain tumor," *Frontiers in Neuroscience*, vol. 11, p. 747, 2017.

[97] A. B. Einarsdottir, S. H. Hardarson, J. V. Kristjansdottir, D. T. Bragason, J. Snaedal, and E. Stefansson, "Retinal oximetry imaging in Alzheimer's disease," *Journal of Alzheimer's Disease*, vol. 49, no. 1, pp. 79–83, 2016.

[98] G. Alcarraz-Vizan, P. Casini, L. Cadavez et al., "Inhibition of BACE2 counteracts hIAPP-induced insulin secretory defects in pancreatic beta-cells," *FASEB Journal*, vol. 29, no. 1, pp. 95–104, 2015.

[99] R. Simo, A. Ciudin, O. Simo-Servat, and C. Hernandez, "Cognitive impairment and dementia: a new emerging complication of type 2 diabetes-the diabetologist's perspective," *Acta Diabetologica*, vol. 54, no. 5, pp. 417–424, 2017.

[100] A. Ciudin, O. Simo-Servat, C. Hernandez et al., "Retinal microperimetry: a new tool for identifying patients with type 2 diabetes at risk for developing Alzheimer disease," *Diabetes*, vol. 66, no. 12, pp. 3098–3104, 2017.

[101] M. B. Rougier, J. F. Korobelnik, F. Malet et al., "Retinal nerve fibre layer thickness measured with SD-OCT in a population-based study of French elderly subjects: the Alienor study," *Acta Ophthalmologica*, vol. 93, no. 6, pp. 539–545, 2015.

[102] C. Schweitzer, J. F. Korobelnik, M. Le Goff et al., "Diagnostic performance of peripapillary retinal nerve fiber layer thickness for detection of glaucoma in an elderly population: the Alienor study," *Investigative Ophthalmology and Visual Science*, vol. 57, no. 14, pp. 5882–5891, 2016.

[103] L. Tellouck, M. Durieux, P. Coupe et al., "Optic radiations microstructural changes in glaucoma and association with

severity: a study using 3 tesla-magnetic resonance diffusion tensor imaging," *Investigative Ophthalmology and Visual Science*, vol. 57, no. 15, pp. 6539–6547, 2016.

[104] J. L. Mendez-Gomez, M. B. Rougier, L. Tellouck et al., "Peripapillary retinal nerve fiber layer thickness and the evolution of cognitive performance in an elderly population," *Frontiers in Neurology*, vol. 8, p. 93, 2017.

[105] K. G. Goozee, T. M. Shah, H. R. Sohrabi et al., "Examining the potential clinical value of curcumin in the prevention and diagnosis of Alzheimer's disease," *British Journal of Nutrition*, vol. 115, no. 3, pp. 449–465, 2016.

[106] M. Chen, Z. Y. Du, X. Zheng, D. L. Li, R. P. Zhou, and K. Zhang, "Use of curcumin in diagnosis, prevention, and treatment of Alzheimer's disease," *Neural Regeneration Research*, vol. 13, no. 4, pp. 742–752, 2018.

[107] A. Ning, J. Cui, E. To, K. H. Ashe, and J. Matsubara, "Amyloid-beta deposits lead to retinal degeneration in a mouse model of Alzheimer disease," *Investigative Ophthalmology and Visual Science*, vol. 49, no. 11, pp. 5136–5143, 2008.

[108] S. E. Perez, S. Lumayag, B. Kovacs, E. J. Mufson, and S. B. Xu, "β-amyloid deposition and functional impairment in the retina of the APPswe/PS1 delta E9 transgenic mouse model of Alzheimer's disease," *Investigative Ophthalmology and Visual Science*, vol. 50, no. 2, pp. 793–800, 2009.

[109] K. Chiu, T. F. Chan, A. Wu, I. Y. P. Leung, K. F. So, and R. C. C. Chang, "Neurodegeneration of the retina in mouse models of Alzheimer's disease: what can we learn from the retina?," *Age*, vol. 34, no. 3, pp. 633–649, 2012.

[110] J. C. Vickers, R. A. Lazzarini, B. M. Riederer, and J. H. Morrison, "Intraperikaryal neurofilamentous accumulations in a subset of retinal ganglion-cells in aged mice that express a human neurofilament gene," *Experimental Neurology*, vol. 136, no. 2, pp. 266–269, 1995.

[111] A. I. Ramirez, R. de Hoz, E. Salobrar-Garcia et al., "The role of microglia in retinal neurodegeneration: Alzheimer's disease, Parkinson, and glaucoma," *Frontiers in Aging Neuroscience*, vol. 9, p. 214, 2017.

[112] D. J. Mordant, I. Al-Abboud, G. Muyo, A. Gorman, A. R. Harvey, and A. I. McNaught, "Oxygen saturation measurements of the retinal vasculature in treated asymmetrical primary open-angle glaucoma using hyperspectral imaging," *Eye*, vol. 28, no. 10, pp. 1190–1200, 2014.

[113] A. M. Shahidi, S. R. Patel, J. G. Flanagan, and C. Hudson, "Regional variation in human retinal vessel oxygen saturation," *Experimental Eye Research*, vol. 113, pp. 143–147, 2013.

[114] K. Rose, S. I. Kulasekara, and C. Hudson, "Intervisit repeatability of retinal blood oximetry and total retinal blood flow under varying systemic blood gas oxygen saturations," *Investigative Ophthalmology and Visual Science*, vol. 57, no. 1, pp. 188–197, 2016.

[115] K. Herrup, "The case for rejecting the amyloid cascade hypothesis," *Nature Neuroscience*, vol. 18, no. 6, pp. 794–799, 2015.

[116] S. S. More and R. Vince, "Hyperspectral imaging signatures detect amyloidopathy in Alzheimer's mouse retina well before onset of cognitive decline," *ACS Chemical Neuroscience*, vol. 6, no. 2, pp. 306–315, 2015.

[117] S. S. More, J. M. Beach, and R. Vince, "Early detection of amyloidopathy in Alzheimer's mice by hyperspectral endoscopy," *Investigative Ophthalmology and Visual Science*, vol. 57, no. 7, pp. 3231–3238, 2016.

[118] C. Schon, N. A. Hoffmann, S. M. Ochs et al., "Long-term in vivo imaging of fibrillar tau in the retina of P301S transgenic mice," *PLoS One*, vol. 7, no. 12, Article ID e53547, 2012.

[119] P. A. Williams, R. A. Thirgood, H. Oliphant et al., "Retinal ganglion cell dendritic degeneration in a mouse model of Alzheimer's disease," *Neurobiology of Aging*, vol. 34, no. 7, pp. 1799–1806, 2013.

[120] H. Zhao, R. Chang, H. Che et al., "Hyperphosphorylation of tau protein by calpain regulation in retina of Alzheimer's disease transgenic mouse," *Neuroscience Letters*, vol. 551, pp. 12–16, 2013.

[121] C. Y. Ho, J. C. Troncoso, D. Knox, W. Stark, and C. G. Eberhart, "Beta-amyloid, phospho-tau and alpha-synuclein deposits similar to those in the brain are not identified in the eyes of Alzheimer's and Parkinson's disease patients," *Brain Pathology*, vol. 24, no. 1, pp. 25–32, 2014.

[122] D. E. Barnes and K. Yaffe, "The projected effect of risk factor reduction on Alzheimer's disease prevalence," *Lancet Neurology*, vol. 10, no. 9, pp. 819–828, 2011.

[123] C. Reitz, C. Brayne, and R. Mayeux, "Epidemiology of Alzheimer disease," *Nature Reviews Neurology*, vol. 7, no. 3, pp. 137–152, 2011.

[124] C. Kerbage, C. H. Sadowsky, D. Jennings, G. D. Cagle, and P. D. Hartung, "Alzheimer's disease diagnosis by detecting exogenous fluorescent signal of ligand bound to beta amyloid in the lens of human eye: an exploratory study," *Frontiers in Neurology*, vol. 4, 2013.

[125] K. L. Thomson, J. M. Yeo, B. Waddell, J. R. Cameron, and S. Pal, "A systematic review and meta-analysis of retinal nerve fiber layer change in dementia, using optical coherence tomography," *Alzheimer's and Dementia*, vol. 1, no. 2, pp. 136–143, 2015.

[126] L. P. Cunha, L. C. Lopes, L. V. F. Costa-Cunha et al., "Macular thickness measurements with frequency domain-OCT for quantification of retinal neural loss and its correlation with cognitive impairment in Alzheimer's disease," *PLoS One*, vol. 11, no. 4, Article ID e0153830, 2016.

[127] J. den Haan, S. F. Janssen, J. A. van de Kreeke, P. Scheltens, F. D. Verbraak, and F. H. Bouwman, "Retinal thickness correlates with parietal cortical atrophy in early-onset Alzheimer's disease and controls," *Alzheimer's and Dementia*, vol. 10, pp. 49–55, 2018.

[128] S. Frost, Y. Kanagasingam, H. Sohrabi et al., "Retinal vascular biomarkers for early detection and monitoring of Alzheimer's disease," *Translational psychiatry*, vol. 3, article e233, 2013.

[129] H. Jiang, Y. Wei, Y. Shi et al., "Altered macular microvasculature in mild cognitive impairment and Alzheimer disease," *Journal of Neuro-Ophthalmology*, 2017, In press.

[130] K. Kotliar, C. Hauser, M. Ortner et al., "Altered neurovascular coupling as measured by optical imaging: a biomarker for Alzheimer's disease," *Scientific Reports*, vol. 7, no. 1, article 12906, 2017.

[131] M. Bulut, F. Kurtulus, O. Gozkaya et al., "Evaluation of optical coherence tomography angiographic findings in Alzheimer's type dementia," *British Journal of Ophthalmology*, vol. 102, no. 2, pp. 233–237, 2018.

[132] G. Seidel, G. Aschinger, C. Singer et al., "Estimating retinal blood flow velocities by optical coherence tomography," *JAMA Ophthalmology*, vol. 134, no. 10, pp. 1104–1110, 2016.

[133] G. C. Aschinger, L. Schmetterer, K. Fondi et al., "Effect of diffuse luminance flicker light stimulation on total retinal blood flow assessed with dual-beam bidirectional Doppler OCT," *Investigative Ophthalmology and Visual Science*, vol. 58, no. 2, pp. 1167–1178, 2017.

[134] B. Baumann, A. Woehrer, G. Ricken et al., "Visualization of neuritic plaques in Alzheimer's disease by polarization-sensitive optical coherence microscopy," *Scientific Reports*, vol. 7, article 43477, 2017.
[135] M. Ang, M. Baskaran, R. M. Werkmeister et al., "Anterior segment optical coherence tomography," *Progress in Retinal and Eye Research*, 2018, In press.
[136] G. Kallo, M. Emri, Z. Varga et al., "Changes in the chemical barrier composition of tears in Alzheimer's disease reveal potential tear diagnostic biomarkers," *PLoS One*, vol. 11, no. 6, Article ID e0158000, 2016.
[137] N. Ornek, E. Dag, and K. Ornek, "Corneal sensitivity and tear function in neurodegenerative diseases," *Current Eye Research*, vol. 40, no. 4, pp. 423–428, 2015.
[138] T. L. Spires-Jones, W. H. Stoothoff, A. de Calignon, P. B. Jones, and B. T. Hyman, "Tau pathophysiology in neurodegeneration: a tangled issue," *Trends in Neurosciences*, vol. 32, no. 3, pp. 150–159, 2009.
[139] A. Mudher and S. Lovestone, "Alzheimer's disease-do tauists and baptists finally shake hands?," *Trends in Neurosciences*, vol. 25, no. 1, pp. 22–26, 2002.
[140] P. Rusu, A. Jansen, P. Soba et al., "Axonal accumulation of synaptic markers in APP transgenic Drosophila depends on the NPTY motif and is paralleled by defects in synaptic plasticity," *European Journal of Neuroscience*, vol. 25, no. 4, pp. 1079–1086, 2007.
[141] R. M. Dutescu, Q. X. Li, J. Crowston, C. L. Masters, P. N. Baird, and J. G. Culvenor, "Amyloid precursor protein processing and retinal pathology in mouse models of Alzheimer's disease," *Graefe's Archive for Clinical and Experimental Ophthalmology*, vol. 247, no. 9, pp. 1213-1221, 2009.
[142] L. Gao, X. Chen, Y. Tang et al., "Neuroprotective effect of memantine on the retinal ganglion cells of APPswe/PS1DeltaE9 mice and its immunomodulatory mechanisms," *Experimental Eye Research*, vol. 135, pp. 47–58, 2015.
[143] F. Berisha, G. T. Feke, C. L. Trempe, J. W. McMeel, and C. L. Schepens, "Retinal abnormalities in early Alzheimer's disease," *Investigative Ophthalmology and Visual Science*, vol. 48, no. 5, pp. 2285–2289, 2007.
[144] A. Trebbastoni, F. D'Antonio, A. Bruscolini et al., "Retinal nerve fibre layer thickness changes in Alzheimer's disease: results from a 12-month prospective case series," *Neuroscience Letters*, vol. 629, pp. 165–170, 2016.
[145] G. Coppola, A. Di Renzo, L. Ziccardi et al., "Optical coherence tomography in Alzheimer's disease: a meta-analysis," *PLoS One*, vol. 10, no. 8, Article ID e0134750, 2015.
[146] C. B. Saper, D. C. German, and C. L. White, "Neuronal pathology in the nucleus basalis and associated cell groups in senile dementia of the Alzheimer's type: possible role in cell loss," *Neurology*, vol. 35, no. 8, pp. 1089–1095, 1985.
[147] W. J. Burke, H. D. Chung, J. S. Huang et al., "Evidence for retrograde degeneration of epinephrine neurons in Alzheimer's disease," *Annals of Neurology*, vol. 24, no. 4, pp. 532–536, 1988.
[148] M. T. Heneka, M. J. Carson, J. El Khoury et al., "Neuroinflammation in Alzheimer's disease," *Lancet Neurology*, vol. 14, no. 4, pp. 388–405, 2015.
[149] A. Swanson, T. Wolf, A. Sitzmann, and A. A. Willette, "Neuroinflammation in Alzheimer's disease: pleiotropic roles for cytokines and neuronal pentraxins," *Behavioural Brain Research*, vol. 347, pp. 49–56, 2018.
[150] H. Fillit, W. H. Ding, L. Buee et al., "Elevated circulating tumor necrosis factor levels in Alzheimer's disease," *Neuroscience Letters*, vol. 129, no. 2, pp. 318–320, 1991.
[151] D. Paris, N. Patel, A. DelleDonne, A. Quadros, R. Smeed, and M. Mullan, "Impaired angiogenesis in a transgenic mouse model of cerebral amyloidosis," *Neuroscience Letters*, vol. 366, no. 1, pp. 80–85, 2004.
[152] G. T. Feke, B. T. Hyman, R. A. Stern, and L. R. Pasquale, "Retinal blood flow in mild cognitive impairment and Alzheimer's disease," *Alzheimer's and Dementia*, vol. 1, no. 2, pp. 144–151, 2015.
[153] C. S. Tsai, R. Ritch, B. Schwartz et al., "Optic nerve head and nerve fiber layer in Alzheimer's disease," *Archives of Ophthalmology*, vol. 109, no. 2, pp. 199–204, 1991.
[154] A. Kesler, V. Vakhapova, A. D. Korczyn, E. Naftaliev, and M. Neudorfer, "Retinal thickness in patients with mild cognitive impairment and Alzheimer's disease," *Clinical Neurology and Neurosurgery*, vol. 113, no. 7, pp. 523–526, 2011.
[155] M. P. Bambo, E. Garcia-Martin, F. Gutierrez-Ruiz et al., "Analysis of optic disk color changes in Alzheimer's disease: a potential new biomarker," *Clinical Neurology and Neurosurgery*, vol. 132, pp. 68–73, 2015.
[156] S. S. Liu and S. Q. Zhu, "Correlation between Alzheimer disease and cataract," *Chinese Journal of Ophthalmology*, vol. 53, no. 4, pp. 314–316, 2017.
[157] T. Tian, B. Zhang, Y. Jia, and Z. Li, "Promise and challenge: the lens model as a biomarker for early diagnosis of Alzheimer's disease," *Disease Markers*, vol. 2014, Article ID 826503, 5 pages, 2014.
[158] E. L. Granholm, M. S. Panizzon, J. A. Elman et al., "Pupillary responses as a biomarker of early risk for Alzheimer's disease," *Journal of Alzheimer's Disease*, vol. 56, no. 4, pp. 1419–1428, 2017.
[159] R. A. Sperling, P. S. Aisen, L. A. Beckett et al., "Toward defining the preclinical stages of Alzheimer's disease: recommendations from the National Institute on Aging-Alzheimer's Association workgroups on diagnostic guidelines for Alzheimer's disease," *Alzheimer's and dementia*, vol. 7, no. 3, pp. 280–292, 2011.
[160] A. Trebbastoni, M. Marcelli, F. Mallone et al., "Attenuation of choroidal thickness in patients with Alzheimer Disease: evidence from an Italian prospective study," *Alzheimer Disease and Associated Disorders*, vol. 31, no. 2, pp. 128–134, 2017.
[161] P. Jirarattanasopa, S. Ooto, I. Nakata et al., "Choroidal thickness, vascular hyperpermeability, and complement factor H in age-related macular degeneration and polypoidal choroidal vasculopathy," *Investigative Ophthalmology and Visual Science*, vol. 53, no. 7, pp. 3663–3672, 2012.
[162] T. Inoue, T. Kawaji, and H. Tanihara, "Elevated levels of multiple biomarkers of Alzheimer's disease in the aqueous humor of eyes with open-angle glaucoma," *Investigative Ophthalmology and Visual Science*, vol. 54, no. 8, pp. 5353–5358, 2013.
[163] S. Janciauskiene, K. Westin, O. Grip, and T. Krakau, "Detection of Alzheimer peptides and chemokines in the aqueous humor," *European Journal of Ophthalmology*, vol. 21, no. 1, pp. 104–111, 2011.
[164] G. C. Gilmore and J. A. Levy, "Spatial contrast sensitivity in Alzheimer's disease: a comparison of two methods," *Optometry and Vision Science*, vol. 68, no. 10, pp. 790–794, 1991.
[165] V. Polo, M. J. Rodrigo, E. Garcia-Martin et al., "Visual dysfunction and its correlation with retinal changes in patients with Alzheimer's disease," *Eye*, vol. 31, no. 7, pp. 1034–1041, 2017.

[166] S. N. Thiyagesh, T. F. Farrow, R. W. Parks et al., "The neural basis of visuospatial perception in Alzheimer's disease and healthy elderly comparison subjects: an fMRI study," *Psychiatry Research*, vol. 172, no. 2, pp. 109–116, 2009.
[167] F. K. Cormack, M. Tovee, and C. Ballard, "Contrast sensitivity and visual acuity in patients with Alzheimer's disease," *International Journal of Geriatric Psychiatry*, vol. 15, no. 7, pp. 614–620, 2000.
[168] M. Mapstone, K. Dickerson, and C. J. Duffy, "Distinct mechanisms of impairment in cognitive ageing and Alzheimer's disease," *Brain*, vol. 131, no. 6, pp. 1618–1629, 2008.
[169] G. C. Gilmore, H. E. Wenk, L. A. Naylor, and E. Koss, "Motion perception and Alzheimer's disease," *Journal of Gerontology*, vol. 49, no. 2, pp. P52–P57, 1994.
[170] M. Rizzo and M. Nawrot, "Perception of movement and shape in Alzheimer's disease," *Brain*, vol. 121, no. 12, pp. 2259–2270, 1998.
[171] A. Cronin-Golomb, R. Sugiura, S. Corkin, and J. H. Growdon, "Incomplete achromatopsia in Alzheimer's disease," *Neurobiology of Aging*, vol. 14, no. 5, pp. 471–477, 1993.
[172] H. Bridge, "Effects of cortical damage on binocular depth perception," *Philosophical Transactions of the Royal Society B: Biological Sciences*, vol. 371, no. 1697, article 20150254, 2016.
[173] W. Mittenberg, E. J. Choi, and C. C. Apple, "Stereoscopic visual impairment in vascular dementia," *Archives of Clinical Neuropsychology*, vol. 15, no. 7, pp. 561–569, 2000.
[174] R. Feng, L. Li, H. Yu, M. I. N. Liu, and W. E. I. Zhao, "Melanopsin retinal ganglion cell loss and circadian dysfunction in Alzheimer's disease (review)," *Molecular Medicine Reports*, vol. 13, no. 4, pp. 3397–3400, 2016.
[175] C. La Morgia, F. N. Ross-Cisneros, A. A. Sadun, and V. Carelli, "Retinal ganglion cells and circadian rhythms in Alzheimer's disease, Parkinson's disease, and beyond," *Frontiers in Neurology*, vol. 8, p. 162, 2017.
[176] E. S. Musiek, D. D. Xiong, and D. M. Holtzman, "Sleep, circadian rhythms, and the pathogenesis of Alzheimer Disease," *Experimental and Molecular Medicine*, vol. 47, no. 3, article e148, 2015.
[177] A. Tales, T. Troscianko, D. Lush, J. Haworth, G. K. Wilcock, and S. R. Butler, "The pupillary light reflex in aging and Alzheimer's disease," *Aging*, vol. 13, no. 6, pp. 473–478, 2001.
[178] "Familial aggregation and prevalence of myopia in the Framingham offspring eye study," *Archives of Ophthalmology*, vol. 114, no. 3, pp. 326–332, 1996.
[179] J. A. Moncaster, R. Pineda, R. D. Moir et al., "Alzheimer's disease amyloid-beta links lens and brain pathology in Down syndrome," *PLoS One*, vol. 5, no. 5, Article ID e10659, 2010.
[180] I. Sotiropoulos, C. Catania, T. Riedemann et al., "Glucocorticoids trigger Alzheimer disease-like pathobiochemistry in rat neuronal cells expressing human tau," *Journal of Neurochemistry*, vol. 107, no. 2, pp. 385–397, 2008.
[181] A. I. Pogue, P. Dua, J. M. Hill, and W. J. Lukiw, "Progressive inflammatory pathology in the retina of aluminum-fed 5xFAD transgenic mice," *Journal of Inorganic Biochemistry*, vol. 152, pp. 206–209, 2015.

Association of Genes in the High-Density Lipoprotein Metabolic Pathway with Polypoidal Choroidal Vasculopathy in Asian Population

Ming-zhen Yuan, Ruo-an Han, Chen-xi Zhang, and You-xin Chen

Department of Ophthalmology, Peking Union Medical College Hospital, Chinese Academy of Medical Sciences and Peking Union Medical College, Beijing, China

Correspondence should be addressed to You-xin Chen; chenyouxinpumch@163.com

Academic Editor: Lev Prasov

Purpose. To assess the association of genes in the high-density lipoprotein metabolic pathway (HDLMP) with polypoidal choroidal vasculopathy (PCV) and the genetic difference in the HDLMP between PCV and age-related macular degeneration (AMD). *Methods.* We performed a literature search in EMBASE, PubMed, and Web of Science for genetic studies on 7 single nucleotide polymorphisms (SNPs) from 5 genes in the HDLMP including cholesteryl ester transfer protein (CETP), hepatic lipase (LIPC), lipoprotein lipase (LPL), ATP-binding cassette transporter A1 (ABCA1), and ATP-binding cassette transporter G1 (ABCG1) in PCV. All studies were published before September 30, 2017, without language restriction. Pooled odds ratios (ORs) and 95% confidence intervals (CIs) of each polymorphism were estimated. We also compared the association profiles between PCV and AMD and performed a sensitivity analysis. *Results.* Our result is based on 43 articles. After excluding duplicates and articles without complete information, 7 studies were applicable to meta-analysis. 7 polymorphisms were meta-analyzed: CETP rs2303790/rs3764261, LIPC rs10468017/rs493258, LPL rs12678919, ABCA1 rs1883025, and ABCG1 rs57137919. We found that in Asian population, CETP rs3764261 (T allele; OR = 1.46; 95% CI: 1.28–1.665, $P < 0.01$), CETP rs2303790 (G allele; OR = 1.57; 95% CI: 1.258–1.96, $P < 0.01$), and ABCG1 rs57137919 (A allele; OR = 1.168; 95% CI: 1.016–1.343, $P < 0.01$) were significantly associated with PCV, and ABCG1 rs57137919 (A allele; OR = 1.208, 95% CI: 1.035–1.411, $P < 0.01$) has different effects in PCV and AMD. The other 4 polymorphisms in LIPC/LPL/ABCA1 had no significant association with PCV ($P > 0.05$). The sensitivity analysis validated the significance of our analysis. *Conclusions.* Our study revealed 7 polymorphisms in 5 genes. Among them, CETP (rs3764261/rs2303790) and ABCG1 (rs57137919) were the major susceptibility genes for PCV in Asian population and ABCG1 (rs57137919) showed allelic diversity between PCV and AMD. Since the size for PCV and AMD was small, we need to study these genes genotyping in larger samples.

1. Introduction

Polypoidal choroidal vasculopathy (PCV) is a choroidal vascular disease of first described in the early 1980s as polypoidal subretinal vascular lesions associated with serous or hemorrhagic detachment of the retinal pigment epithelium (RPE) [1]. Later, PCV is regarded as a particular type of choroidal neovascularization (CNV) characterized by the distinct presence of polypoidal vascular lesions and a branching vascular network. PCV can be clearly demonstrated and diagnosed by indocyanine green angiography [2]. From a clinical perspective, PVC is considered as a subtype of AMD because of some similarities like neovascularization, subretinal hemorrhage and fluid, pigment epithelial detachment (PED), vision loss owing to bleeding, leakage, scar formation, and other similarities in phenotypic features [3–6]. Genetically, PCV and AMD also have the common susceptible genes, such as high temperature required factor A1 gene (HTRA1) and the complementary factor H gene (CFH) [7]. However, many controversial studies demonstrate that PCV should be classified as a distinct disease entity of AMD for their different epidemiological, clinical characteristics, natural history, and treatment outcomes [8–11]. Moreover, recent researches in the field of genetics suggest that

PCV may not be as closely related to AMD, such as its differential risk to a mutation in FGD6, viralicidic activity 2-like (SKIV2L), complement component 3 (C3), elastin (ELN), and apolipoprotein E (APOE) [12–16]. These literatures make for a question whether PCV is a subtype of AMD or a distant disease from AMD.

Many studies have indicated lipid deposition in Bruch's membrane and soft drusen, and the amount of lipid was lower in the peripheral area than in the macula of human eyes [17]. A number of population-based studies revealed the association between drusen and the AMD, and drusen are regarded as one of the determinant factors of both early and late AMD [18, 19]. In addition, some studies indicated that the prevalence of drusen under RPE was lower in PCV than in AMD [20, 21], which pointed out that absence of drusen may be one of the important criteria to diagnose PCV. However, some clinical studies insisted that drusen were frequently seen in PCV [22, 23], and several studies reported that drusen were observed in 20% to 27% of unaffected [21, 24]. Therefore, whether drusen plays a functional role in the occurrence and development is still up for debate. As we know, lipids stand for over 40% of the drusen volume [25]; therefore, many academics studied the vital function of lipids in the pathogenesis of PCV and AMD. Due to the different ethnic groups and lifestyles of individuals, the strength of such relevances is widely variable [26–28]; therefore, many studies investigated the effect between gene variations in the HDLMP and risk factors on PCV and AMD. Genetic studies in the HDLMP with PCV and AMD have identified susceptibility single nucleotide polymorphisms (SNPs) in multiple genes, including rs3764261/rs2303790 in CETP, rs493258/rs10468017 in LIPC, rs12678919 in LPL, rs1883025 in ABCA1, and rs57137919 in ABCG1.

Thus far, some studies have studied the impact of lipid metabolism-related and systemic lipoprotein genes in PCV. Here, in order to give the comprehensive analysis of effects and solve the controversies, we conduct meta-analysis and report a systematic review by summing up all published articles of genetic associations in the HDLMP of PCV. This study (1) conducted an investigation of which genetic variants of the HDLMP are meaningfully associated with PCV and their effect sizes and (2) analyzed whether there were differences between genetic risks of the HDLMP in PCV and AMD.

2. Methods

2.1. Search Strategy. We searched EMBASE, PubMed, and Web of Science using the following MeSH terms and free words: (polypoidal choroidal vasculopathy or polypoidal choroidal vascular disease or polypoidal choroidal vascular diseases or PCV) and (cholesteryl ester transfer protein or CETP or hepatic lipase or LIPC or lipoprotein lipase or LPL or ATP-binding cassette transporter A1 or ABCA1 or ATP-binding cassette transporter G1 or ABCG1). All searched articles were published before September 30, 2017, without language restriction. We also screened the reference lists of all eligible studies, reviews, and meta-analyses to ensure that any relevant studies were not omitted. We also searched all reported genome-wide association studies of PCV including the supplementary materials to maximize the usable data. The detail of search strategy is revealed in Table S1.

2.2. Inclusion and Exclusion Criteria. We included those studies that satisfied the following criteria in the meta-analysis: (1) case-control studies, cohort studies, or population-based studies that evaluated the association of gene variants of CETP/LIPC/LPL/ABCA1/ABCG1 with PCV or its subtypes and (2) allele or genotype counts and/or frequencies being presented or able to be calculated from the data in the study. Case reports, conference reports, reviews, animal studies, and reports with insufficient information were excluded (Table S2).

2.3. Data Extraction and Quality Assessment. Two reviewers (Y. M. z. and Y. J. y.) independently reviewed and extracted data from studies on the association between CETP/LIPC/LPL/ABCA1/ABCG1 SNPs and PCV. If there were any differences between them, another two reviewers would help to resolve it (Z. C. x. and H. R. a.) after thorough discussion. The following information was extracted from each article: the name of first author, publication year, ethnicity of the study population, study design, genotyping method, sample size, demographics, allele and genotype distribution (Table 1), and the results of the Hardy–Weinberg equilibrium (HWE) test in controls (Table S3). We assessed the quality of individual studies using the Newcastle–Ottawa Scale [29]. Briefly, 9 quality indicators were used; if a study fulfilled 1 indicator, we assigned a "yes" under this item or a "no." Thus, the quality score for each study might be between 0 and 9 (Table S4).

2.4. Statistical Analysis. We conducted meta-analysis for each polymorphism which had been reported in ≥2 studies or cohorts. The association was evaluated by different genetic models, including allelic, heterozygous, and homozygous models. For each study, the odds ratio (OR) with 95% confidence interval (95% CI) was calculated to evaluate the strength of association between the each SNP and PCV risk. Moreover, we used the I^2 value to quantify the proportion of the variability in effect estimates, which is due to heterogeneity rather than sampling error. The I^2 value was shown as of no (0–25%), low (25–50%), moderate (50–75%), or high heterogeneity (75–100%) [30]. The I^2 test was to assess heterogeneity among studies. The potential publication bias was assessed visually in a funnel plot of log (OR) against its standard error, and the degree of asymmetry was evaluated using Begg's test and Egger's test ($P < 0.05$ was considered to be statistically significant). We undertook the sensitivity analysis to examine the influence by removing the unreliable study [31]. The software STATA (version 12.0, StataCorp LP, College Station, TX) was used for the meta-regression analysis. A pooled P value of less than 0.05 was considered statistically significant.

3. Results

3.1. Eligibility and Characteristics of Included Studies. Figure 1 illustrates the study inclusion of this meta-analysis. A total of 43 articles published before September 30, 2017,

Table 1: Characteristics of the included studies in the meta-analysis.

First author and reference	Year	Ethnicity	Study design	Genotyping method	HWE reported	PCV			AMD			Control			Gene/loci investigated
						N	Male ratio	Mean age ± SD (yrs)	N	Male ratio	Mean age ± SD (yrs)	N	Male ratio	Mean age ± SD (yrs)	
Nakata et al. [32]	2013	Japanese	1	TaqMan and Beadchip	Yes	581	0.73	72.59 ± 8.13	—	—	—	793	0.41	65.99 ± 4.33	CETP, LIPC, LPL
Zhang et al. [33]	2013	Chinese	1	PCR	Yes	250	0.66	65 ± 8.6	157	0.64	67 ± 9.21	204	0.61	69 ± 9	LIPC, ABCA1, CETP, LPL,
Li et al. [34]	2014	Chinese	1	PCR	Yes	298	0.62	66.8 ± 9.7	300	0.63	69.4 ± 8.9	296	0.48	65.1 ± 9.5	ABCA1
Liu et al. [13]	2014	Chinese	1	PCR	Yes	233	0.7	68.5 ± 5.9	200	0.55	75.3 ± 7.7	275	0.44	74.3 ± 7.6	ABCA1, LIPC, CETP, ABCG1
Meng et al. [36]	2015	Chinese	1	PCR	Yes	291	0.79	66.6 ± 9.6	230	0.63	69.3 ± 8.8	221	0.48	67.2 ± 9.6	CETP, LIPC, LPL
	2016	Chinese (Hong Kong)	1	TaqMan and PCR	Yes	236	0.69	68.5 ± 9	235	0.55	75.3 ± 7.6	365	0.42	74.4 ± 7.7	ABCG1
Li et al. [37]	2016	Chinese (Shantou)	1	TaqMan and PCR	Yes	187	0.72	63.1 ± 10.5	189	0.69	67.3 ± 10.1	670	0.43	73.8 ± 6.8	ABCG1
	2016	Japanese (Osaka)	1	TaqMan and PCR	Yes	204	0.77	72.2 ± 8.0	192	0.67	74.3 ± 7.3	157	0.33	47.9 ± 15.1	ABCG1
Qiao et al. [38]	2017	Chinese (Hong Kong)	1	Beadchip	Yes	156	—	—	310	—	—	1006	—	—	CETP

The characteristics of the eligible studies are shown. PCV: polypoidal choroidal vasculopathy; AMD: age-related macular degeneration; HWE: Hardy–Weinberg equilibrium.

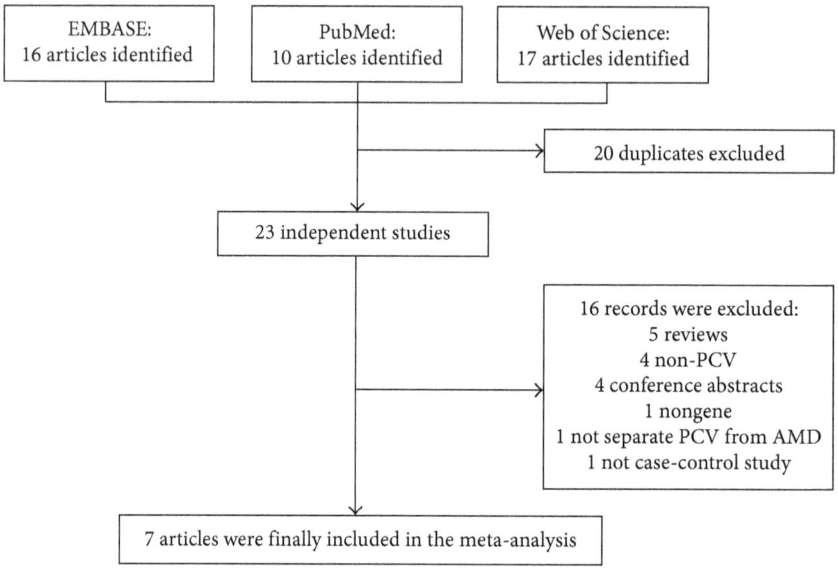

Figure 1: Flow diagram and results of literature review. The flow diagram describes the filtering process of related articles, including the number and reason of exclusion. PCV: polypoidal choroidal vasculopathy; AMD: age-related macular degeneration.

were identified in the EMBASE, PubMed, and Web of Science databases. Of these, we excluded 20 articles because they were duplicates. For the remaining 23 studies, the full texts were retrieved. After reviewing the full texts, we excluded another 16 reports, among which 5 studies were reviews, 4 were not related to PCV, 4 were conference abstracts, 1 was not about the genetic studies, 1 did not separate PCV from AMD, and 1 was not the case-control study. Finally, 7 articles were eligible for the meta-analysis [32–38], involving 3342 PCV cases versus 8256 controls and 2761 PCV cases versus 2660 AMD cases. The main traits of the included studies are summed up in Table 1. Patients from each study received complete ophthalmic examinations, including fluorescein angiography and ICGA. Polypoidal choroidal vasculopathy was diagnosed on the basis of choroidal polypoidal lesions shown by ICGA. All studies adopted a case-control design. These studies were performed in various populations, including Chinese (6 studies), Japanese (3 studies), and Korean (1 study). In all studies, valid genotyping approaches were used, including polymerase chain reaction, TaqMan genotyping assay, and BeadChip.

3.2. Risk of Bias Assessment in Eligible Studies. As shown in Table S4, all eligible studies clearly described the diagnostic criteria for PCV and AMD. Patients with other macular diseases like central serous chorioretinopathy, myopic choroidal neovascularization, angioid streaks, presumed ocular histoplasmosis, or with CNV and PCV in the same or fellow eye were excluded. In all studies, comprehensive ophthalmic examinations were performed on the control subjects. One study used control subjects recruited from the community [32], and the others used hospital-recruited controls. Two studies were diverse-ethnic population study [37, 38]. One study did not provide the sex and age of cohorts. There was no ethnic difference between cases and controls. Confounding factors were matched between cases and controls in 7 studies. The scores for the quality assessment ranged from 5 to 7. All the studies informed HWE in controls.

3.3. Meta-Analysis of CETP/LIPC/LPL/ABCA1/ABCG1 Polymorphisms in PCV. Totally 17 SNPs had been studied in PCV in the literature (Figure 2). However, only 7 SNPs (CETP rs2303790/rs3764261, LIPC rs10468017/rs493258, LPL rs12678919, ABCA1 rs1883025, and ABCG1 rs57137919) in PCV were reported in more than one study and thus eligible for meta-analysis (details can be seen in Table S5). Summary of the allelic associations of these polymorphisms is shown in Table 2. The other 10 SNPs reported in only one report but performed no association with PCV [33, 36].

CETP rs3764261 is the most widely investigated SNP in PCV, with a number of 1355 cases and 1493 controls studied for the meta-analysis [32, 33, 35, 36]. The results showed statistically significant association between CETP rs3764261 and PCV in Asian population (Table 2). As for the allelic model, the odds ratio (OR) for the risk allele T was 1.46 (95% confidence interval (CI): 1.28–1.665, $P < 0.01$, $I^2 = 0\%$). In the subgroup analysis by ethnicity, still significant association was detected in Chinese (OR = 1.528, 95% CI: 1.268–1.841, $P < 0.01$, $I^2 = 0\%$). Also, CETP rs2303790 [33, 38] and ABCG1 rs57137919 [35, 37] showed significant associations with PCV in the allelic model. As for CETP rs2303790, the frequency of the G allele was significantly higher in PCV patients than in controls, conferring a 1.57-fold increased risk toward PCV (95% CI: 1.258–1.96, $P < 0.01$, $I^2 = 0$). As for ABCG1 rs57137919, the frequency of the A allele was significantly higher in PCV patients than in controls, conferring a 1.168-fold increased risk (95% CI: 1.016–1.343, $P = 0.029$, $I^2 = 61.5\%$). Through quality assessment and sensitivity analysis, we found the heterogeneity derived from the data of Shantou population [37]. After excluding the data of Shantou population, the result showed that the pooled allelic OR was significantly elevated (A allele; OR = 1.313,

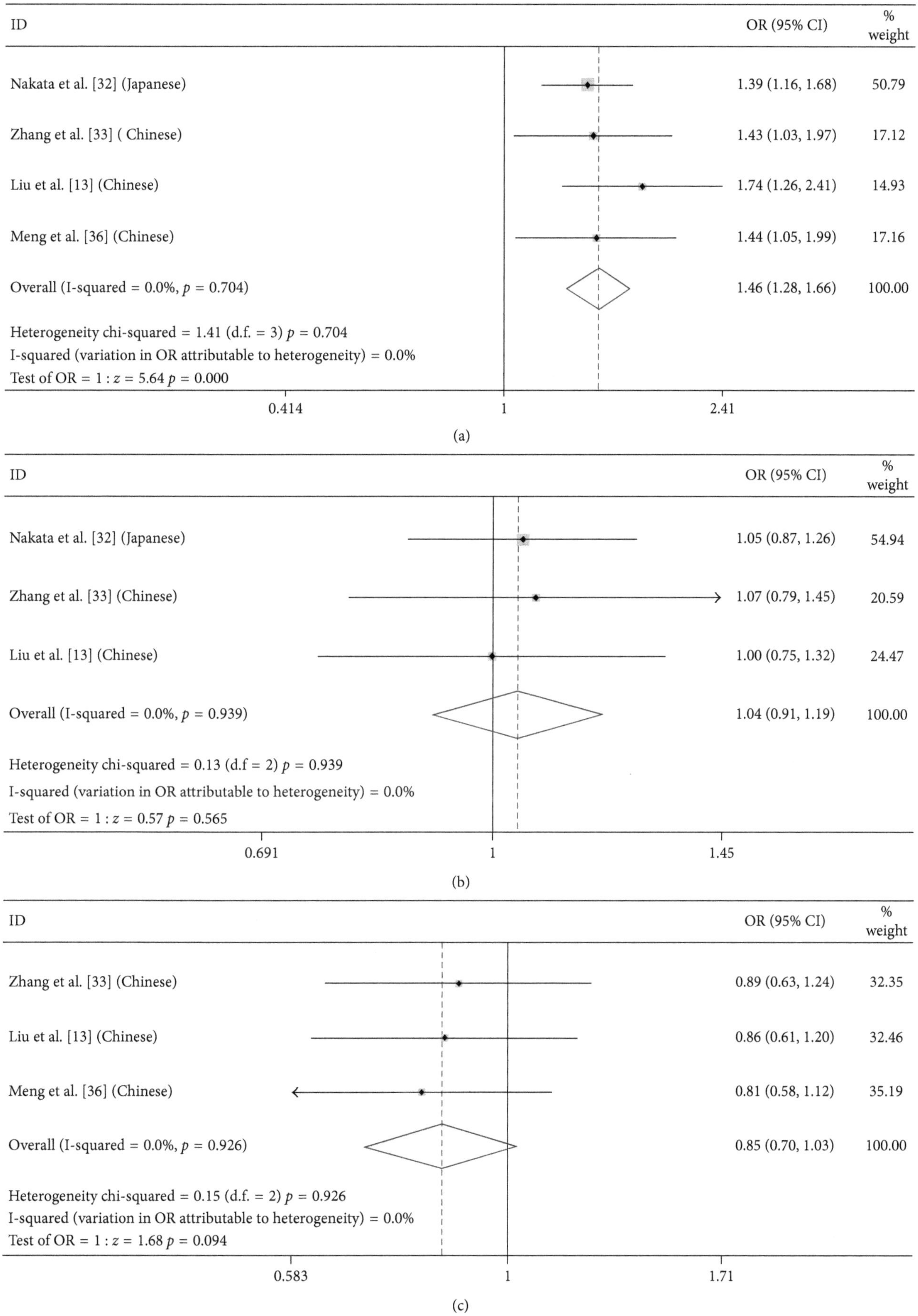

Figure 2: Continued.

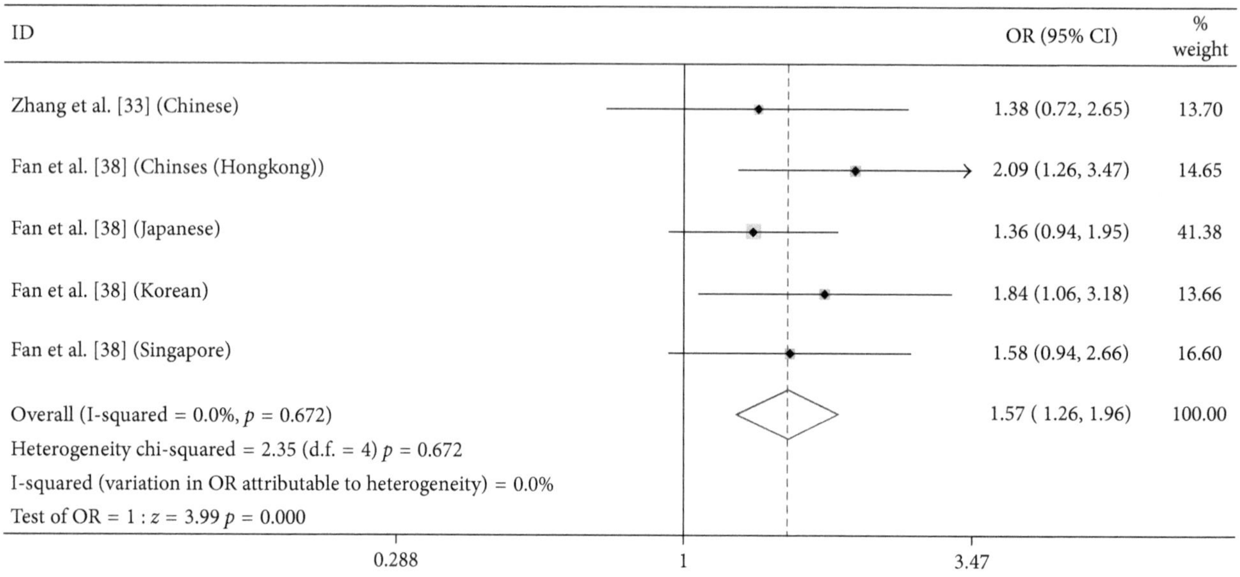

(d)

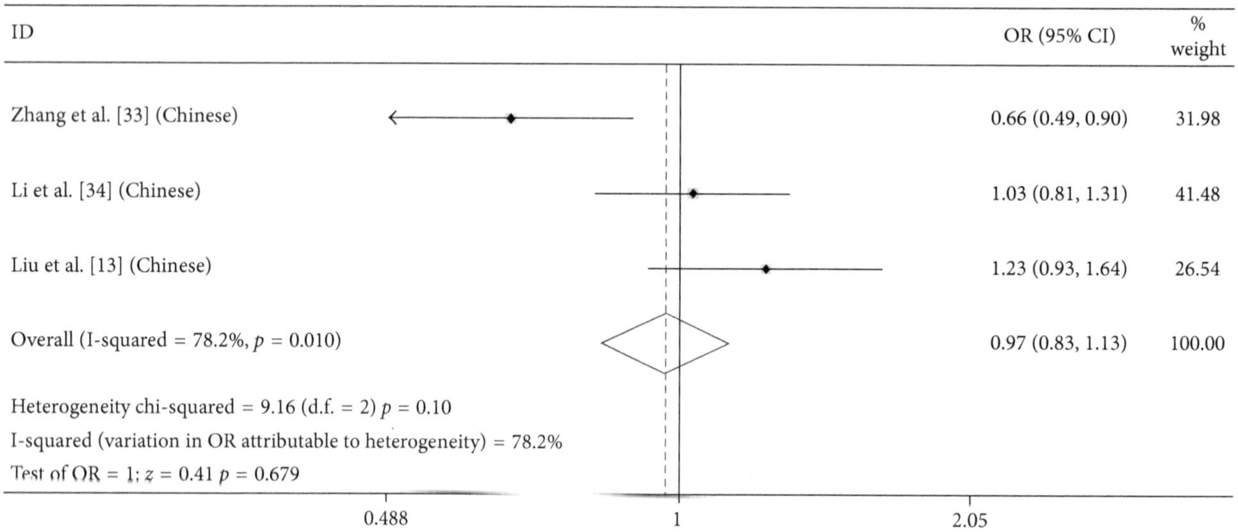

(e)

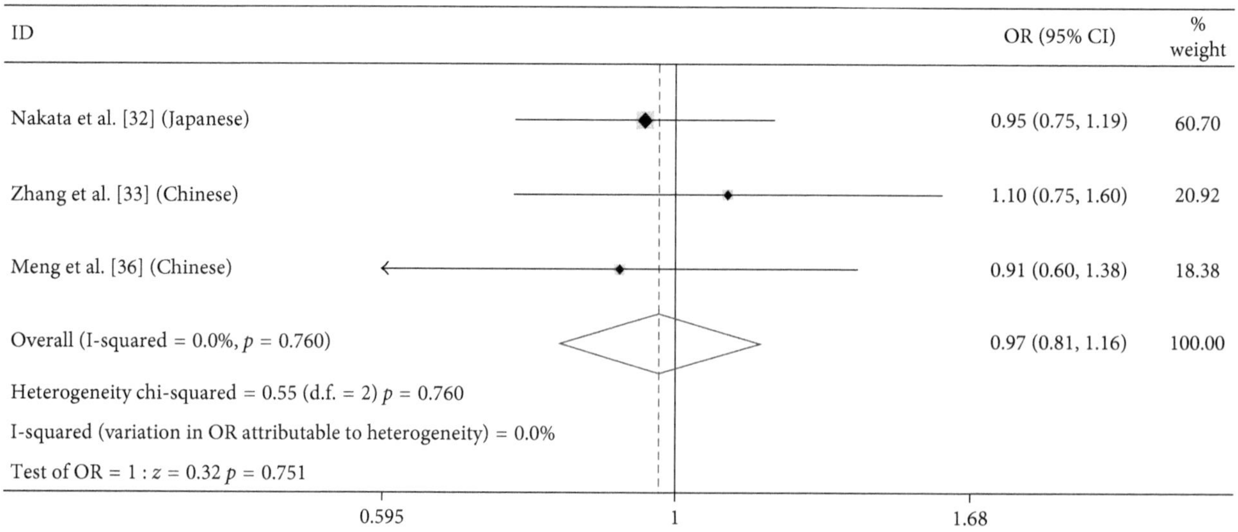

(f)

Figure 2: Continued.

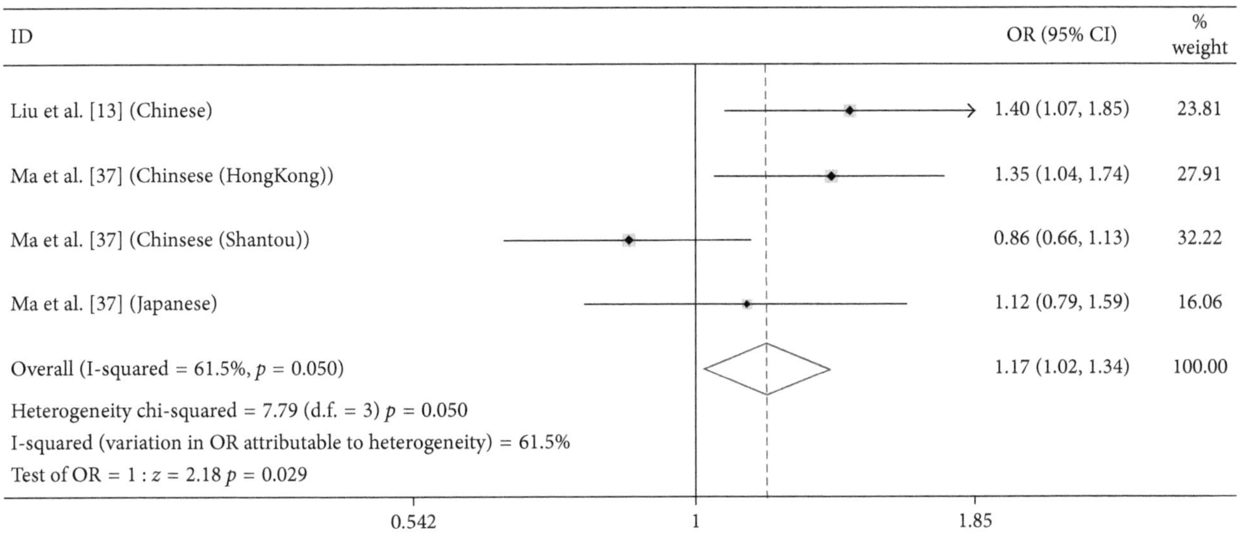

(g)

FIGURE 2: Forest plot of 7 SNPs in PCV in allelic model. The figure shows specific odds ratios (ORs) for study. The size of the box is proportional to the weight of the study. Horizontal lines represent 95% confidence intervals (CIs). A diamond is on behalf of the summary OR with its corresponding 95% CI. (a) CETP rs3764261 (T); (b) LIPC rs493258 (G); (c) LIPC rs10468017 (T); (d) CETP rs2303790 (G); (e) ABVA1 rs1883025 (T); (f) LPL rs12678919 (G); (g) ABCG1 rs57137919 (A).

TABLE 2: Meta-analysis of CETP/LIPC/LPL/ABCA1/ABCG1 polymorphisms in PCV.

Region	Gene	Polymorphism	Ethnicity	Associated versus reference allele	Number of cohorts	Sample size (case/control)	OR (95% CI)	Z score	P value	I^2 (%)	P value of Begg's test	P value of Egger's test
16q21	*CETP*	rs3764261	Asia	T versus G	4	1355/1493	1.46 (1.28–1.665)	5.64	0	0	0.308	0.415
			Chinese	T versus G	3	774/700	1.528 (1.268–1.841)	4.46	0	0	>0.999	0.071
9q31	*ABCA1*	rs1883025	Chinese	T versus C	3	781/775	0.968 (0.828–1.131)	0.41	0.679	78.2	>0.999	0.745
9q31	*LIPC*	rs493258	Asia	G versus A	3	1064/1272	1.041 (0.907–1.195)	0.57	0.565	0	>0.999	0.867
15q22	*LIPC*	rs10468017	Chinese	T versus C	3	774/700	0.849 (0.7–1.028)	1.68	0.094	0	>0.999	0.465
15q22	*LPL*	rs12678919	Asia	G versus A	3	1122/1218	0.972 (0.814–1.161)	0.32	0.751	0	>0.999	0.799
21q22	*ABCG1*	rs57137919	Asia	A versus G	4	860/1467	1.168 (1.016–1.343)	2.18	0.029	61.5	>0.999	0.808
16q21	CETP	rs2303790	Asia	G versus A	5	1312/5479	1.57 (1.258–1.96)	3.99	0	0	>0.999	0.527

Summary of the allelic associations of CETP/LIPC/LPL/ABCA1/ABCG1 polymorphisms in PCV. PCV: polypoidal choroidal vasculopathy; AMD: age-related macular degeneration; OR: odds ratio; CI: confidence intervals.

95% CI: 1.113–1.548, $P < 0.01$, $I^2 = 0\%$). Regarding the other 4 SNPs, LIPC rs10468017/rs493258, LPL rs12678919, and ABCA1 rs1883025, the pooled ORs were not statistically significant in PCV in the allelic ($P > 0.05$). As for ABCA1 rs1883025 (T allele; OR = 0.968, 95% CI: 0.828–1.131, $P = 0.679$, $I^2 = 78.2\%$), quality assessment and sensitivity analysis showed that the study of Zhang et al. was of higher risk of causing bias than the other cohorts [33]. Therefore, we excluded the study and also found that the pooled allelic OR was not significant (T allele; OR = 1.1, 95% CI: 0.926–1.335, $P = 0.257$, $I^2 = 0\%$).

3.4. Meta-Analysis of CETP/LIPC/LPL/ABCA1/ABCG1 Polymorphisms Compared between PCV and AMD. We identified 6 studies in which both PCV and AMD were assessed for associations with a total of 7 SNPs in 5 genes (i.e., CETP rs2303790/rs3764261, LIPC rs10468017/rs493258, LPL rs12678919, ABCA1 rs1883025, and ABCG1 rs57137919) (Table 3 and Figure 3). Only 1 SNP (ABCG1 rs57137919) showed significant difference between PCV and AMD (A allele; OR = 1.208, 95% CI: 1.035–1.411, $P = 0.017$, $I^2 = 0\%$) [35, 37]. The other 6 SNPs, namely, CETP rs2303790/rs3764261, LIPC rs10468017/rs493258, LPL rs12678919, and ABCA1 rs1883025,

Table 3: Meta-analysis of CETP/LIPC/LPL/ABCA1/ABCG1 polymorphisms compared between PCV and AMD.

Region	Gene	Polymorphism	Ethnicity	Associated versus reference allele	Number of cohorts	Sample size (PCV/AMD)	OR (95% CI)	Z score	P value	I^2 (%)	P value of Begg's test	P value of Egger's test
16q21	*CETP*	rs3764261	Chinese	T versus G	3	774/587	1.17 (0.971–1.409)	1.65	0.178	33.6	>0.999	0.572
9q31	*ABCA1*	rs1883025	Chinese	T versus C	3	781/775	1.025 (0.869–1.208)	0.29	0.77	0	>0.999	0.832
9q31	*LIPC*	rs493258	Chinese	G versus A	2	483/357	1.123 (0.897–1.407)	1.01	0.312	0	>0.999	—
15q22	*LIPC*	rs10468017	Chinese	T versus C	3	774/587	1.101 (0.892–1.359)	0.89	0.371	0	0.296	0.483
15q22	*LPL*	rs12678919	Asia	G versus A	2	541/387	1.163 (0.861–1.572)	0.98	0.325	0	>0.999	—
21q22	*ABCG1*	rs57137919	Asia	A versus G	4	860/816	1.208 (1.035–1.411)	2.39	0.017	0	0.734	0.156
16q21	CETP	rs2303790	Asia	G versus A	5	1312/1314	1.067 (0.825–1.378)	0.49	0.622	0	0.462	0.299

Summary of the genetic difference in CETP/LIPC/LPL/ABCA1/ABCG1 polymorphisms between PCV and AMD is shown. PCV: polypoidal choroidal vasculopathy; AMD: age-related macular degeneration; OR: odds ratio; CI: confidence interval.

were evaluated in 2 to 3 cohorts and showed no significant differences between PCV and AMD ($P > 0.05$). As for CETP rs3764261 (T allele; OR = 1.17, 95% CI: 0.971–1.409, $P = 0.178$, $I^2 = 33.6\%$), quality assessment and sensitivity analysis showed that the study of Liu et al. was of higher risk of causing bias than the other cohorts [35]. Therefore, we ruled out the cohort, and then the pooled allelic OR of the result was significant (T allele; OR = 1.301, 95% CI: 1.033–1.638, $P = 0.025$, $I^2 = 0\%$) [33, 36].

3.5. Publication Bias Analysis. In theory, due to the limited number of available studies, it is not suitable for publication bias analysis. But in order to make this meta-analysis more powerful and more creditable, we used funnel plots and Begg's/Egger's test to detect publication bias. Begg's test and Egger's test suggested an absence of publication bias in the all SNPs ($P > 0.05$) (Tables 2 and 3). The shape of the funnel plots did not reveal any evidence of obvious asymmetry (Figures S1 and S2).

4. Discussion

In the systematic review and meta-analysis, we have summarized the association profiles of genes in the HDLMP in PCV and assessed the genetic difference in the HDLMP between PCV and AMD for the first time (i.e., CETP, LIPC, LPL, ABCA1, and ABCG1). We found significant association between reported CETP rs2303790/rs3764261, ABCG1 rs57137919, and PCV. Also, we identified ABCG1 rs57137919 showing significant differences between PCV and AMD. In contrast, LIPC rs10468017/rs493258, LPL rs12678919, and ABCA1 rs1883025 were not statistically significant in PCV and reported SNPs in 4 genes in the HDLMP (i.e., CETP, LIPC, LPL, and ABCA1) showed no significant differences between PCV and AMD.

CETP can make oxidized lipids transfer from the outer segments of the photoreceptors or other membranes to HDL-like lipoprotein particles. The particles are internalized by RPE and excreted back into the circulation via ABCG1 transporters through Bruch's membrane [39]. ABCG1 was relevant to an increased macrophage apoptosis, which may be due to the accumulation of oxysterol in macrophages caused by decreased ABCG1-mediated cholesterol efflux [40]. ABCA1 was expressed in the retina and retinal pigment epithelium [41], and ABCA1 can form nascent HDL by mediating the efflux of cholesterol and phospholipids to lipid-poor apolipoproteins [42, 43]. Also, several studies have demonstrated ABCA1 was significantly related to the progression of drusen, but the association between large drusen and geographic atrophy/neovascular was not significant [44]. Besides, LIPC gene is a critical enzyme in HDL metabolism which has the function of encoding hepatic triglyceride lipase and catalyzing the hydrolysis of phospholipids, monoglycerides, diglycerides, triglycerides, and acylCoA thioesters [45, 46]. LPL gene encodes LPL which can play an important role in HDL metabolism. LPL can not only facilitate triglyceride hydrolysis but also serve as a ligand/bridging factor for receptor-mediated lipoprotein uptake [47]. Besides, lipoproteins derived from plasma have been proved to be the crucial upstream source of fatty acids within Bruch's membrane and supply an energy source to the retina [48–50] as well as perform significant roles in the transportation of vitamin C, vitamin E, lutein, and zeaxanthin for use by photoreceptors [51, 52]. Therefore, dysfunction of CETP, LIPC, LPL, ABCA1, and ABCG1 may cause accumulation of oxidized lipids in the retina, and the unreasonable products could induce inflammation and vascular anomaly, which play a crucial role in the development of PCV and AMD via lipid metabolism [53, 54].

In the studies (including 3 in Chinese [33, 35, 36] and 1 in Japanese [32]), we found that CETP rs3764261 was to be associated with PCV in Asian population with an odds ratio of 1.46 (95% CI: 1.28–1.665, $P = 0$, $I^2 = 0\%$) for the T allele. Apart from CETP rs3764261, we also found that CETP

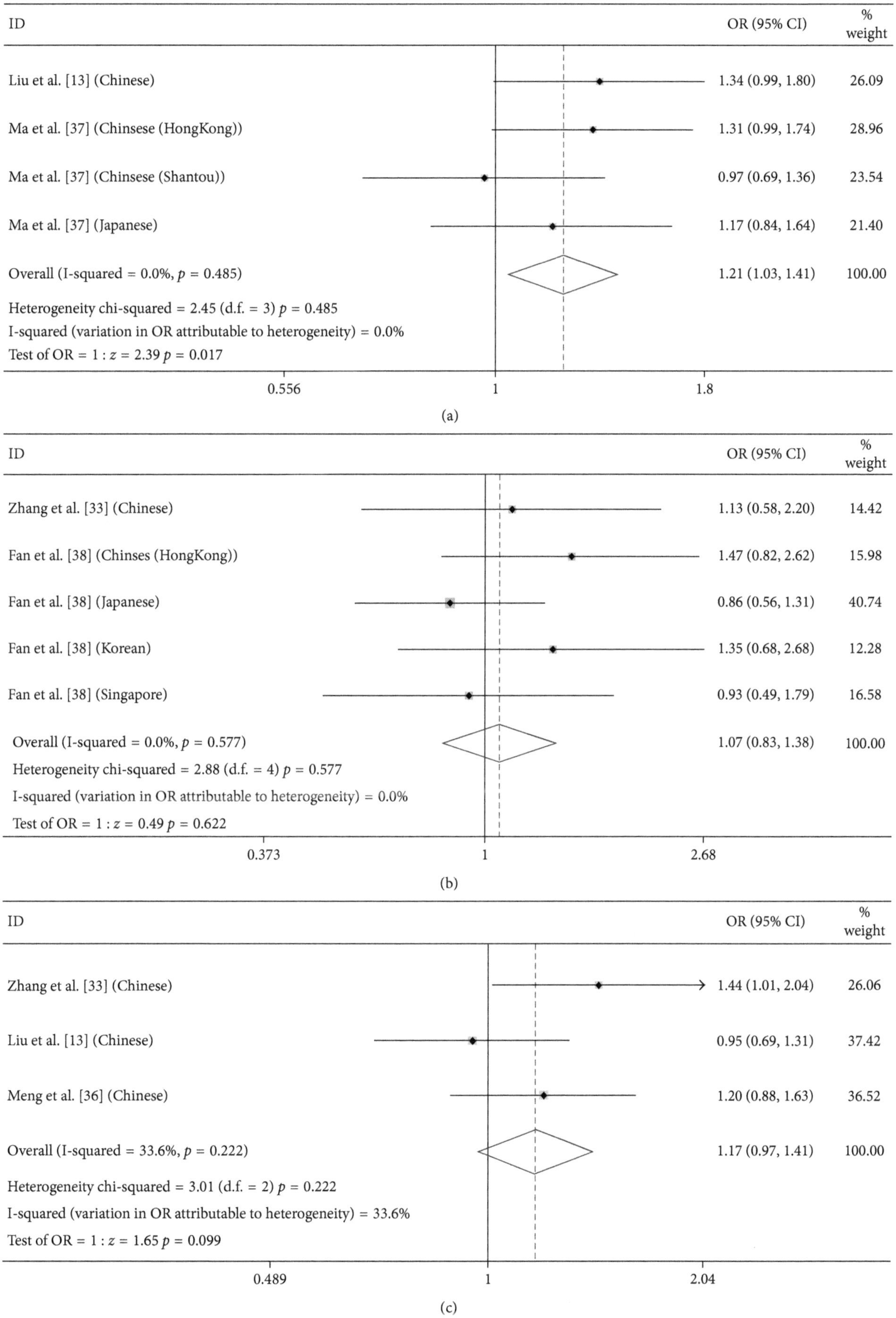

Figure 3: Continued.

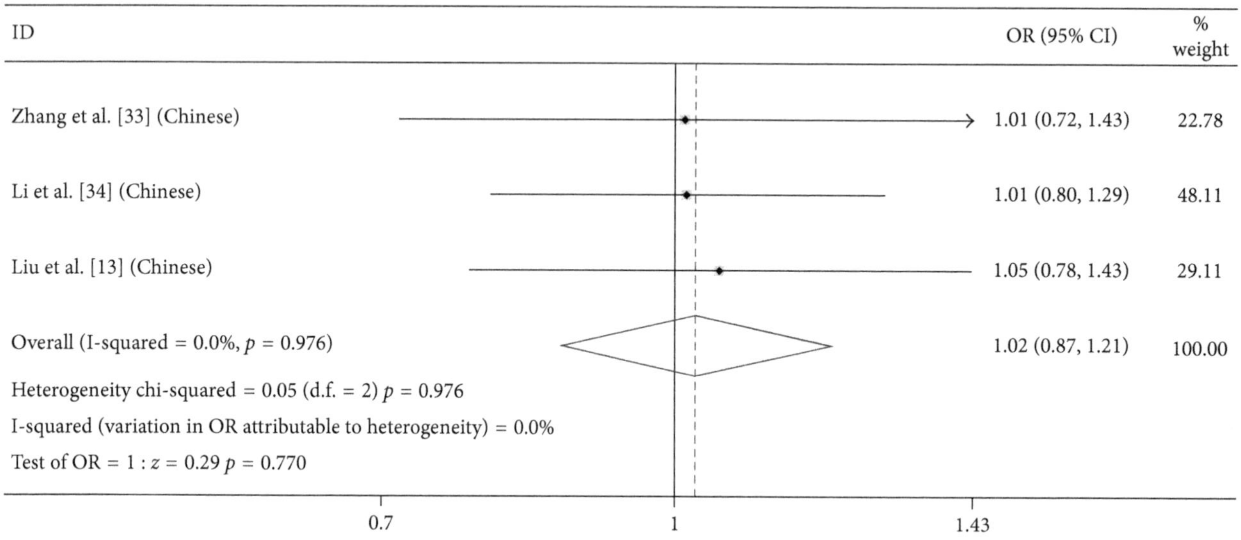

(d)

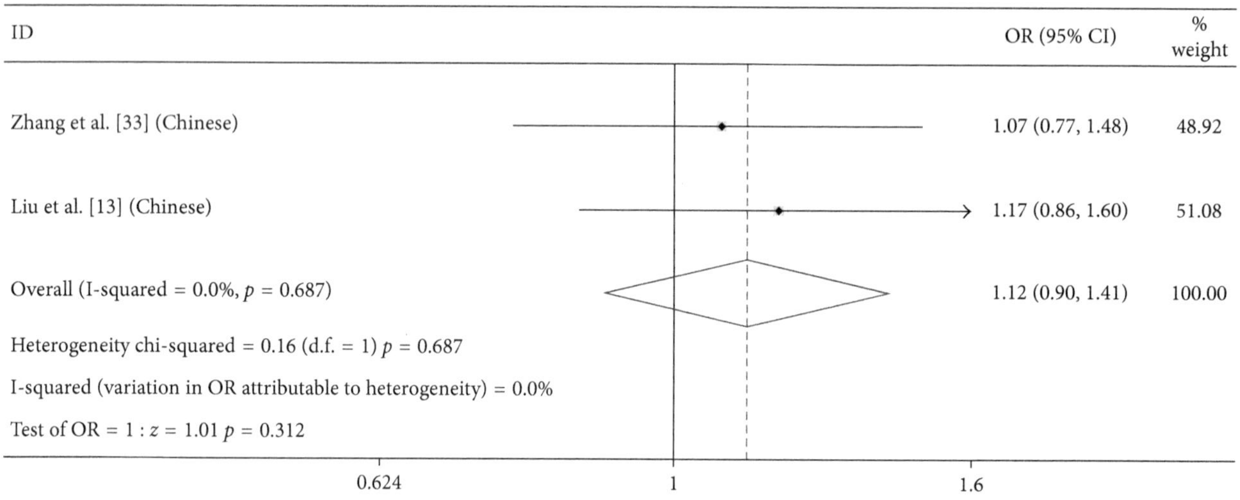

(e)

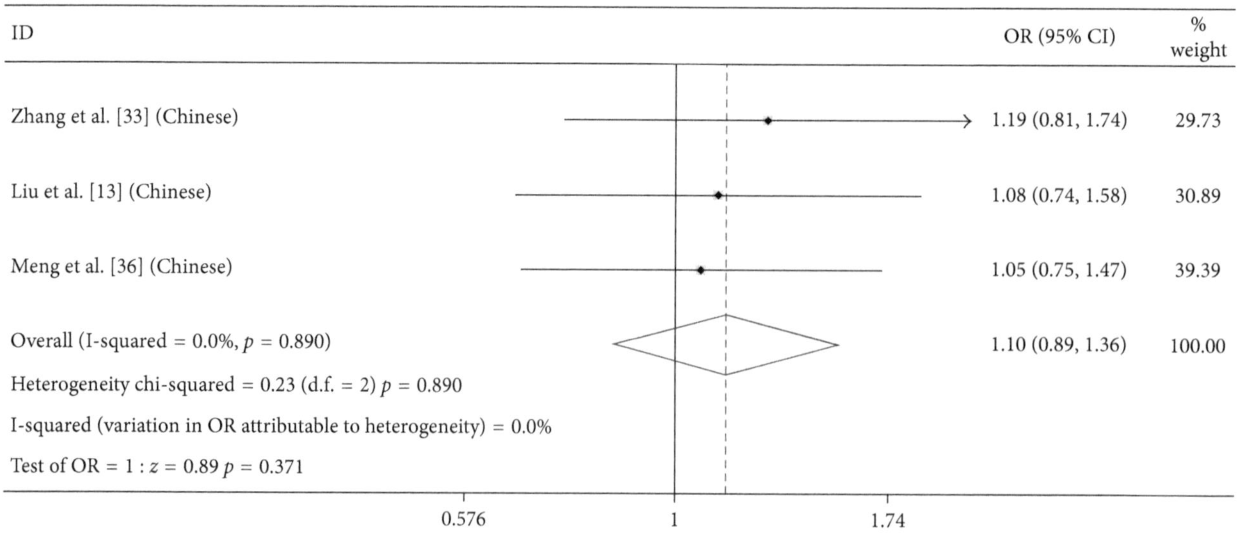

(f)

Figure 3: Continued.

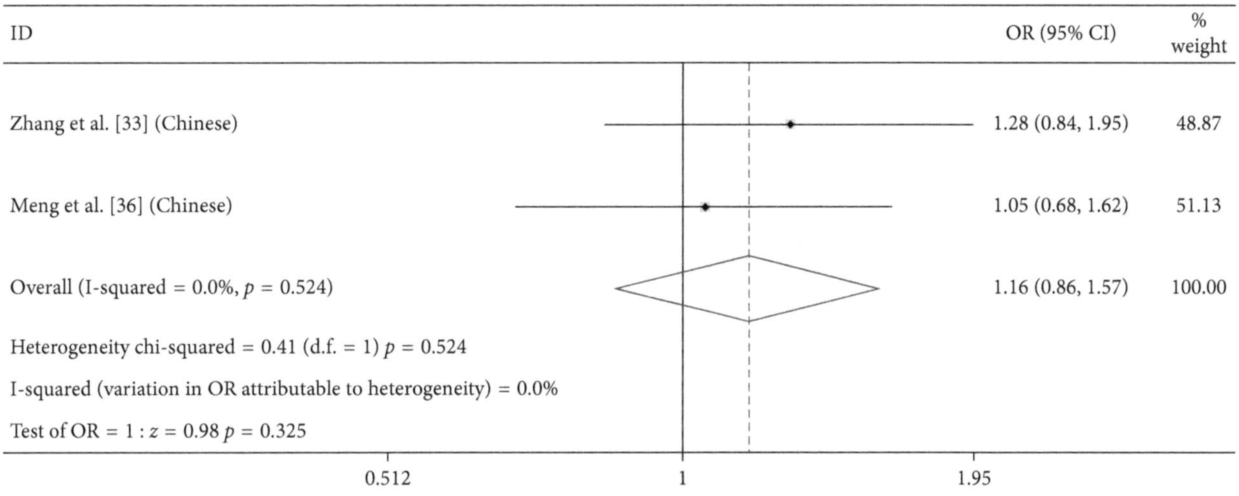

(g)

FIGURE 3: Forest plot of SNPs compared between PCV and AMD in allelic model. The figure shows specific odds ratios (ORs) for study. The size of the box is proportional to the weight of the study. Horizontal lines represent 95% confidence intervals (CIs). A diamond is on behalf of the summary OR with its corresponding 95% CI. (a) ABCG1 rs57137919 (A); (b) CETP rs2303790 (G); (c) CETP rs3764261 (T); (d) ABCA1 rs1883025 (T); (e) LIPC rs493258 (G); (f) LIPC rs10468017 (T); (g) LPL rs12678919 (G).

rs2303790 was associated with PCV in Asian population [33, 38] (G allele; OR = 1.57, 95% CI: 1.258–1.96, $P < 0.01$, $I^2 = 0$). Therefore, CETP rs3764261/rs2303790 provided an increased risk for PCV in Asian population. Through the analysis of the studies in which both PCV and AMD were assessed for associations with CETP, we found CETP rs2303790 showed no significant difference between PCV and AMD. However, as for CETP rs3764261, two studies dedicated that CETP rs3764261 was significantly associated with an increased risk for PCV, but no association was found with AMD(T allele; OR = 1.301, 95% CI: 1.033–1.638, $P = 0.025$, $I^2 = 0\%$) [33, 40], but one study showed that CETP rs3764261 is a susceptibility gene for PCV and AMD [35]. According to the article of GWAS and meta-analysis published by Cheng et al., the minor allele at CETP rs3764261 variant was proved to be a risk factor to the development of AMD in Asian population [55]. However, several recent studies indicated that CETP rs3764261 was related to a decreased risk of AMD in Chinese population and Lithuanian population [56, 57]. Therefore, it is still disputed whether CETP rs3764261 has different effects in PCV and AMD, and we need further studies in which both PCV and AMD are assessed for associations with CETP to confirm it.

From the studies [35, 37], for ABCG1 rs57137919, the frequency of the A allele in PCV patients was significantly higher than in controls (OR = 1.168, 95% CI: 1.016–1.343, $P = 0.029$, $I^2 = 61.5\%$). Interestingly, we found the result had the heterogeneity. Through quality assessment and sensitivity analysis, we found the heterogeneity derived from the data of Shantou population. After reading the related articles, we found all the studies used TaqMan genotyping assays, as well as the same inclusion criteria and exclusion criteria. Therefore, we speculate that there may be racial differences between Shantou population and others, but we need further studies to prove the view and find the causes of heterogeneity. Also, we found the significant difference between PCV and AMD in ABCG1 rs57137919 (G allele; OR = 1.208, 95% CI: 1.035–1.411, $P = 0.017$, $I^2 = 0\%$). In one of the studies, Li et al. studied the relevance of ABCG1 rs57137919 to PCV and AMD in Hong Kong, Shantou, and Osaka study subjects, and the results showed that the association of ABCG1 rs57137919 with PCV was significant in the Hong Kong cohort, but not in the Shantou or the Osaka cohort. Also, they indicated that the association of ABCG1 rs57137919 with AMD was not significant in the Hong Kong, Shantou, and Osaka cohorts. In another study, Liu et al. provided putative evidence of a role of ABCG1 rs57137919 in the vascularized complication of PCV. Because there were only two studies about relevance of ABCG1 rs57137919 to PCV and AMD, we need further replication studies in other ethnic populations to confirm the role of ABCG1 in PCV and AMD.

From our meta-analysis, we found other 4 SNPs (LIPC rs10468017/rs493258, LPL rs12678919, and ABCA1 rs1883025) were not statistically significant in PCV and AMD. Besides, the associations of eleven SNPs in CETP/LIPC/ABCA1/ABCG1 were reported in only 1 study [33, 36–38] (details can be seen in Table S5). Among these SNPs, Zhang et al. discovered that the rs5882 variant in CETP was significantly associated with PCV (G allele; $P = 0.73E-04$), but not with AMD (G allele; $P = 0.297$), and suggested the need to find biological clues about the different underlying HDL pathways by separating PCV from AMD so as to explore the pathogenesis of PCV and AMD [33].

Another recent study reported that LIPC rs1532085 conferred an increased risk for PCV (A allele; $P = 0.0094$), but not AMD (A allele; $P = 0.0938$). Also, this study found hyperlipidemia is a risk factor for PCV [36]. Recently, Li et al. have newly identified ABCG1 rs225396 to be associated with

PCV (T allele; $P = 0.026$) and AMD (T allele; $P = 0.048$) in Chinese and Japanese subjects, which pointed out ABCG1 as a new susceptibility gene for PCV and AMD [37]. In 2017, Qiao et al. reported that the strongest PCV-associated SNP, CETP rs183130 (T allele; $P = 3.07E - 07$), was in high LD with the currently studied SNP rs3764261 in Europeans, and similar association patterns were shown in AMD at CETP rs183130 (T allele; $P = 4.31E - 05$). Also, they found that the most significant association signals recognized in Europeans were at rs5817082, rs1864163, and rs17231506 in CETP, but only rs17232506 showed significant association with PCV and AMD [38]. However, all the results above were reported in only 1 study, and they were challenged by pretty small sample sizes, so we need more researches with independent cohorts to verify these association findings.

In conclusion, our systematic review and meta-analysis has provided an overview of the association profiles of genes in the HDLMP in PCV for the first time and assessed the genetic difference in the HDLMP between PCV and AMD. The results suggest that CETP (rs3764261/rs2303790) and ABCG1 (rs57137919) are the major susceptibility genes for PCV in the Asian population, and ABCG1 (rs57137919) has different effects in PCV and AMD in the Asian population. However, due to the small pooled sample size for PCV and AMD, further studies of these genes in larger samples are warranted to confirm the association of gene variations in the HDLMP with PCV in other populations such as Caucasian and Australian. Moreover, further studies should focus on the genotype-phenotype correlations and the relevance of genotype to therapy in PCV, which may provide us the clues about the pathogenesis of PCV.

Conflicts of Interest

The authors declare that there are no conflicts of interest regarding the publication of this paper.

References

[1] L. A. Yannuzzi, J. Sorenson, R. F. Spaide et al., "Idiopathic polypoidal choroidal vasculopathy (IPCV)," *Retina*, vol. 10, no. 1, pp. 1–8, 1990.

[2] C. S. Tan, W. K. Ngo, L. W. Lim et al., "A novel classification of the vascular patterns of polypoidal choroidal vasculopathy and its relation to clinical outcomes," *British Journal of Ophthalmology*, vol. 98, no. 11, pp. 1528–1533, 2014.

[3] S. Honda, W. Matsumiya, and A. Negi, "Polypoidal choroidal vasculopathy: clinical features and genetic predisposition," *Ophthalmologica*, vol. 231, no. 2, pp. 59–74, 2014.

[4] A. Laude, P. D. Cackett, E. N. Vithana et al., "Polypoidal choroidal vasculopathy and neovascular age-related macular degeneration: same or different disease?," *Progress in Retinal and Eye Research*, vol. 29, no. 1, pp. 19–29, 2010.

[5] L. A. Yannuzzi, D. W. Wong, B. S. Sforzolini et al., "Polypoidal choroidal vasculopathy and neovascularized age-related macular degeneration," *Archives of Ophthalmology*, vol. 117, no. 11, pp. 1503–1510, 1999.

[6] J. Z. Kuo, T. Y. Wong, and F. S. Ong, "Genetic risk, ethnic variations and pharmacogenetic biomarkers in age-related macular degeneration and polypoidal choroidal vasculopathy," *Expert Review of Ophthalmology*, vol. 8, no. 2, pp. 127–140, 2013.

[7] X. Y. Liang, T. Y. Lai, D. T. Liu et al., "Differentiation of exudative age-related macular degeneration and polypoidal choroidal vasculopathy in the ARMS2/HTRA1 locus," *Investigative Opthalmology and Visual Science*, vol. 53, no. 6, pp. 3175–3182, 2012.

[8] D. R. Goldman, K. B. Freund, C. A. McCannel et al., "Peripheral polypoidal choroidal vasculopathy as a cause of peripheral exudative hemorrhagic chorioretinopathy: a report of 10 eyes," *Retina*, vol. 33, no. 1, pp. 48–55, 2013.

[9] I. Mantel, A. Schalenbourg, and L. Zografos, "Peripheral exudative hemorrhagic chorioretinopathy: polypoidal choroidal vasculopathy and hemodynamic modifications," *American Journal of Ophthalmology*, vol. 153, no. 5, pp. 910–922, 2012.

[10] S. Honda, H. Imai, K. Yamashiro et al., "Comparative assessment of photodynamic therapy for typical age-related macular degeneration and polypoidal choroidal vasculopathy: a multicenter study in Hyogo prefecture, Japan," *Ophthalmologica*, vol. 223, no. 5, pp. 333–338, 2009.

[11] W. Matsumiya, S. Honda, S. Kusuhara et al., "Effectiveness of intravitreal ranibizumab in exudative age-related macular degeneration (AMD): comparison between typical neovascular AMD and polypoidal choroidal vasculopathy over a 1 year follow-up," *BMC Ophthalmology*, vol. 13, no. 1, p. 10, 2013.

[12] L. Huang, H. Zhang, C. Y. Cheng et al., "A missense variant in FGD6 confers increased risk of polypoidal choroidal vasculopathy," *Nature Genetics*, vol. 48, no. 6, pp. 640–647, 2016.

[13] K. Liu, T. Y. Lai, S. W. Chiang et al., "Gender specific association of a complement component 3 polymorphism with polypoidal choroidal vasculopathy," *Scientific Reports*, vol. 4, no. 1, p. 7018, 2014.

[14] K. Liu, L. J. Chen, P. O. Tam et al., "Associations of the C2-CFB-RDBP-SKIV2L locus with age-related macular degeneration and polypoidal choroidal vasculopathy," *Ophthalmology*, vol. 120, no. 4, pp. 837–843, 2013.

[15] N. Gotoh, S. Kuroiwa, T. Kikuchi et al., "Apolipoprotein E polymorphisms in Japanese patients with polypoidal choroidal vasculopathy and exudative age-related macular degeneration," *American Journal of Ophthalmology*, vol. 138, no. 4, pp. 567–573, 2004.

[16] N. Kondo, S. Honda, K. Ishibashi et al., "Elastin gene polymorphisms in neovascular age-related macular degeneration and polypoidal choroidal vasculopathy," *Investigative Opthalmology and Visual Science*, vol. 49, no. 3, pp. 1101–1105, 2008.

[17] F. G. Holz, G. Sheraidah, D. Pauleikhoff et al., "Analysis of lipid deposits extracted from human macular and peripheral Bruch's membrane," *Archives of Ophthalmology*, vol. 112, no. 3, pp. 402–406, 1994.

[18] R. Reynolds, B. Rosner, and J. M. Seddon, "Serum lipid biomarkers and hepatic lipase gene associations with age-related macular degeneration," *Ophthalmology*, vol. 117, no. 10, pp. 1989–1995, 2010.
[19] L. Hyman, A. P. Schachat, Q. He et al., "Hypertension, cardiovascular disease, and age-related macular degeneration. Age-related macular degeneration risk factors study group," *Archives of Ophthalmology*, vol. 118, no. 3, pp. 351–358, 2000.
[20] Y. Hirami, M. Mandai, M. Takahashi et al., "Association of clinical characteristics with disease subtypes, initial visual acuity, and visual prognosis in neovascular age-related macular degeneration," *Japanese Journal of Ophthalmology*, vol. 53, no. 4, pp. 396–407, 2009.
[21] I. Maruko, T. Iida, M. Saito et al., "Clinical characteristics of exudative age-related macular degeneration in Japanese patients," *American Journal of Ophthalmology*, vol. 144, no. 1, pp. 15–22, 2007.
[22] T. Mathis, L. Kodjikian, M. Mauget-Faysse et al., "Polypoidal choroidal vasculopathy occurring in the context of large colloid drusen," *Ophthalmic Surgery, Lasers and Imaging Retina*, vol. 47, no. 12, pp. 1154–1156, 2016.
[23] D. Iwama, A. Tsujikawa, M. Sasahara et al., "Polypoidal choroidal vasculopathy with drusen," *Japanese Journal of Ophthalmology*, vol. 52, no. 2, pp. 116–121, 2008.
[24] I. D. Ladas, A. A. Rouvas, M. M. Moschos et al., "Polypoidal choroidal vasculopathy and exudative age-related macular degeneration in Greek population," *Eye*, vol. 18, no. 5, pp. 455–459, 2004.
[25] L. Wang, M. E. Clark, D. K. Crossman et al., "Abundant lipid and protein components of drusen," *PLoS One*, vol. 5, no. 4, article e10329, 2010.
[26] R. Klein, T. Peto, A. Bird et al., "The epidemiology of age-related macular degeneration," *American Journal of Ophthalmology*, vol. 137, no. 3, pp. 486–495, 2004.
[27] U. Chakravarthy, T. Y. Wong, A. Fletcher et al., "Clinical risk factors for age-related macular degeneration: a systematic review and meta-analysis," *BMC Ophthalmology*, vol. 10, no. 1, p. 31, 2010.
[28] B. J. Cho, J. W. Heo, T. W. Kim et al., "Prevalence and risk factors of age-related macular degeneration in Korea: the Korea National Health and Nutrition Examination Survey 2010-2011," *Investigative Opthalmology and Visual Science*, vol. 55, no. 2, pp. 1101–1108, 2014.
[29] D. Yuan, D. Yuan, S. Yuan et al., "The age-related maculopathy susceptibility 2 polymorphism and polypoidal choroidal vasculopathy in Asian populations: a meta-analysis," *Ophthalmology*, vol. 120, no. 10, pp. 2051–2057, 2013.
[30] J. P. Higgins, S. G. Thompson, J. J. Deeks et al., "Measuring inconsistency in meta-analyses," *BMJ*, vol. 327, no. 7414, pp. 557–560, 2003.
[31] A. Thakkinstian, G. J. McKay, M. McEvoy et al., "Systematic review and meta-analysis of the association between complement component 3 and age-related macular degeneration: a HuGE review and meta-analysis," *American Journal of Epidemiology*, vol. 173, no. 12, pp. 1365–1379, 2011.
[32] I. Nakata, K. Yamashiro, T. Kawaguchi et al., "Association between the cholesteryl ester transfer protein gene and polypoidal choroidal vasculopathy," *Investigative Opthalmology and Visual Science*, vol. 54, no. 9, pp. 6068–6073, 2013.
[33] X. Zhang, M. Li, F. Wen et al., "Different impact of high-density lipoprotein-related genetic variants on polypoidal choroidal vasculopathy and neovascular age-related macular degeneration in a Chinese Han population," *Experimental Eye Research*, vol. 108, pp. 16–22, 2013.
[34] F. Li, Y. Li, M. Li et al., "ABCA1 rs1883025 polymorphism shows no association with neovascular age-related macular degeneration or polypoidal choroidal vasculopathy in a Northern Chinese population," *Ophthalmic Research*, vol. 51, no. 4, pp. 210–215, 2014.
[35] K. Liu, L. J. Chen, T. Y. Lai et al., "Genes in the high-density lipoprotein metabolic pathway in age-related macular degeneration and polypoidal choroidal vasculopathy," *Ophthalmology*, vol. 121, no. 4, pp. 911–916, 2014.
[36] Q. Meng, L. Huang, Y. Sun et al., "Effect of high-density lipoprotein metabolic pathway gene variations and risk factors on neovascular age-related macular degeneration and polypoidal choroidal vasculopathy in China," *PLoS One*, vol. 10, no. 12, article e143924, 2015.
[37] L. Ma, K. Liu, M. Tsujikawa et al., "Association of ABCG1 with neovascular age-related macular degeneration and polypoidal choroidal vasculopathy in Chinese and Japanese," *Investigative Opthalmology and Visual Science*, vol. 57, no. 13, pp. 5758–5763, 2016.
[38] Q. Fan, C. Cheung, L. J. Chen et al., "Shared genetic variants for polypoidal choroidal vasculopathy and typical neovascular age-related macular degeneration in East Asians," *Journal of Human Genetics*, vol. 62, no. 12, pp. 1049–1055, 2017.
[39] I. R. Rodriguez and I. M. Larrayoz, "Cholesterol oxidation in the retina: implications of 7KCh formation in chronic inflammation and age-related macular degeneration," *Journal of Lipid Research*, vol. 51, no. 10, pp. 2847–2862, 2010.
[40] F. Liu, W. Wang, Y. Xu et al., "ABCG1 rs57137919G>a polymorphism is functionally associated with varying gene expression and apoptosis of macrophages," *PLoS One*, vol. 9, no. 6, article e97044, 2014.
[41] K. G. Duncan, K. Hosseini, K. R. Bailey et al., "Expression of reverse cholesterol transport proteins ATP-binding cassette A1 (ABCA1) and scavenger receptor BI (SR-BI) in the retina and retinal pigment epithelium," *British Journal of Ophthalmology*, vol. 93, no. 8, pp. 1116–1120, 2009.
[42] G. Schmitz and T. Langmann, "Structure, function and regulation of the ABC1 gene product," *Current Opinion in Lipidology*, vol. 12, no. 2, pp. 129–140, 2001.
[43] S. Yokoyama, "ABCA1 and biogenesis of HDL," *Journal of Atherosclerosis and Thrombosis*, vol. 13, no. 1, pp. 1–15, 2006.
[44] Y. Yu, R. Reynolds, B. Rosner et al., "Prospective assessment of genetic effects on progression to different stages of age-related macular degeneration using multistate Markov models," *Investigative Opthalmology and Visual Science*, vol. 53, no. 3, pp. 1548–1556, 2012.
[45] B. M. Neale, J. Fagerness, R. Reynolds et al., "Genome-wide association study of advanced age-related macular degeneration identifies a role of the hepatic lipase gene (LIPC)," *Proceedings of the National Academy of Sciences*, vol. 107, no. 16, pp. 7395–7400, 2010.
[46] J. Lee, J. Zeng, G. Hughes et al., "Association of LIPC and advanced age-related macular degeneration," *Eye*, vol. 27, no. 2, pp. 265–270, 2013.
[47] W. Chen, D. Stambolian, A. O. Edwards et al., "Genetic variants near TIMP3 and high-density lipoprotein-associated loci influence susceptibility to age-related macular degeneration," *Proceedings of the National Academy of Sciences*, vol. 107, no. 16, pp. 7401–7406, 2010.
[48] I. A. Pikuleva and C. A. Curcio, "Cholesterol in the retina: the best is yet to come," *Progress in Retinal and Eye Research*, vol. 41, pp. 64–89, 2014.
[49] L. Bretillon, G. Thuret, S. Gregoire et al., "Lipid and fatty acid profile of the retina, retinal pigment epithelium/choroid, and

the lacrimal gland, and associations with adipose tissue fatty acids in human subjects," *Experimental Eye Research*, vol. 87, no. 6, pp. 521–528, 2008.

[50] L. Wang, C. M. Li, M. Rudolf et al., "Lipoprotein particles of intraocular origin in human Bruch membrane: an unusual lipid profile," *Investigative Opthalmology and Visual Science*, vol. 50, no. 2, pp. 870–877, 2009.

[51] E. Loane, J. M. Nolan, and S. Beatty, "The respective relationships between lipoprotein profile, macular pigment optical density, and serum concentrations of lutein and zeaxanthin," *Investigative Opthalmology and Visual Science*, vol. 51, no. 11, pp. 5897–5905, 2010.

[52] C. A. Curcio, M. Johnson, J. D. Huang et al., "Aging, age-related macular degeneration, and the response-to-retention of apolipoprotein B-containing lipoproteins," *Progress in Retinal and Eye Research*, vol. 28, no. 6, pp. 393–422, 2009.

[53] J. G. Hollyfield, V. L. Bonilha, M. E. Rayborn et al., "Oxidative damage-induced inflammation initiates age-related macular degeneration," *Nature Medicine*, vol. 14, no. 2, pp. 194–198, 2008.

[54] P. X. Shaw, L. Zhang, M. Zhang et al., "Complement factor H genotypes impact risk of age-related macular degeneration by interaction with oxidized phospholipids," *Proceedings of the National Academy of Sciences*, vol. 109, no. 34, pp. 13757–13762, 2012.

[55] C. Y. Cheng, K. Yamashiro, L. J. Chen et al., "New loci and coding variants confer risk for age-related macular degeneration in East Asians," *Nature Communications*, vol. 6, p. 6063, 2015.

[56] D. Wang, J. Zhou, X. Hou et al., "CETP gene may be associated with advanced age-related macular degeneration in the Chinese population," *Ophthalmic Genetics*, vol. 36, no. 4, pp. 303–308, 2015.

[57] R. Liutkeviciene, A. Vilkeviciute, G. Streleckiene et al., "Associations of cholesteryl ester transfer protein (CETP) gene variants with predisposition to age-related macular degeneration," *Gene*, vol. 636, pp. 30–35, 2017.

26

Vascular Endothelial Growth Factor, Basic Fibroblast Growth Factor, and Pigment Epithelium-Derived Factor Expression in the Neovascular Iris in Retinal Diseases

Heng Miao,[1] Xianru Hou,[1] De-Kuang Hwang,[2,3] and Yong Tao[4]

[1]*Department of Ophthalmology, People's Hospital, Peking University, Beijing, China*
[2]*Department of Ophthalmology, Taipei Veterans General Hospital, Taipei, Taiwan*
[3]*Department of Ophthalmology, School of Medicine, National Yang-Ming University, Taipei, Taiwan*
[4]*Department of Ophthalmology, Beijing Chaoyang Hospital, Capital Medical University, Beijing, China*

Correspondence should be addressed to De-Kuang Hwang; m95gbk@gmail.com and Yong Tao; drtaoyong@163.com

Academic Editor: Lisa Toto

Objective. To determine the expression of cytokines in the iris of patients with neovascular glaucoma (NVG). *Methods.* Patients with NVG associated with proliferative diabetic retinopathy (PDR, group 1) or central retinal vein occlusion (CRVO, group 2) who had undergone surgical treatment were enrolled. Patients with primary open-angle glaucoma requiring surgical treatment were included in the control group (group 3). All iris specimens were obtained during trabeculectomy, 7 days after intravitreal injections of ranibizumab. The messenger RNA (mRNA) and protein levels of three target cytokines—vascular endothelial growth factor (VEGF), basic fibroblast growth factor (bFGF), and pigment epithelium-derived factor (PEDF)—in the iris were analyzed and compared. *Results.* We included 39 eyes from 39 patients (12, 15, and 12 in groups 1, 2, and 3, resp.). The protein and mRNA levels of PEDF were higher in two NVG groups. The protein levels, but not mRNA level, of bFGF were higher in the two NVG groups. The protein and mRNA levels of VEGF were similar in the three groups. *Conclusions.* The protein level of bFGF increased in the irises of the NVG patients was not expressed by the iris itself, whereas PEDF may be expressed by the iris tissue in these patients.

1. Introduction

Neovascular glaucoma (NVG) is a type of glaucoma in which progressive optic nerve damage and intraocular pressure elevation are mainly caused by the mechanical blockage of the aqueous outflow of neovascularization from the iris and anterior chamber angle [1]. Compared with primary glaucoma, NVG is relatively difficult to treat, and its visual outcomes are poorer [2]. Various pro- and antiangiogenic factors and inflammatory cytokines participate in the formation of iris neovascularization, including vascular endothelial growth factor (VEGF), basic fibroblast growth factor (bFGF), and pigment epithelium-derived factor (PEDF) [3, 4].

Patients with intraocular ischemic or inflammatory conditions, such as diabetic retinopathy, retinal vein occlusion, and retinopathy of prematurity, commonly develop NVG [1, 5, 6]. In these patients, the pathogenesis of iris neovascularization may be ascribed to the anterior diffusion of cytokines that are expressed by hypoxic retinal tissues; hence, standard treatment options focus on the blockage of cytokines and the treatment of the ischemic retina, such as retinal photocoagulation and cryotherapy [3]. However, despite repeated treatments, iris neovascularization may continuously progress in clinical settings. After chronic intraocular inflammation and ischemia, the iris tissue may itself secrete various factors and cytokines to compensate for the imbalance.

In the present study, we measured the messenger RNA (mRNA) and protein levels of VEGF, bFGF, and PEDF in the iris tissue of patients who had NVG associated with retinal diseases and had undergone surgical treatment. By determining the difference between the mRNA and protein levels,

Table 1: Primers for quantitation of VEGF, bFGF, and PEDF.

Target	Primer's sequence (5′-3′) (forward and reverse) and length (bp)	Amplicon size (bp)
VEGF	(F) AGATCGAGTACATCTTCAAGCCATC (25) (R) CGTCATTGCAGCAGCCC (17)	66
bFGF	(F) CCGACGGCCGAGTTGAC (17) (R) TAACGGTTAGCACACACTCCTTTG (24)	112
PEDF	(F) CGACCAACGTGCTCCTGTCT (20) (R) GATGTCTGGGCTGCTGATCA (20)	131
GAPDH	(F) CATCCATGACAACTTTGGTATCGT (24) (R) CAGTCTTCTGGGTGGCAGTGA (21)	74

VEGF: vascular endothelial growth factor; bFGF: basic fibroblast growth factor; PEDF: pigment epithelium-derived factor; GAPDH: glyceraldehyde-3-phosphate dehydrogenase.

we examined whether these cytokines are expressed by the iris itself in these patients to gain an in-depth understanding of the pathogenesis of NVG.

2. Methods

2.1. Study Patients. This prospective case-control study was approved by the Institutional Review Board of Peking University People's Hospital and was conducted in adherence to the tenets of the Declaration of Helsinki. Patients with NVG secondary to proliferative diabetic retinopathy (PDR, group 1) and central retinal vein occlusion (CRVO, group 2) were enrolled in this study after receiving the explanation of and signing the informed consent form. In addition, patients with primary open-angle glaucoma (POAG, group 3) were selected and enrolled in the control group. Patients' age, sex, best-corrected visual acuity, and preoperative intraocular pressure were recorded. Patients with multiple mechanisms or etiologies for glaucoma were excluded from the study.

2.2. Sample Collection and Measurement. Approximately 7 days before surgery, 0.5 mg of ranibizumab was intravitreally injected in all operated NVG eyes [7]. All patients underwent standard trabeculectomy with mitomycin-C. During the operation, peripheral iridectomy was performed, and the iris tissue specimen was collected. The specimen was then divided into two parts and stored at −70°C for measurement [7].

The first part of the specimen of each patient was used for determining the mRNA level in triplicate. Total RNA was extracted using the spin or vacuum total RNA isolation system (Promega Corp., Madison, USA) and reverse transcribed using a complementary DNA (cDNA) synthesis kit (RevertAid First Strand cDNA Synthesis Kit, Fermentas, Burlington, ON, Canada) [8]. Real-time polymerase chain reaction (PCR) was conducted using the Thermo Scientific PikoReal real-time PCR system (Thermo Fisher Scientific Corp., USA) with SYBR green I (GoTaq qPCR Master Mix, Promega Corp.). The average threshold cycle (Ct) values of targeted molecules were calculated on the basis of three repeated measurements for each sample [8]. Because we used the solid iris tissue, instead of soluble liquids such as the aqueous humor, as the sample in this study and because the sizes of the excised tissues varied, we used the relative amount, instead of the absolute amount, after normalization. The mRNA levels of VEGF, bFGF, and PEDF were determined and compared after being normalized to the mRNA level of glyceraldehyde-3-phosphate dehydrogenase (GAPDH) by using the $2^{-\triangle\triangle Ct}$ method. Primer sequences used in the analysis are listed in Table 1 [7].

For protein analysis, all of the remaining iris tissue specimens in each group were mixed together and compared because the amount of the remaining tissue specimens was too low to be used for determining the protein level of each growth factor individually. Each sample was mixed with 500 μL of cell lysis buffer (P0013, Beyotime Biotech, Jiangsu, China) and homogenized using a glass homogenizer. After centrifugation, the supernatant was used for Western blot analysis. Before electrophoresis, the bicinchoninic acid protein assay (Beyotime Biotech, Jiangsu, China) was used and 20 μg of the protein was loaded onto each lane [9]. The concentration of each cytokine protein was measured using the Western blot technique. The primary antibodies VEGF (ab1316, 1:200 dilution, Abcam Inc., Cambridge, MA, USA), bFGF (ab181, 1:250 dilution, Abcam Inc.), and PEDF (bs-0731R, 1:100 dilution, Bioss Co., Beijing, China) were used for the analysis. Protein levels were quantified through densitometry and normalized to the GAPDH level (Gel-Pro analyzer 4.0, Media Cybernetics, USA) [10].

2.3. Statistical Analyses. The baseline characteristics of the patients in the three groups were compared using the one-way analysis of variance (ANOVA) and chi-square tests. The mRNA levels in each specimen and the pooled protein level of the 3 target cytokines (VEGF, bFGF, and PEDF) were calculated 3 times. The average results of mRNA levels are reported as the mean ± standard deviation. The chi-square test and the one-way ANOVA test with Bonferroni correction were used to compare categorical and continuous variables, respectively, between the disease and control groups. All statistical analyses were performed using the Statistical Package for Social Sciences (version 19.0) for Windows (SPSS Inc., Chicago, IL, USA). The two-sided significance level was set at 0.05.

Table 2: Summary of clinical findings (mean ± standard deviation).

Group	Total	POAG	NVG secondary to PDR	NVG secondary to CRVO	p value
Age	50.88 ± 10.76	54.38 ± 8.50	50.13 ± 8.97	48.13 ± 12.80	0.378*
Gender (male/female)	23/16	6/6	8/4	9/6	0.641**
BCVA (logMAR)	2.15 ± 1.18	1.27 ± 0.92	2.59 ± 1.33	2.59 ± 0.79	0.018*
IOP at the time of surgery (mmHg)	37.04 ± 13.25	33.38 ± 14.54	38.63 ± 14.67	39.13 ± 11.24	0.358*

We included 39 eyes from 39 patients (12 eyes from 12 patients with POAG, 12 eyes from 12 patients with NVG secondary to PDR, and 15 eyes from 15 patients with NVG secondary to CRVO). *One-way ANOVA; ** χ^2 test. NVG: neovascular glaucoma; POAG: primary open-angle glaucoma; PDR: proliferative diabetic retinopathy; CRVO: central retinal vein occlusion; BCVA: best-corrected visual acuity; IOP: intraocular pressure.

3. Results

At the end of enrollment, 39 eyes from 39 patients were included. Of the 39 eyes, 12, 15, and 12 were associated with PDR, CRVO, and POAG and accordingly included in the PDR, CRVO, and control groups, respectively. No significant difference in age, sex, or intraocular pressure was observed among the three groups. However, visual acuity was better in patients with POAG (Table 2).

The mean mRNA levels of VEGF and bFGF did not differ significantly among the three groups ($p = 0.436$ and 0.621, resp.). However, the mRNA level of PEDF was significantly higher in the PDR and CRVO groups than in the control group ($p = 0.005$ for PDR versus POAG groups and $p = 0.045$ for CRVO versus POAG groups). The difference in the mRNA level of PEDF was not significant between the PDR and CRVO groups ($p = 0.584$, Figure 1).

The results of the Western blot analysis indicated that the protein level of VEGF did not differ significantly among the three groups (all $p > 0.05$); however, the levels of bFGF and PEDF were significantly higher in both the PDR and CRVO groups than in the control group ($p = 0.045$ and 0.010 for bFGF, respectively; both $p < 0.001$ for PEDF). The protein levels of bFGF and PEDF did not significantly differ between the PDR and CRVO groups ($p = 0.738$ for bFGF; $p = 0.322$ for PEDF, Figure 2).

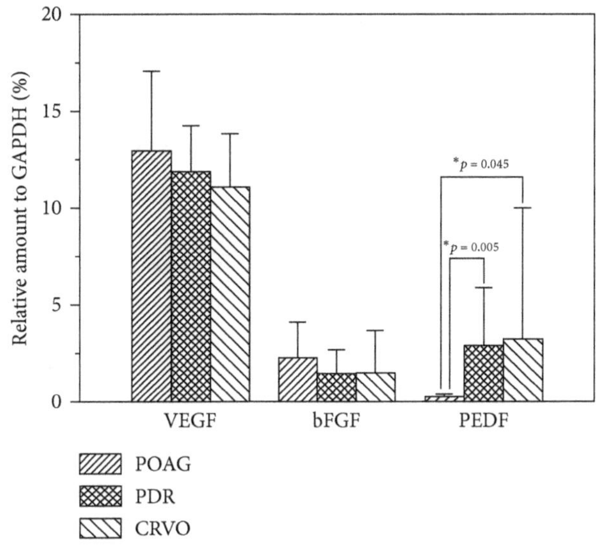

Figure 1: mRNA level normalized to that of glyceraldehyde-3-phosphate dehydrogenase (GAPDH) in the iris. The mRNA levels of vascular endothelial growth factor (VEGF) and basic fibroblast growth factor (bFGF) did not differ among patients with neovascular glaucoma (NVG) secondary to proliferative diabetic retinopathy (PDR), central retinal vein occlusion (CRVO), and primary open-angle glaucoma (POAG) ($p = 0.436$ and 0.621, resp.). The mRNA level of pigment epithelium-derived factor (PEDF) was significantly higher in patients with NVG secondary to PDR ($p = 0.005$) and CRVO ($p = 0.045$) than in patients with POAG. No significant difference was observed between the two NVG groups ($p = 0.584$).

4. Discussion

Neovascularization is a complex process in which many pro- and antiangiogenic factors are involved [7, 11]. Among these factors, VEGF, bFGF, and PEDF are the three most crucial cytokines that participate in retinal neovascular diseases [3, 4]. Studies have reported an increase in the VEGF level in the aqueous humor of patients with age-related macular degeneration, diabetic retinopathy, CRVO, and NVG [12, 13]. In patients with NVG, the intraocular VEGF level has been reported to be associated with not only intraocular pressure control but also surgical success rates and visual outcomes [13–16]. Therefore, intravitreal anti-VEGF therapy has now become one of the mainstream treatments for NVG. In patients with NVG, tangential traction and mechanical obstruction of the trabecular meshwork by the fibrovascular tissue on the iris play a crucial role in the pathogenesis of NVG [17, 18]. bFGF is one of the other crucial regulators suggested to be involved in tissue fibrosis. In addition, bFGF has been shown to enhance endothelial cell proliferation, migration, and angiogenic differentiation [4, 19].

PEDF can be identified and isolated from retinal pigment epithelial cells and has been found to have potent antiangiogenic activity. PEDF expression has been indicated to be negatively correlated with VEGF expression in the aqueous humor and blood of patients with PDR [20–24]. Elayappan et al. reported that PEDF can inhibit the migration and tube formation of retinal endothelial cells in the presence of VEGF [25]. However, Matsuyama demonstrated no change in the intraocular PEDF level after the administration of anti-VEGF agents intravitreally [26].

Theoretically, a tissue would express and secrete a protein through the translation and synthesis of mRNA. If the

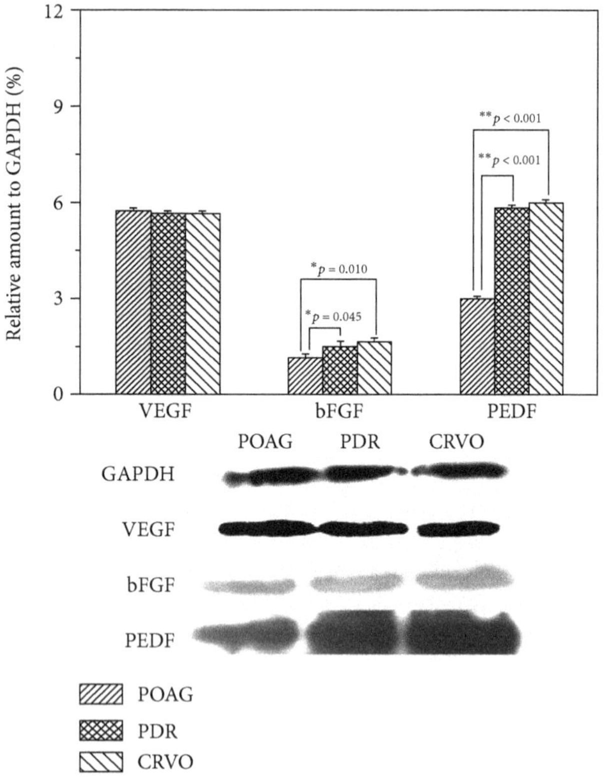

FIGURE 2: Protein levels of vascular endothelial growth factor (VEGF), basic fibroblast growth factor (bFGF), and pigment epithelium-derived factor (PEDF) measured through Western blotting and normalized to the glyceraldehyde-3-phosphate dehydrogenase (GAPDH) level. VEGF levels did not differ among patients with neovascular glaucoma (NVG) secondary to proliferative diabetic retinopathy (PDR), central retinal vein occlusion (CRVO), and primary open-angle glaucoma (POAG). bFGF and PEDF levels were significantly higher in patients with NVG secondary to PDR and CRVO than in patients with POAG (control) ($p = 0.045$ and 0.010 for bFGF, resp.; all $p < 0.001$ for PEDF). No significant difference was found between the two NVG groups ($p = 0.738$ and 0.322 for bFGF and PEDF, resp.).

protein and mRNA levels of the tissue have both been elevated, then that protein would be considered to be secreted by the tissue itself. However, if the protein level has increased but the mRNA level has remained low, as in a control, then the tissue might have been influenced by this protein, and the tissue itself might not have secreted the protein. In the present study, we analyzed the mRNA and protein levels of the three cytokines and found that the mRNA and protein levels of VEGF were not significantly higher in the irises of the patients with NVG associated with PDR or CRVO than in those of the patients with POAG. This finding can be attributed to the preoperative injection of ranibizumab, which may have markedly downregulated the intraocular protein level of VEGF. However, the equivalence of mRNA levels suggests that the neovascular iris tissue of the patients with PDR and CRVO did not itself express excessive VEGF.

The protein level of bFGF was significantly higher in the patients with NVG than in the patients with POAG. This finding signifies that the increase in the bFGF level may play a role in the neovascularization of the iris in patients with PDR or CRVO. However, the mRNA level of bFGF in the patients with PDR and CRVO was similar to that in the patients with POAG. Thus, it can be hypothesized that the increased bFGF protein was expressed by and diffused from the posterior segment of the eyeball, mainly the retina, and was not secreted by the iris stroma. This finding demonstrates that iris neovascularization in patients with NVG secondary to retinal diseases is primarily caused by proangiogenic cytokines triggered or expressed by only the ischemic retina.

In this study, we found that the mRNA and protein levels of PEDF were significantly higher in the irises of the patients with NVG than in those of the patients with POAG. This result suggests that not only the retina but also the iris itself may be able to produce this antiangiogenic factor. Although the protein level of VEGF was not high in our study due to anti-VEGF therapy, the overexpression of the mRNA and protein levels of PEDF in the iris tissue might have constituted a negatively controlled process that balanced the persistently increasing levels of angiogenic factors in the anterior chamber. The iris tissue did not overexpress proangiogenic factors, even in the patients with PDR. Because the iris has complex blood circulation and higher blood flow than that in the retina, the iris tissue may more easily receive sufficient oxygen or nutrition and seldom triggers the expression of these cytokines.

This study has several limitations. First, we compared the mRNA and protein levels of the patients with NVG with only those of the patients with POAG, rather than with those of the normal population. Although we excluded patients with any other possible mechanisms for glaucoma from the control group, no evidence supports that VEGF, bFGF, and PEDF expression in the irises of patients with POAG is similar to that in the irises of healthy people. Additional studies comparing representative controls should be conducted to confirm our results. Second, our study examined only three typical angiogenic factors, which may not represent all changes that occur in the irises of patients with NVG. More angiogenic and inflammatory cytokines should be analyzed to verify our conclusions. Third, in this study, we hypothesized that the protein levels in the iris tissue are highly correlated with those in the aqueous humor. However, future studies should examine the protein levels of various cytokines in aqueous or vitreous specimens and compare them with the levels in the iris tissue. Fourth, the small sample size of this study led to a relatively large standard deviation in our results. For example, the mRNA level of PEDF of the two patients in the CRVO group was considerably lower than the other data in the same group, which resulted in a low mean value with high standard deviation in the results. Although we found statistical significance, the clinical significance of this variation should be considered, and an additional study with a larger sample size should be conducted. Finally, after anti-VEGF treatment, the situation inside the eye may become more complex than that after the treatment of naïve eyes.

In summary, our study results reveal that the protein levels of bFGF and PEDF were elevated in the irises of the patients with retinal-disease-associated NVG. The protein levels of VEGF in these patients were similar to those in the patients with POAG 7 days after intravitreal injections of ranibizumab. Increased mRNA levels of PEDF were found in the irises of the patients with NVG. By contrast, the mRNA levels of bFGF were not increased in the irises of the patients with NVG. Our results suggest that the iris tissue itself may secrete PEDF but not bFGF in these diseases. The treatment of these patients should focus on the origin of proangiogenic cytokine expression rather than the neovascular iris.

Additional Points

Summary Statement. Retinal-disease-related neovascular glaucoma is a vision-threatening condition. The authors measured the messenger RNA (mRNA) and protein levels of cytokines and found that the basic fibroblast growth factor and pigment epithelium-derived factor (PEDF) were mainly expressed in other tissues rather than the iris. On the other hand, the iris might express PEDF because its mRNA level in the iris was high.

Conflicts of Interest

All authors declare that they have no conflicts of interests.

Authors' Contributions

Yong Tao and De-Kuang Hwang participated in the study design. Heng Miao and Xianru Hou performed the literature search. Yong Tao and De-Kuang Hwang helped in the data interpretation. Heng Miao, Xianru Hou, and De-Kuang Hwang wrote the paper. Heng Miao and Xianru Hou contributed equally to this study.

Acknowledgments

This work was supported by the National High Technology Research and Development Program of China (no. 2015AA020949), the Beijing Nova Program (Z151110000030000), the Fok Ying Tong Education Foundation (no. 141038), and Peking University People's Hospital Research and Development Funds (no. RDB2009-16).

References

[1] S. Gartner and P. Henkind, "Neovascularization of the iris (rubeosis iridis)," *Survey of Ophthalmology*, vol. 22, no. 5, pp. 291–312, 1978.

[2] L. C. Olmos and R. K. Lee, "Medical and surgical treatment of neovascular glaucoma," *International Ophthalmology Clinics*, vol. 51, no. 3, pp. 27–36, 2011.

[3] G. B. Rodrigues, R. Y. Abe, C. Zangalli et al., "Neovascular glaucoma: a review," *International Journal of Retina and Vitreous*, vol. 2, no. 1, p. 26, 2016.

[4] S. Watanabe, N. Morisaki, M. Tezuka et al., "Cultured retinal pericytes stimulate in vitro angiogenesis of endothelial cells through secretion of a fibroblast growth factor-like molecule," *Atherosclerosis*, vol. 130, no. 1-2, pp. 101–107, 1997.

[5] G. C. Brown, L. E. Magargal, A. Schachat, and H. Shah, "Neovascular glaucoma. Etiologic considerations," *Ophthalmology*, vol. 91, no. 4, pp. 315–320, 1984.

[6] G. Spaulding, "Rubeosis iridis in retinoblastoma and pseudoglioma," *Transactions of the American Ophthalmological Society*, vol. 76, pp. 584–609, 1978.

[7] X. R. Hou, H. Miao, Y. Tao, X. X. Li, and I. Y. Wong, "Expression of cytokines on the iris of patients with neovascular glaucoma," *Acta Ophthalmologica*, vol. 93, no. 2, pp. e100–e104, 2015.

[8] T. Schagat, L. Kiak, and M. Mandrekar, "RNA purification kit: comparison, yield, quality, and real-time, RT-PCR performance," *Promega Notes*, vol. 99, pp. 12–15, 2008.

[9] Y. Wei, D. Weng, F. Li et al., "Involvement of JNK regulation in oxidative stress-mediated murine liver injury by microcystin-LR," *Apoptosis*, vol. 13, no. 8, pp. 1031–1042, 2008.

[10] T. Ozaki, T. Yamashita, and S. Ishiguro, "Ca^{2+}-induced release of mitochondrial m-calpain from outer membrane with binding of calpain small subunit and Grp75," *Archives of Biochemistry and Biophysics*, vol. 507, no. 2, pp. 254–261, 2011.

[11] F. M. Damico, "Angiogenesis and retinal diseases," *Arquivos Brasileiros de Oftalmologia*, vol. 70, no. 3, pp. 547–553, 2007.

[12] T. H. Lim, S. H. Bae, Y. J. Cho, J. H. Lee, H. K. Kim, and Y. H. Sohn, "Concentration of vascular endothelial growth factor after intracameral bevacizumab injection in eyes with neovascular glaucoma," *Korean Journal of Ophthalmology*, vol. 23, no. 3, pp. 188–192, 2009.

[13] Y. G. Kim, S. Hong, C. S. Lee et al., "Level of vascular endothelial growth factor in aqueous humor and surgical results of Ahmed glaucoma valve implantation in patients with neovascular glaucoma," *Journal of Glaucoma*, vol. 18, no. 6, pp. 443–447, 2009.

[14] Y. Sasamoto, Y. Oshima, A. Miki et al., "Clinical outcomes and changes in aqueous vascular endothelial growth factor levels after intravitreal bevacizumab for iris neovascularization and neovascular glaucoma: a retrospective two-dose comparative study," *Journal of Ocular Pharmacology and Therapeutics*, vol. 28, no. 1, pp. 41–48, 2012.

[15] M. Tolentino, "Systemic and ocular safety of intravitreal anti-VEGF therapies for ocular neovascular disease," *Survey of Ophthalmology*, vol. 56, no. 2, pp. 95–113, 2011.

[16] V. Gupta, R. Jha, A. Rao, G. Kong, and R. Sihota, "The effect of different doses of intracameral bevacizumab on surgical outcomes of trabeculectomy for neovascular glaucoma," *European Journal of Ophthalmology*, vol. 19, no. 3, pp. 435–441, 2009.

[17] T. Kubota, A. Tawara, Y. Hata, A. Khalil, and H. Inomata, "Neovascular tissue in the intertrabecular spaces in eyes with neovascular glaucoma," *British Journal of Ophthalmology*, vol. 80, no. 8, pp. 750–754, 1996.

[18] J. Nadal, E. Carreras, B. Kudsieh, and M. I. Canut, "Neovascular glaucoma treatment with extraction of anterior chamber fibrovascular tissue," *JAMA Ophthalmology*, vol. 131, no. 8, pp. 1083–1085, 2013.

[19] A. Bikfalvi, S. Klein, G. Pintucci, and D. B. Rifkin, "Biological roles of fibroblast growth factor-2," *Endocrine Reviews*, vol. 18, no. 1, pp. 26–45, 1997.

[20] J. Tombran-Tink and L. V. Johnson, "Neuronal differentiation of retinoblastoma cells induced by medium conditioned by human RPE cells," *Investigative Ophthalmology & Visual Science*, vol. 30, no. 8, pp. 1700–1707, 1989.

[21] D. W. Dawson, O. V. Volpert, P. Gillis et al., "Pigment epithelium-derived factor: a potent inhibitor of angiogenesis," *Science*, vol. 285, no. 5425, pp. 245–248, 1999.

[22] K. Matsuyama, N. Ogata, M. Matsuoka et al., "Relationship between pigment epithelium-derived factor (PEDF) and renal function in patients with diabetic retinopathy," *Molecular Vision*, vol. 14, pp. 992–996, 2008.

[23] N. Mohan, F. Monickaraj, M. Balasubramanyam, M. Rema, and V. Mohan, "Imbalanced levels of angiogenic and angiostatic factors in vitreous, plasma and postmortem retinal tissue of patients with proliferative diabetic retinopathy," *Journal of Diabetes and its Complications*, vol. 26, no. 5, pp. 435–441, 2012.

[24] P. Murugeswari, D. Shukla, A. Rajendran, R. Kim, P. Namperumalsamy, and V. Muthukkaruppan, "Proinflammatory cytokines and angiogenic and anti-angiogenic factors in vitreous of patients with proliferative diabetic retinopathy and Eales' disease," *Retina*, vol. 28, no. 6, pp. 817–824, 2008.

[25] B. Elayappan, H. Ravinarayannan, S. P. B. S. Pasha, K. Lee, and S. Gurunathan, "PEDF inhibits VEGF- and EPO- induced angiogenesis in retinal endothelial cells through interruption of PI_3K/Akt phosphorylation," *Angiogenesis*, vol. 12, no. 4, pp. 313–324, 2009.

[26] K. Matsuyama, N. Ogata, N. Jo, C. Shima, M. Matsuoka, and M. Matsumura, "Levels of vascular endothelial growth factor and pigment epithelium-derived factor in eyes before and after intravitreal injection of bevacizumab," *Japanese Journal of Ophthalmology*, vol. 53, no. 3, pp. 243–248, 2009.

27

The Evolution of Central Retinal and Choroidal Thickness in Acute Anterior Uveitic Patients with Spondyloarthropathy

Zsuzsanna Szepessy,[1] Árpád Barsi,[2] Kinga Kránitz,[1] and Zoltán Zsolt Nagy[1]

[1]*Department of Ophthalmology, Semmelweis University, Budapest, Hungary*
[2]*Department of Photogrammetry and Geoinformatics, Budapest University of Technology and Economics, Budapest, Hungary*

Correspondence should be addressed to Zsuzsanna Szepessy; szepzsu@yahoo.com

Academic Editor: Alessandro Lambiase

Purpose. To describe and correlate the degree of anterior segment inflammation with central retinal and choroidal thickness throughout the treatment period (in the course of follow-up) in the eyes affected with acute anterior uveitis in the patients with seronegative spondyloarthropathy (subgroup: ankylosing spondylitis). *Methods.* Thirty eyes of 30 consecutive Caucasian patients with HLA-B27-associated acute anterior uveitis were included in this study. The flare, AC cell number, and central retinal/choroidal thickness were determined at each visit by optical coherence tomography and laser flare photometry. Treatment consisted of topical corticosteroids. Statistical analysis was performed by MathWorks Matlab software. *Results.* In the follow-up period, central retinal thickness was increased in the first 9-10 days and then decreased until stabilization (after 5-6 weeks). The flare and AC cell number decreased rapidly at the beginning of the treatment, in the first 10 days, and thereafter, slower decrease could be observed until complete resolution of inflammation. Statistically significant, positive correlation was found between initial laser flare value and maximal central retinal thickness ($r = 0.881$, $p < 0.001$). Positive correlation between flare and retinal thickening was observable throughout the treatment period. Central choroidal thickness was decreased also significantly during the follow-up ($p < 0.001$). *Conclusions.* The retina and choroid may play a biomarker function in the anterior segment inflammation of the eye in the patients with seronegative spondyloarthropathy.

1. Introduction

Spondyloarthropathy (SpA) is a group of chronic inflammatory rheumatic diseases, which are characterized by common clinical symptoms and genetic similarities [1]. Spondyloarthropathy is genetically linked (90% of cases), and the strongest contributing factor is the HLA B27 antigen [1, 2]. Ocular inflammation is a common extra-articular manifestation of seronegative spondyloarthropathy. Anterior uveitis is one of the most important features with a prevalence of 25–30% in the SpA patients [1, 2]. Five major subtypes of SpA are recognized on the basis of recently proposed classification criteria (European Spondyloarthropathy Study Group). In this study, one of the most common subtypes of SpA ankylosing spondylitis (AS) was studied intentionally.

Acute inflammatory process in the anterior segment, as opposed to chronic anterior uveitis, is rarely associated with significant macular edema, but subclinical retinal thickening has already been described [3, 4]. Our earlier results showed also close linear correlation between central foveal thickness and anterior segment inflammation (laser flare photometry values) at the beginning of the first anterior uveitic attack in the patients with HLA-B27-related spondyloarthropathy [3].

In recent years, some studies have used EDI-OCT to evaluate choroidal changes in ocular inflammatory disorders [5, 6]. Some authors have reported that the patients with active Vogt–Koyanagi–Harada disease [5] and Behçet disease [6] exhibit a markedly thickened choroid. Currently, there are a limited number of reports on choroidal thickness change in anterior uveitis [7].

The aim of this study was to describe the evolution of retinal and choroidal thickness in eyes affected with acute anterior uveitis in the course of follow-up in the patients with seronegative spondyloarthropathy. Our goal was to evaluate the correlation between flare and retinal/choroidal thickening throughout the treatment period.

2. Materials and Methods

This prospective study was performed at the Department of Ophthalmology of the Semmelweis University (Budapest, Hungary) on 30 eyes of 30 consecutive Caucasian patients (24 males and 6 females; age: 27–50 years; mean age: 35 years) with acute anterior uveitis for the first time.

Before their first uveitic attack, rheumatic diseases, seronegative spondyloarthropathy (subtype: ankylosing spondylitis), have been diagnosed by rheumatologist. All patients were HLA-B27 positive. The patients with a history of psoriatic arthritis (PsA), reactive arthritis (ReA), arthritis associated with inflammatory bowel disease (AIBD), other systemic diseases, intermediate uveitis, posterior uveitis, intraocular surgery, macular disease (e.g., epiretinal fibrosis and diabetic maculopathy), and amblyopic eyes were excluded from the study. Ankylosing Spondylitis Disease Activity Score (ASDAS) of the patients in this study was less than 2.0 to define "moderate disease activity." All of them were treated with systemic nonsteroidal anti-inflammatory drugs by rheumatologist.

All participants were treated in accordance with the tenets of the Declaration of Helsinki. Written informed consent was obtained from all participants in this study.

All patients underwent a comprehensive eye examination, including best corrected visual acuity (BCVA), measurement of the intraocular pressure, and slit-lamp and indirect fundus examination after pupil dilation. The axial length (AL) of the eyes was measured using optical biometry (Lenstar LS 900 Haag-Streit AG, Switzerland).

OCT examinations were performed on each eye using EDI-OCT (Optovue Inc., Fremont, CA, USA) and swept-source optical coherence tomograph (DRI OCT Triton, Topcon Co., Tokyo, Japan) by the same operator through dilated pupils at least 5 mm in diameter. The retinal and choroidal thickness measurements for the central ETDRS region of the macula were recorded at each visit throughout the treatment period (Figure 1).

Quantitative measurements of anterior segment aqueous flare and inflammatory cells were conducted using a laser flare meter (Kowa FC-600). Flare values and cell counts were measured at 30 minutes after pupillary dilation. The same examiner has obtained five measurements from each eye, and the results were averaged after excluding all measurements with artefacts.

SUN (Standardization of Uveitis Nomenclature) Working Group standardized the grading of anterior segment cells and flare. For anterior segment cells, in a field size of 1 × 1 mm slit beam, the following grades were described: 0 (<1 cell), 0.5+ (1–5 cells), 1+ (6–15 cells), 2+ (16–25 cells), 3+ (26–50 cells), and 4+ (>50 cells). The number of the anterior segment cells was also determined, counted using SUN criteria.

All uveitic eyes were initially managed with topical corticosteroid drops (prednisolone acetate 1%) every 1–6 hours depending on severity and cyclopentolate (5 mg/ml) three times a day. Steroid was withdrawn slowly, and corticosteroid drops were continued until the cellular reaction is absent. Cycloplegics were discontinued when the cellular reaction is subsiding. The patients were followed daily until manifest response to local treatment was observed (defined as a decrease of anterior segment cells on slit-lamp examination or a decrease of more than 20% from the baseline in laser flare photometry) and weekly thereafter until complete resolution of inflammatory activity.

Statistical analysis was performed by MathWorks Matlab 2012b software and its Statistics Toolbox. A p value of less than 0.05 was considered as statistically significant.

3. Results

The clinical signs data at the beginning of the first inflammatory episode (best corrected visual acuity (BCVA), flare, anterior segment cells (AC), intraocular pressure, central retinal thickness, and central choroidal thickness) are shown in Table 1.

As expected, flare and anterior segment cell number are significantly lower between initial flare/AC cell number and final flare/AC cell number ($p < 0.001$).

Figure 2 presents the evolution of the mean laser flare value in the course of follow-up. AC cell number in the anterior uveitic eyes is significantly decreased during the treatment period ($p < 0.001$), as shown in Figure 3. The mean initial laser flare value is reduced by 50% after 12 days. Flare and AC cell number are decreased rapidly at the beginning of the treatment, in the first 10 days, and thereafter decreased slowly until complete resolution of inflammation.

The central retinal thickness was significantly decreased ($p < 0.001$) between the beginning and the end of the follow-up period. Figure 4 shows the evolution of mean central retinal thickness in the treatment period. In the follow-up period, central retinal thickness increased a little in the first 9-10 days, followed by a progressive decrease until stabilization (after 5-6 weeks). The mean difference between the initial and maximal retinal thickness was 8.367 μm.

Statistically significant, positive correlation was found between initial laser flare value and maximal central retinal thickness ($r = 0.881$, $p < 0.001$) in this homogenous group of uveitic eyes, as shown in Figure 5. Figure 6 demonstrates that the positive correlation between flare and retinal thickness remained throughout the treatment period.

Finally, the central (subfoveal) choroidal thickness was significantly decreased ($p < 0.001$) in the treatment period, as shown in Figures 7 and 8.

4. Discussion

Our study demonstrated a pattern of evolution of the retinal and choroidal thickness and flare values throughout the treatment period in the eyes affected by HLA-B27-associated acute anterior uveitis (AAU) (subgroup: ankylosing spondylitis).

The most common posterior segment findings in AAU are subclinical increase in retinal thickness, choroidal thickness, and macular edema. A number of studies have investigated

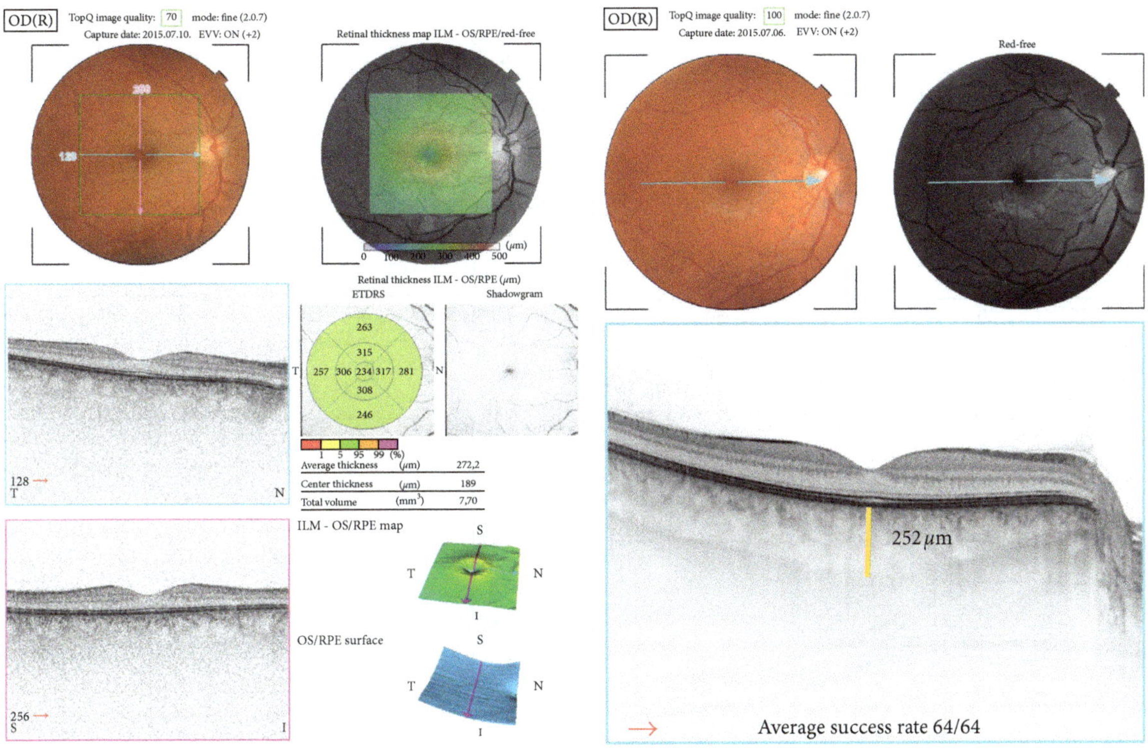

(a) (b)

Figure 1: Retinal (a) and choroidal (b) thickness measurements by swept-source optical coherence tomograph (DRI OCT Triton, Topcon Co., Tokyo, Japan).

Table 1: Clinical signs of the first anterior uveitic attack in ankylosing spondylitis patients.

	BCVA (Snellen)	Flare (photon/unit)	AC cell number (SUN)	IOP (Hgmm)	Central retinal thickness (μm)	Central choroidal thickness (μm)
Minimum	0.6	66.63	12	11	189.00	245.00
Maximum	1.0	135.23	35	18	262.00	312.00
Mean	0.90	90.52	15.56	14.24	220.171	278.166
Standard deviation	0.120	25.315	7.695	2.450	21.056	21.475
Median	0.9	90.23	16	14	219.3	275.5

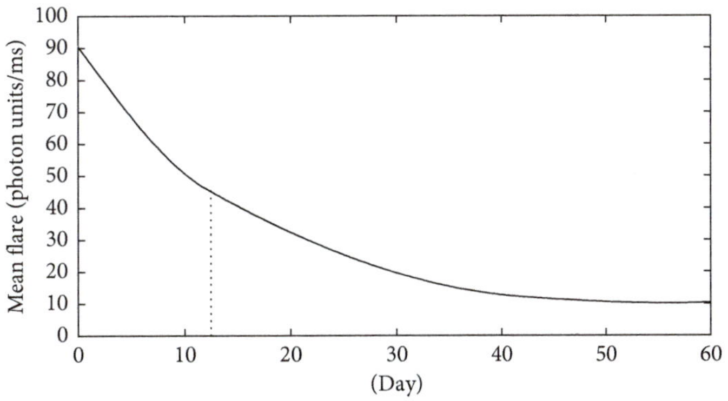

Figure 2: The evolution of the mean laser flare value in the course of follow-up of the acute anterior uveitic patient with ankylosing spondylitis. The mean initial laser flare value is reduced by 50% after 12 days.

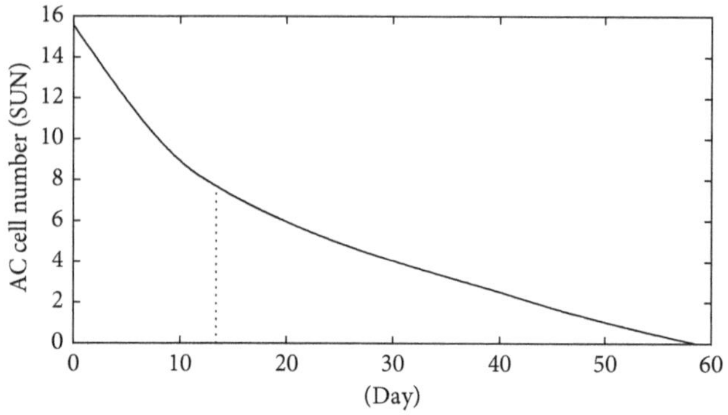

FIGURE 3: The evolution of AC cell number (SUN) during the treatment period of the acute anterior uveitic patient with ankylosing spondylitis.

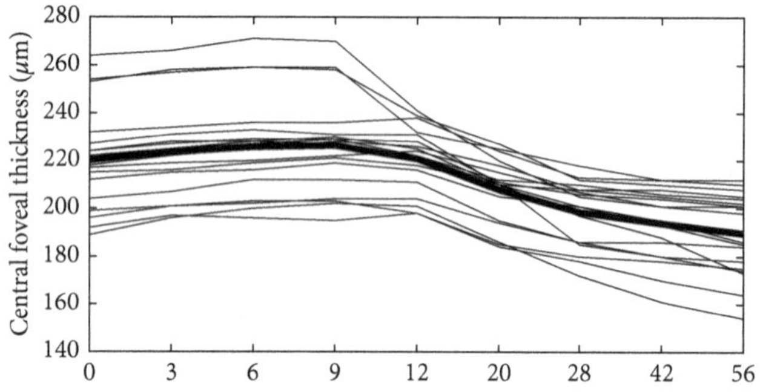

FIGURE 4: The evolution of mean central retinal thickness in the treatment period of the acute anterior uveitic patient with ankylosing spondylitis (the mean central retinal thickness value is represented by a bold line).

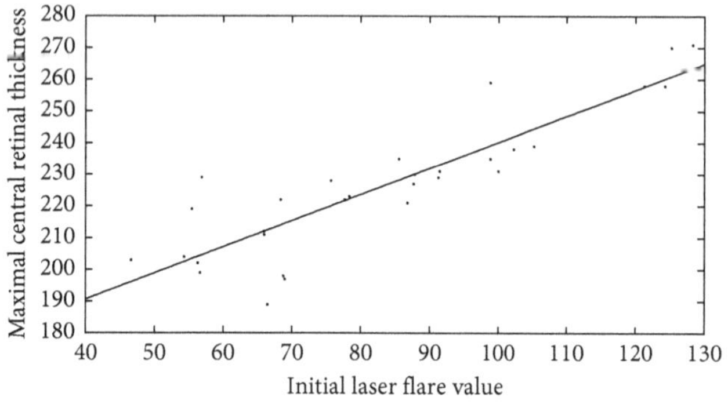

FIGURE 5: Statistically significant, positive correlation was found between initial laser flare value and maximal central retinal thickness ($r = 0.881$, $p < 0.001$) in the acute anterior uveitic eyes.

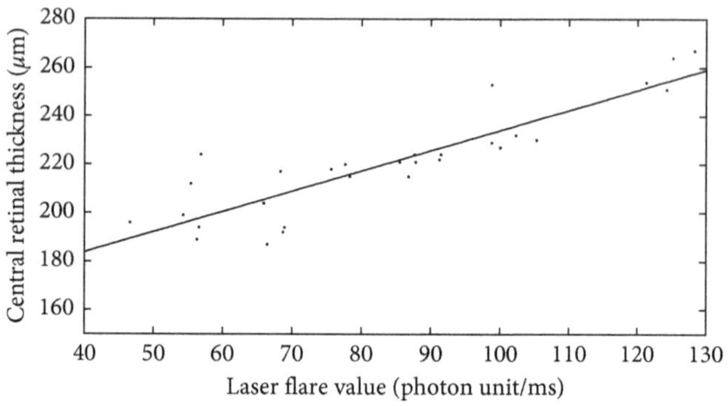

(a)

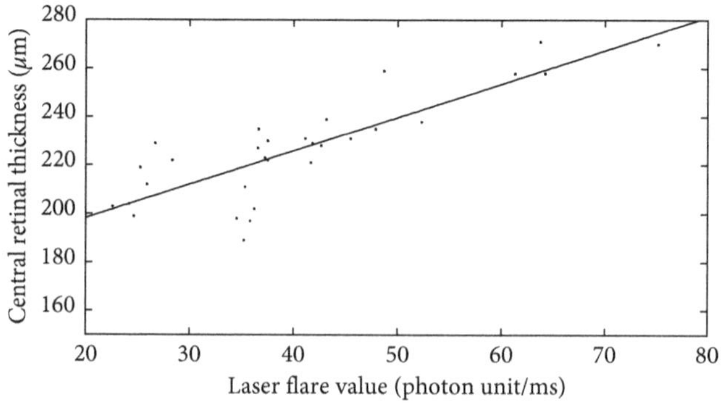

(b)

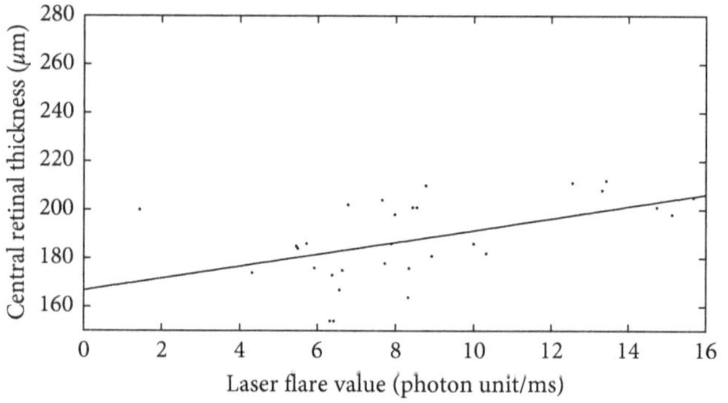

(c)

FIGURE 6: Positive linear correlation between flare and retinal thickness remained throughout the treatment period: (a) 0 days; (b) 10 days; (c) 30 days.

retinal thickness of the anterior uveitic patients at the onset of the inflammation [3, 4, 8–10]. For instance, Moreno-Arrones et al. [4], Balaskas et al. [8], and our earlier study [3] also described statistically significant difference in retinal thickness between the uveitic eyes and the fellow eyes for all OCT subfields. In contrast, de Lahitte et al. described only perifoveolar, pericentral thickening in the patients with juvenile idiopathic arthritis-associated chronic anterior uveitis [11].

Our earlier results have shown that changes of the anterior segment inflammation might cause subclinical retinal changes [3]. We suppose that ocular inflammation may produce a breakdown of the blood-retinal barrier and increase vascular permeability which generates retinal thickening.

In our current study, the evolution of the mean central foveal thickness and anterior segment flare values in the treatment period was shown. In this follow-up period, central retinal thickness increased a little in the first 10 days, followed by a progressive decrease until stabilization (after 5-6 weeks). The mean difference between the initial and maximal retinal thickness was 8.367 μm in our study. The maximal retinal thickness of the affected eyes was observed on day 9-10 from the beginning of the inflammation.

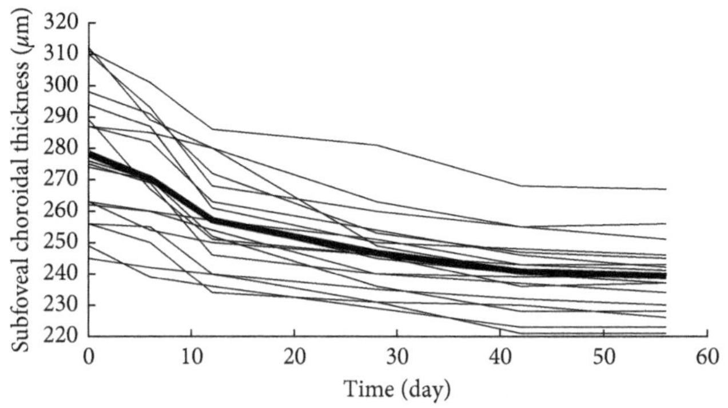

Figure 7: The evolution of mean central (subfoveal) choroidal thickness in the treatment period of the acute anterior uveitic patient with ankylosing spondylitis. The mean central choroidal thickness value is represented by a bold line.

This time lag between the retinal thickening and the onset of inflammation may be the explanation of the development of Irvine–Gass syndrome, whereas macular edema presents several weeks following cataract surgery (inflammatory agents). The other typical phenomenon is diabetic macular edema, which develops slowly as an accumulative response of the retina for multiple factors, that is, inflammation. The main factor triggering macular edema is the release of inflammatory mediators. In chronic uveitis, the repeated/long-lasting inflammatory stimuli could result in additive effects on the retinal thickening. In alignment, Balaskas et al. presented also an increase in retinal thickness over a period of 17 to 25 days in the AAU patients [8]. An important result is that retinal thickness, as measured by OCT, is a useful clinical parameter to monitor response to treatment. Changes in retinal thickness in the AAU patients demonstrate the characteristic pattern of the retinal response to inflammation and therapy. The reply of the retina for the inflammatory agents seems to be delayed.

Anterior segment cells were counted using SUN criteria, but we have used also laser flare photometry (LFP) to eliminate the subjectivity in measurements of anterior segment cells by slit-lamp biomicroscopy [12, 13]. LFP results were always interpreted in conjunction with the clinical observations. Flare and AC cell number were decreased rapidly at the beginning of the treatment, in the first 10 days, and thereafter, slower decrease could be observed until complete resolution of inflammation. While the inflammation values decreased rapidly in the first 10 days, the retinal thickness increased slightly in this period; however, after 10 days, both parameters decreased during the follow-up period.

The mean initial laser flare value was reduced by 50% after 12 days in our study. In the literature, Balaskas et al. [8] described a 50% reduction of flare after 14 days, and de Ancos et al. [14] observed the same drop after 2 days. Contradictory results may come from a different initial severity of the anterior segment inflammation in the studies. According to our results, retinal thickness increased slightly in the first 10 days when flare reduction was remarkable; however, significant changes in retinal thickness values could be observed later in the treatment period.

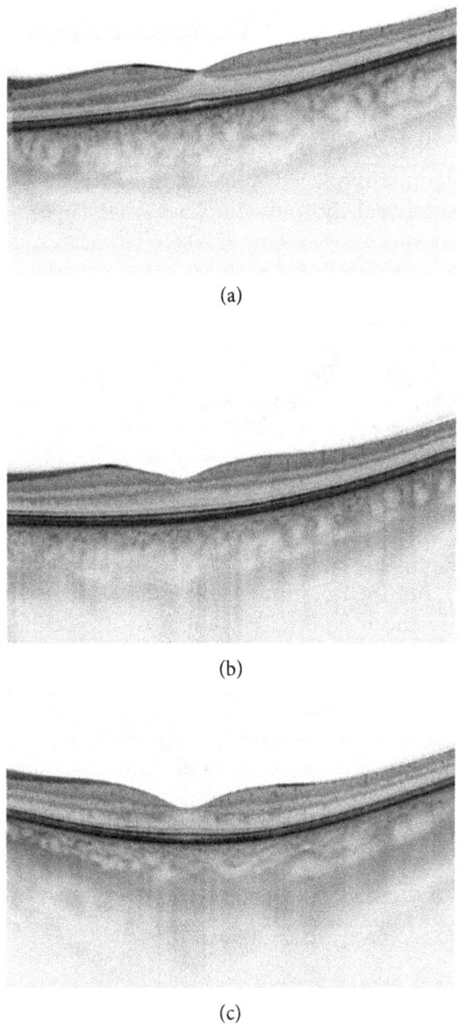

Figure 8: Swept-source OCT cross-sectional images of a 35-year-old male anterior uveitic patient with seronegative spondyloarthropathy: (a) at the beginning of the anterior uveitis (0 days, central retinal thickness: 234 μm, central choroidal thickness: 298 μm); (b) after 10 days in the treatment period (10 days, central retinal thickness: 248 μm, central choroidal thickness: 267 μm); (c) after a month (30 days, central retinal thickness: 219 μm, central choroidal thickness: 242 μm).

As shown in our earlier study, positive correlation was found between initial central foveal thickness and initial laser flare values of the uveitic patient with HLA-B27-related spondyloarthropathy [3]. Gonzales et al. also described that flare was significantly higher in the uveitic patients with macular edema than in patients without macular edema [12].

In this study, positive correlation was demonstrated between flare and central retinal thickness throughout the treatment period, and also, close correlation was shown between initial laser flare values and maximal central retinal thickness. Accordingly, the retina may be an indicator not only of posterior segment inflammation activity but also the anterior segment inflammation.

This study also showed a significant decrease in choroidal thickness in the eyes with active anterior uveitis following anti-inflammatory treatment. It is widely known that the choroid is influenced by ocular inflammatory conditions. Several authors have suggested increased vascular permeability in the posterior segment and choroidal effusion as the mechanisms of choroidal thickening during ocular inflammation [15, 16]. In the present study, the mean values of subfoveal choroidal thickness in the eyes with AAU changed significantly from 278.166 to 239.222 μm. This study showed a significant decrease in choroidal thickness in the eyes with active anterior uveitis after treatment.

Our results indicate that subclinical choroidal inflammation may also be present in active anterior uveitis. These findings suggest that choroidal evaluation may be useful for monitoring disease activity.

Nevertheless, a larger case series could contribute to a more sophisticated statistical evaluation of the patients with AAU, but their common inflammatory pattern enables us to study the inflammation effect of the retina and the choroid.

In conclusion, swept-source OCT is also a useful tool in monitoring subclinical retinal and choroidal thickening in anterior uveitis with the SpA patients in the treatment period. It may indicate that the retina and choroid play a biomarker function in anterior segment inflammation but the reply of the retina for the inflammatory agents seems to be delayed.

Conflicts of Interest

The authors declare that there are no conflicts of interest.

References

[1] G. Wilson and D. D. Folzenlogen, "Spondyloarthropathies: new directions in etiopathogenesis, diagnosis and treatment," *Missouri Medicine*, vol. 109, no. 1, pp. 69–74, 2012.

[2] J. T. Rosenbaum, "Characterization of uveitis associated with spondyloarthritis," *Journal of Rheumatology*, vol. 16, no. 6, pp. 792–796, 1989.

[3] Z. Szepessy, A. Barsi, and J. Németh, "Macular changes correlate with the degree of acute anterior uveitis in patients with spondyloarthropathy," *Ocular Immunology and Inflammation*, vol. 24, no. 2, pp. 153–158, 2016.

[4] J. P. Moreno-Arrones, M. B. Gorrono-Echebarría, and M. A. Teus, "OCT in acute anterior uveitis," *Archivos de la Sociedad Española de Oftalmología*, vol. 84, no. 4, pp. 185–190, 2009.

[5] I. Maruko, T. Iida, Y. Sugano et al., "Subfoveal choroidal thickness after treatment of Vogt-Koyanagi-Harada disease," *Retina*, vol. 31, no. 3, pp. 510–517, 2011.

[6] N. Yesilirmak, W. H. Lee, S. Gur Gungor, E. Yaman Pinarci, I. Akkoyun, and G. Yilmaz, "Enhanced depth imaging optical coherence tomography in patients with different phases of Behcet's panuveitis," *Canadian Journal of Ophthalmology*, vol. 52, no. 1, pp. 48–53, 2017.

[7] B. Basarir, U. Celik, C. Altan, and N. B. Celik, "Choroidal thickness changes determined by EDI-OCT on acute anterior uveitis in patients with HLA-B27-positive ankylosing spondylitis," *International Ophthalmology*, vol. 38, no. 1, pp. 307–312, 2017.

[8] K. Balaskas, P. Ballabeni, and Y. Guex-Crosier, "Retinal thickening in HLA-B27-associated acute anterior uveitis: evolution with time and association with severity of inflammatory activity," *Investigative Opthalmology and Visual Science*, vol. 53, no. 10, pp. 6171–6177, 2012.

[9] A. Traill, R. Stawell, A. Hall, and E. Zamir, "Macular thickening in acute anterior uveitis," *Ophthalmology*, vol. 114, p. 402, 2007.

[10] C. G. Castellano, S. S. Stinnett, P. S. Mettu, R. M. McCallum, and G. J. Jaffe, "Retinal thickening in iridocyclitis," *American Journal of Ophthalmology*, vol. 148, no. 3, pp. 341.e1–349.e1, 2009.

[11] G. D. de Lahitte, C. Terrada, T. H. Tran et al., "Maculopathy in uveitis of juvenile idiopathic arthritis: an optical coherence tomography study," *British Journal of Ophthalmology*, vol. 92, no. 1, pp. 64–69, 2008.

[12] C. A. Gonzales, J. G. Ladas, J. L. Davis et al., "Relationships between laser flare photometry values and complications of uveitis," *Archives of Ophthalmology*, vol. 119, no. 12, pp. 1763–1769, 2001.

[13] C. P. Herbort, Y. Guex-Crosier, E. de Ancos, and N. Pittet, "Use of laser flare photometry to assess and monitor inflammation in uveitis," *Ophthalmology*, vol. 104, no. 1, pp. 64–71, 1997.

[14] E. de Ancos, N. Pitter, and C. P. Herbort, "Quantitative measurement of inflammation in HLA-B27 acute anterior uveitis using the Kowa FC-100 laser flare-cell meter," *Klinische Monatsblätter für Augenheilkunde*, vol. 204, no. 5, pp. 330–333, 1994.

[15] M. Kim, S. Y. Choi, and Y. H. Park, "Analysis of choroidal and central foveal thicknesses in acute anterior uveitis by enhanced-depth imaging optical coherence tomography," *BMC Ophthalmology*, vol. 17, p. 225, 2017.

[16] M. Kola, A. Kalkisim, M. Karkucak et al., "Evaluation of choroidal thickness in ankylosing spondylitis using optical coherence tomography," *Ocular Immunology and Inflammation*, vol. 22, no. 6, pp. 434–438, 2014.

28

Total Penetrating Keratoplasty: Indications, Therapeutic Approach, and Long-Term Follow-Up

Katarzyna Krysik,[1] Ewa Wroblewska-Czajka,[2] Anita Lyssek-Boron,[1] Edward A. Wylegala,[2,3,4] and Dariusz Dobrowolski[1,2,3]

[1]*Department of Ophthalmology with Pediatric Unit, St. Barbara Hospital, Trauma Center, Medykow Square 1, 41-200 Sosnowiec, Poland*
[2]*Department of Ophthalmology, District Railway Hospital, Panewnicka 65 St., 40-760 Katowice, Poland*
[3]*Chair and Clinical Department of Ophthalmology, School of Medicine with the Division of Dentistry in Zabrze, Medical University of Silesia in Katowice, Panewnicka 65 St., 40-760 Katowice, Poland*
[4]*Hebei Provincial Eye Hospital, Xingtai, China*

Correspondence should be addressed to Dariusz Dobrowolski; dardobmd@wp.pl

Academic Editor: Zisis Gatzioufas

Purpose. Evaluation of the indications, anatomical and functional results, and complications of total penetrating keratoplasty (TPK) in disorders involving whole cornea. *Materials and Methods.* We analyzed outcomes of the surgical treatment of 47 eyes of 46 patients that underwent TPK. Indications were infectious keratitis, autoimmune disease, injury of the eyeball (mainly chemical burns), and other combined disorders. The surgical technique involved dissection of affected tissues with a margin of 1.0 mm. The size of the corneal graft ranged from 10.0 to 14.0 mm. We analyzed indications, outcomes, and complications of surgery. *Results.* Final restoration of the ocular integrity and maintenance of the globe were achieved in 27 eyes (57%). More than one surgery was necessary in a total of 29 eyes (62%). The frequency of retransplantations did not vary significantly between the groups with different causes of corneal melting/perforation (63% of eyes with infection, 66% of eyes after trauma and 70% of eyes of patients with autoimmune disorders). Surgical treatment failed in 20 eyes (43%). Evisceration was necessary in 13 eyes (28%), phthisis occurred in 7 cases (15%). *Conclusion.* TPK should be considered as a last line treatment in huge corneal destruction to restore integrity of the eye globe.

1. Introduction

Serious corneal disorders like ulcers or perforations frequently give rise to difficult clinical situations, with rapid consecutive threatening of vision and disintegrity of the eye globe. Despite current advances in pharmacological and surgical treatment, severe corneal infections, injuries, or systemic diseases can lead to corneal perforations, which frequently require surgery "à chaud."

Urgent reconstructive surgical interventions may be necessary to avoid consecutive endophthalmitis and the formation of the anterior and posterior synechiae and secondary glaucoma and to prevent the spread of pathogens toward the posterior pole of the eye globe or to avoid other severe complications [1–4]. The optical result of urgent surgical treatment is less important; if possible, visual restoration or rehabilitation may be accomplished in the future. Initial difficult and complicated medical status, despite a wide spectrum of pharmacological and surgical treatments, may result in fatal treatment failure with loss of the eye. The poor visual outcome of rapid corneal surgery may require further surgery [1, 4–6].

The surgical approach to retain corneal integrity may vary, depending on size, localization, depth of corneal tissue damage, and the state of other internal globe tissues. Also, coexistent or causative infection or inflammation may determine the choice and timing of surgical decisions. Additional surgical procedures like amniotic membrane transplants, conjunctival flaps, tarsorrhaphy, and botulin toxin-induced ptosis may be applied in moderate tissue damage or as the initial treatment method [5, 7, 8].

Urgent penetrating keratoplasty (PK), total penetrating keratoplasty (TPK), and corneal or corneoscleral patch graft (CSPG) combination of surgical approaches or keratoprosthesis are usually reserved for progressive, end-stage corneal pathology or last-chance medical treatment [1, 2, 9–13].

The first total penetrating keratoplasty was described in 1951 by Ramon Castroviejo as a method for replacing a large area of diseased cornea and adjacent sclera with donor tissue [14]. The primary aim of this procedure is the tectonic repair of large perforations or other extensive corneal pathologies and restoration of integrity of the globe. Because of its size, frequently involving adjacent sclera and indications for surgery (infections, corneal ulcerations, injuries, and immune disorders), total penetrating keratoplasties are associated with a high risk of complications [15–17]. The use of steroids and other immunosuppressive agents significantly reduces the rate of immunological graft rejections. Causative and complimentary intensive medication is necessary to avoid surgical treatment failure, which would lead to severe visual loss or even loss of the eye globe [5, 12, 17, 18].

The purpose of this study is to report treatment results of patients, who received a total penetrating keratoplasty for corneal diffuse destructive diseases. We review the surgical treatment, anatomical and functional results, and complications of treatment in this group of patients.

2. Material and Methods

We retrospectively reviewed the outcomes of the surgical treatment of 47 eyes of 46 patients that were operated on using the total penetrating keratoplasty technique. All surgeries were performed between January 1, 2010 and July 31, 2017. Patients were recruited from the Ophthalmology Department of Saint Barbara Hospital, Trauma Center, Sosnowiec, Poland, and the Chair and Clinical Department of Ophthalmology, School of Medicine with the Division of Dentistry in Zabrze, Medical University of Silesia, District Railway Hospital, Katowice, Poland. Data from the medical records included demographics, medical history, preoperative and postoperative best spectacle-corrected visual acuity (BSCVA) measured using the Snellen visual acuity (VA) chart, outcome and complications of surgery, results of accessory examinations (microbial tests), postoperative intraocular pressure, graft rejection, and other comorbidities and complications. All patients signed the informed consent form before any surgical procedure. This retrospective, observational study, according to Polish law, does not require acceptance of a local bioethical committee.

Indications for total penetrating keratoplasty were infectious keratitis, autoimmune disease, injury of the eyeball (mainly chemical burns), and other combined disorders. The main goal of the surgical treatment was the total removal of the infected or destroyed cornea and restoration of ocular integrity. After a complete ocular examination, total penetrating keratoplasty (diameter ≥ 10.0 mm) was performed (Figure 1). The surgical technique involved dissection of affected tissues with a margin of minimum 1.0 mm of nonaffected tissue. The size of the corneal graft ranged from 10.0 to 14.0 mm, depending on the extent of corneal necrosis or melting and infiltration of corneal stroma or adjacent ocular tissues. Great care was taken to avoid affecting any structures of the iridocorneal angle while preparing the recipient tissues. The oversize of the graft was 0.5 to 1.0 mm. Optimal graft size was determined by placing various-sized trephines on the recipient cornea to encompass the entire area of pathology. A 360-degree peritomy was performed at the limbus before trephination to facilitate suturing. The donor tissues (corneoscleral rings) were preserved in a cold storage media of Eusol-C solution (Alchimia, S.r.I., Ponte S. Nicolo, Italy). All surgeries were performed under general anaesthesia. To avoid consecutive glaucoma, all patients received peripheral iridectomy, unless an iridotomy or iridectomy had been performed during a preceding surgical intervention. For TPK, we used a Hanna vacuum trephine system (Moria Inc., Antony, France) or freehand trephines, if globe integrity was seriously damaged. All grafts were sutured with single 10-0 nylon sutures into the recipient sclerocorneal bed; the knots were buried. Because of the high risk of rejection in large grafts, both topical and systemic steroid medication was administrated individually, postoperatively. Also, intensive topical and general medical management for the primary ocular pathology was continued, according to its aethiology: immunosuppression, anti-inflammatory, broad-spectrum antibiotic, and antifungal or antiprotozoal therapy, respectively. Patients were also treated with cycloplegics and antiglaucomatous medications, if necessary. Because of the complex nature of underlying pathology, additional one-time or subsequent surgery was performed more than once. We followed up with all patients every two weeks for a period of three months, monthly for a minimum of six months and at differing intervals, thereafter. The mean observation time was 24 months (from 1 to 60 months).

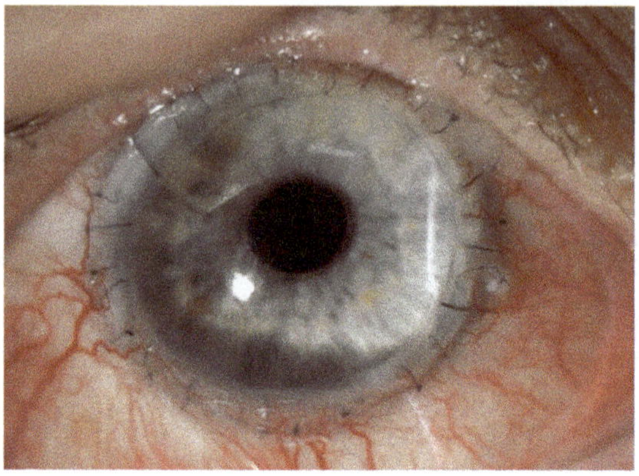

Figure 1: Transparent graft.

The computer software, XLSTAT-Biomed (Addinsoft SARL, France), was used for statistical analysis and to calculate means and standard deviations. The outcome variables were not assumed to have a normal distribution, so one-way analysis of the variance was used to compare the baseline characteristics and postoperative outcomes among subgroups of causes of corneal perforation. A p value of <0.05 was considered statistically significant.

3. Results

Forty-seven eyes of forty-six patients were operated on between January 1, 2010 and July 31, 2017, using the total penetrating keratoplasty technique. This group consisted of 21 females, whose mean age was 66.13 ± 9.94 (range 39 to 80 years), and 25 males, whose mean age was 63.69 ± 14.48 (range 32 to 92 years). There was no statistically significant difference with respect to gender and age between both groups ($p > 0.05$).

All primary causes of corneal destruction and perforation requiring TPK are presented in Table 1. The main cause of this condition was infection. The most frequent infectious factors were bacterial cultures (*Pseudomonas aeruginosa*: 3 eyes (14%); *Enterococcus faecalis*: 2 eyes (9%); *Escherichia coli*: 2 eyes (9%); *Proteus mirabilis*: 3 eyes (14%); *Staphylococcus aureus*: 2 eyes (9%); and *Staphylococcus epidermidis*: 1 eye (5%)) and fungal (*Aspergillus fumigatus*: 3 eyes (14%); *Fusarium solani*: 2 eyes (9%); and *Candida albicans*: 2 eyes (9%)). Autoimmune diseases involved rheumatoid arthritis (7 eyes: 70%), ankylosing spondylitis (2 eyes: 20%), and lupus (1 eye: 10%). Eye injuries were dominated by chemical, mainly alkali, burns of the ocular surface: 8 eyes (67%). Ocular complications of Lyell's syndrome involved 2 patients (2 eyes: 100%). Neurotrophic keratopathy (loss of the neurosensory innervations of the cornea) was responsible for corneal perforation in one eye.

Final restoration of the ocular integrity and maintenance of the globe was achieved in 27 eyes (57%): 15 eyes (32%) of 15 females and 12 eyes (25%) of 12 males. More than one tectonic surgical approach, except primary total penetrating keratoplasty, was necessary in a total of 29 eyes (62%): 13 females (28%) and 16 males (34%). The frequency of repetitive tectonic corneoscleral grafting did not vary significantly between the groups of patients with different causes of corneal perforation (63% of eyes with primary infection, 66% of eyes after ocular trauma, and 70% of eyes of patients with autoimmune disorders). Characteristics of repeated tectonic surgery are reported in Table 2. Surgical treatment failed in 20 eyes (43%): 7 eyes (15%) of 7 females and 13 eyes (28%) of 13 males. Evisceration was necessary in 13 eyes (28%), and phthisis occurred in 7 eyes (15%).

Accessory simultaneous surgical procedures, not always considered before primary tectonic corneoscleral surgery, included intraocular lens explantation: 3 eyes (6%); cataract extraction or spontaneous lens extrusion at the time of surgery: 12 eyes (25%); anterior vitrectomy: 5 eyes (11%); and "open sky" pars plana vitrectomy: 4 eyes (9%).

Preoperative best spectacle-corrected visual acuity ranged from light perception (LP) to 0.05. Because the main purpose of this treatment was to retain ocular integrity, not to improve visual acuity, the final BSCVA was limited and ranged from no light perception to 0.2, after tectonic and successive (if possible) surgical and intensive additional pharmacological treatment. Visual acuity improvement was observed in 10 eyes (21%) after primary tectonic TPK and ranged from hand motion (HM) to 0.1. To achieve better final visual acuity, 11 eyes (23%) had to undergo successive, often complex, surgical treatments. Successive surgical treatment results after primary tectonic TPK are presented in Table 3.

Graft transparency was rated during each follow-up. Final full graft transparency at last controlled visit (Figure 1) was present in 6 eyes (13%) and in 6 eyes after repetitive surgical tectonic treatment. Partial graft transparency (25–50% of corneal tissue area) (Figure 2) was achieved in 11 patients (23%) and totally opaque grafts (Figure 3) appeared in 10 patients (21%), despite repetitive surgical approaches. Postoperative complications of total penetrating keratoplasty are reported in Table 4.

The main cause of surgical treatment failure was persistent epithelial defect, observed in 34 operated eyes (72%), resulting from decreased corneal sensitivity and impaired tear production. There were 22 eyes (65%) with persistent epithelial defect refractory to medical therapy, with consecutive ulceration and perforation of the cornea requiring subsequent tectonic surgery. Repeated total penetrating keratoplasty, penetrating keratoplasty, or corneoscleral patch graft was performed on 11 eyes, including 2 eyes of 2 patients where the tectonic approach was necessary more than twice, as were the eyes of patients with Lyell's syndrome. In one eye of a patient with Lyell's syndrome, despite successive surgical approaches, eyeball atrophy occurred.

Table 1: Causes of the corneal tissue destruction and perforation (% in brackets).

Cause of perforation	Total ($n = 47$) 100%	Female ($n = 22$) 47%	Male ($n = 25$) 53%
Infection	22 (46.8)	11 (23.4)	11 (23.4)
Bacterial	13 (27.6)	6 (10.6)	7 (17)
Fungal	7 (14.9)	4 (8.5)	3 (6.3)
Protozoal	2 (4.25)	1 (2.1)	1 (2.1)
Autoimmune disease	10 (21.3)	6 (12.8)	4 (8.5)
Trauma	12 (25.5)	4 (8.5)	8 (17)
Chemical (burns)	8 (17)	3 (6.3)	5 (10.6)
Penetrating	4 (8.5)	1 (2.1)	3 (6.3)
Other	3 (6.3)	1 (2.1)	2 (4.25)

Table 2: Repeated surgical tectonic treatment after primary TPK (% in brackets).

Characteristics	Total ($n = 29$) (100%)	Females ($n = 13$) (45%)	Males ($n = 16$) (55%)
Regrafts rate			
reTPK	17 (58.6)	7 (53.8)	10 (62.5)
PK	8 (27.6)	5 (38.5)	3 (18.75)
CSPG	4 (13.8)	1 (7.7)	3 (18.75)

TABLE 3: BSCVA after total penetrating keratoplasty and successive optical surgical procedures.

Characteristics	Total n (%) $n = 11$	Preoperative BSCVA (range)	Postoperative BSCVA (range)
Surgical procedure			
PK	4	LP–0.02	CF–0.1
PK + cataract surgery + PCIOL implantation	3	LP–0.01	0.05–0.2
Cataract surgery + PCIOL implantation	2	HM–0.01	0.05–0.2
Secondary PCIOL in-sulcus implantation	1	0.02	0.2
Transscleral IOL fixation	1	0.02	0.1

CF: counting fingers; HM: hand movements.

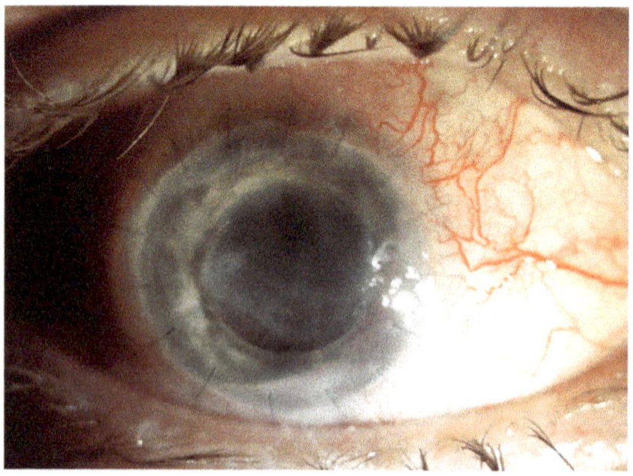

FIGURE 2: Partially transparent graft.

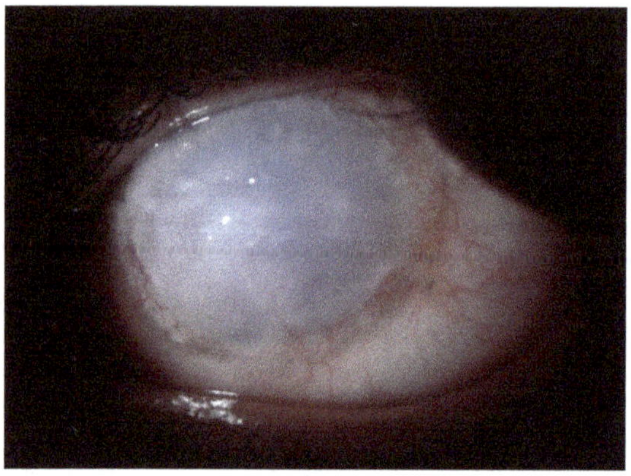

FIGURE 3: Totally opaque graft.

Reinfection was observed in 19 (40%) of eyes that received TPK surgery. Despite vigorous antimicrobial topical and general treatment and repeat tectonic surgery (3 penetrating keratoplasties, 2 total penetrating keratoplasties, and 1 corneoscleral patch graft), 11 (58%) of reinfected eyes developed endophthalmitis, which demanded the radical surgical approach of evisceration. Three eyes developed phthisis.

Graft melting, reported in 16 eyes (34%) and frequently preceded by loosening of the sutures and tissue necrosis resulting from infection or immunological mechanisms, was another important complication of TPK. Primary surgical treatment failed in 12 eyes (25%), and successive surgical treatment was performed: repetitive TPK in 8 eyes and CSPG in 4 eyes. Of this group, 5 eyes (31%) experienced complications from infection, 3 eyes developed phthisis, and evisceration was necessary in 2 eyes.

Early graft rejection, characterised by a whitish, sterile ring or diffuse infiltrates, was present in 5 eyes (11%) and treated for infectious corneal ulcerations. Intensive topical and systemic immunosuppressive and anti-inflammatory treatment was administered, leading to scarring and thinning of the perilimbal tissue. No urgent surgical approach was necessary.

Subsequent consecutive glaucoma or ocular hypertension occurred despite surgically performed iridectomy during tectonic TPK. Peripheral iridectomy was reported in 15 eyes (32%). To normalize refractory to medical treatment in intraocular pressure, 10 eyes (67%) required surgical intervention: 5 trabeculectomies, 3 transscleral cyclophotocoagulation, and 2 Ex-press glaucoma shunt implantations.

4. Discussion

The main purpose of tectonic surgery is restoration and maintenance of ocular integrity. Postoperative visual acuity and graft clarity are related to many complex immunological and physiological conditions. Anatomical integrity of the globe does not guarantee improvement of vision.

Emergency surgical strategies to close a corneal perforation depend on the size and location of the defect, aethiology, and donor corneal tissue availability. When a corneoscleral flap is not available, temporary or definitely amniotic membrane transplantation or conjunctival flap is used to close the perforation. Medical and surgical treatment of large corneal perforations, even with maximal pharmacotherapy of infection, frequently fails.

In our study, we assessed, like other authors [17, 19] that the most frequent indication for rapid tectonic treatment was infection. However, despite maximum broad-spectrum medical and surgical multistage treatment, even when repeated, the final outcome remained frequently unsatisfactory and was considered a therapeutic failure. Endophthalmitis refractory to antimicrobial and anti-inflammatory treatment required the final procedure of evisceration [3, 15].

Large grafts often are regarded as a risk factor for immunologic graft failure [20]. Our results agree with those reported by Ti et al. [15] and Jonas et al. [21]. Corneal graft melting, frequently observed in autoimmune disorders complicated by corneal perforations and usually preceded by

TABLE 4: Postoperative complications of total penetrating keratoplasty (% in brackets).

Primary cause of ocular disease	Infection Total n (%) ($n = 22$)	Autoimmune Total n (%) ($n = 10$)	Trauma Total n (%) ($n = 12$)	Other Total n (%) ($n = 3$)
Complication rate				
Persistent epithelial defect	13 (59.1)	9 (90)	9 (75)	3 (100)
Reinfection	15 (68.2)	3 (30)	1 (8.3)	0
Graft melting	8 (36.4)	7 (70)	2 (16.7)	0
Graft rejection	5 (100)	0	0	0
Glaucoma or ocular hypertension	4 (18.2)	4 (40)	6 (50)	1 (33.3)

loosening of the sutures, is also comparable in frequency, according to the foregoing author's reports.

Delayed epithelialisation or persistent epithelial defect determined a significant graft failure rate and contributed to the higher rate of ocular surface complications [3]. The final result of this complication often leads to repeated tectonic and reconstructive surgery [4, 9, 20].

In the current study, despite the uncertain and frequently inauspicious preliminary prognosis, repeated tectonic surgery and multidrug immunosuppression, overall graft survival, and final globe restoration were achieved in more than half of the eyes treated. This result is comparable with other studies [4, 18]. Groups of patients with extremely large corneoscleral grafts are usually small may be dependent on geographical and ethnic conditions (variability), and statistics may not be representative, which is also emphasized by other authors [2, 4, 15, 19, 20].

Surgical interventions with large corneal perforations frequently result in consecutive glaucoma. Our results for this complication present less frequently than in some studies [6, 15] and are compatible with the reports of Kietzmann et al. [22]. Increased intraocular pressure and secondary glaucoma after total penetrating keratoplasty and other tectonic procedures involving peripheral cornea are more frequent than after procedures involving the central part of the cornea [15, 20].

Total penetrating keratoplasty is still not a standard procedure for the treatment of corneal perforations. Penetrating keratoplasty, lamellar keratoplasties, and corneoscleral patch grafts remain the more frequently used surgical approach. Systemic immunosuppression, and often multidrug therapy, is necessary to minimize the risk of graft rejection and the necessity of repeat tectonic surgical treatment. There are no clear schemes concerning immunosuppressive treatment after CSPG [5, 12, 19, 20].

The sequential, frequently multistage, and combination surgical approach is necessary to achieve final visual acuity improvement [10, 15, 19]. We have to consider primary causative factors of corneal destruction, like severe refractory to antimicrobial treatment infections, autoimmune disorders, or severe burns of the ocular surface, as well as the final result of the tectonic primary and secondary treatment. Elective corneal surgery, like optical keratoplasty, is more secure and its final outcome is more predictable. Also, other surgical techniques, like cataract surgery with IOL implantation and secondary IOL implantation, are crucial to final visual acuity restoration [1, 4, 20, 23].

We demonstrated in this study that results of large corneoscleral grafts are unpredictable. In our opinion, this is frequently the only surgical procedure able to restore ocular integrity with simultaneous removal of infectious material, inflammatory membranes, necrotic tissues, and direct drug administration. Such an approach minimizes the risk of endophthalmitis and the spread of disease to the globe, while simultaneously increasing the probability of graft survival and potential improvement of visual acuity.

Engagement of other specialists like microbiologists and immunologists is important and therapeutically helpful. Such collaboration facilitates the optimal choice of medical treatment and reduces the rate of graft failures and the side effects of pharmacological therapy.

In conclusion, total penetrating keratoplasties, despite the high risk of intra- and postoperative severe complications, constitute a true surgical treatment alternative method for large peripheral cornea and adjacent sclera perforations. Further investigation and development of new surgical techniques are necessary to improve the final results of corneal perforation treatment. The goal should be not only restoration of ocular integrity but also improvement of visual functioning.

Conflicts of Interest

The authors declare that there are no conflicts of interest regarding the publication of this paper.

References

[1] E. de la Torre-Gonzalez and C. Ponce de León Ascencio, "Staged penetrating sclerokeratoplasty and penetrating keratoplasty for management of advanced acquired anterior staphyloma," *Journal of Ophthalmic & Vision Research*, vol. 6, no. 2, pp. 147–150, 2011.

[2] S. W. Rush and R. B. Rush, "Outcomes of infectious versus sterile perforated corneal ulcers after therapeutic penetrating keratoplasty in the United States," *Journal of Ophthalmology*, vol. 2016, Article ID 6284595, 6 pages, 2016.

[3] A. Anshu, A. Parthasarathy, J. S. Mehta, H. M. Htoon, and D. T. H. Tan, "Outcomes of therapeutic deep lamellar keratoplasty and penetrating keratoplasty for advanced infectious keratitis. A comparative study," *Ophthalmology*, vol. 116, no. 4, pp. 615–623, 2009.

[4] H. Parwez, A. K. Tourkmani, D. Kazakos, M. Jones, and D. Anderson, "Emergency corneal grafting in the UK: a

6-year analysis of the UK transplant registry," *British Journal of Ophthalmology*, vol. 102, pp. 26–30, 2018.

[5] R. Różycki, I. Nowak-Gospodarowicz, D. Białas, R. Pawlik, and M. Rękas, "Sclerokeratoplasty as the therapy for corneal perforation due to exposure and neurotrophic keratopathy," *Case Reports in Ophthalmological Medicine*, vol. 2014, Article ID 467249, 4 pages, 2014.

[6] L. W. Hirst and G. A. Lee, "Corneoscleral transplantation for end stage corneal disease," *British Journal of Ophthalmology*, vol. 82, no. 11, pp. 1276–1279, 1998.

[7] S. L. Portnoy, M. S. Insler, and H. E. Kaufman, "Surgical management of corneal ulceration and perforation," *Survey of Ophthalmology*, vol. 34, no. 1, pp. 47–58, 1989.

[8] M. Bouazza, A. A. Bensemlali, M. Elbelhadji et al., "Non-traumatic corneal perforations: therapeutic modalities," *Journal Français d'Ophtalmologie*, vol. 38, no. 5, pp. 395–402, 2015.

[9] A. Viestenz, B. Seitz, H. G. Struck, and A. Viestenz, "Sclerocorneal graft and sequential removal of melted cornea after severe corneal burn with perforation," vol. 31, no. 1, pp. 39–42, 2018.

[10] W. Shi, H. Gao, T. Wang, and L. Xie, "Combined penetrating keratoplasty and keratolimbal allograft transplantation in comparison with corneoscleral transplantation in the treatment of severe eye burns," *Clinical & Experimental Ophthalmology*, vol. 36, no. 6, pp. 501–507, 2008.

[11] D. Derhy, A. Sauer, M. Sabou et al., "Surgical treatment of *Metarhizium anisopliae* sclerokeratitis and endophthalmitis," *Indian Journal of Ophthalmology*, vol. 65, no. 6, pp. 523–526, 2017.

[12] M. Cellini, M. Fresina, E. Strobbe, C. Gizzi, and E. C. Campos, "Corneoscleral graft in Mooren's ulcer: a case report," *Cases Journal*, vol. 2, no. 1, p. 180, 2009.

[13] S. Helsen, S. Ni Dhubhghaill, N. Zakaria, and C. Koppen, "Eckardt keratoprosthesis for tectonic repair of a large corneal perforation," *Cornea*, vol. 35, no. 8, pp. 1147–1149, 2016.

[14] R. Castroviejo, "Total penetrating keratoplasty," *American Journal of Ophthalmology*, vol. 34, no. 12, pp. 1697–1706, 1951.

[15] S.-E. Ti, A. Scott, P. Janardhanan, and D. T. H. Tan, "Therapeutic keratoplasty for advanced suppurative keratitis," *American Journal of Ophthalmology*, vol. 143, no. 5, pp. 755–762.e2, 2007.

[16] M. Cobo, J. R. Ortiz, and S. G. Safran, "Sclerokeratoplasty with maintenance of the angle," *American Journal of Ophthalmology*, vol. 113, no. 5, pp. 533–537, 1992.

[17] R. O. W. Burk and A. M. Joussen, "Corneoscleroplasty with maintenance of the angle in two cases of extensive corneoscleral disease," *Eye*, vol. 14, no. 2, pp. 196–200, 2000.

[18] R. Sundmacher and T. Reinhard, "Central corneolimbal transplantation under systemic ciclosporin a cover for severe limbal stem cell insufficiency," *Graefe's Archive for Clinical and Experimental Ophthalmology*, vol. 234, Supplement 1, pp. S122–S125, 1996.

[19] L. Xie, H. Zhai, X. Dong, and W. Shi, "Primary diseases of corneal perforation in Shandong Province, China: a 10-year retrospective study," *American Journal of Ophthalmology*, vol. 145, no. 4, pp. 662–666.e1, 2008.

[20] M. Ang, J. S. Mehta, C. C. A. Sng, H. M. Htoon, and D. T. H. Tan, "Indications, outcomes, and risk factors for failure in tectonic keratoplasty," *Ophthalmology*, vol. 119, no. 7, pp. 1311–1319, 2012.

[21] J. B. Jonas, R. M. Rank, and W. M. Budde, "Tectonic sclerokeratoplasty and tectonic penetrating keratoplasty as treatment for perforated or predescemetal corneal ulcers," *American Journal of Ophthalmology*, vol. 132, no. 1, pp. 14–18, 2001.

[22] A. S. Kietzmann, K. M. Goins, J. E. Sutphin, and M. D. Wagoner, "Keratoplasty for treatment of *Acanthamoeba* keratitis," *Ophthalmology*, vol. 116, no. 5, pp. 864–869, 2009.

[23] J. J. Ling, D. J. Bays, G. R. Thompson 3rd, A. Moshri, and M. J. Mannis, "Favorable outcome in *coccidioides* endophthalmitis—a combined medical and surgical treatment approach," *Cornea*, vol. 36, no. 11, pp. 1423–1425, 2017.

Permissions

All chapters in this book were first published in JO, by Hindawi Publishing Corporation; hereby published with permission under the Creative Commons Attribution License or equivalent. Every chapter published in this book has been scrutinized by our experts. Their significance has been extensively debated. The topics covered herein carry significant findings which will fuel the growth of the discipline. They may even be implemented as practical applications or may be referred to as a beginning point for another development.

The contributors of this book come from diverse backgrounds, making this book a truly international effort. This book will bring forth new frontiers with its revolutionizing research information and detailed analysis of the nascent developments around the world.

We would like to thank all the contributing authors for lending their expertise to make the book truly unique. They have played a crucial role in the development of this book. Without their invaluable contributions this book wouldn't have been possible. They have made vital efforts to compile up to date information on the varied aspects of this subject to make this book a valuable addition to the collection of many professionals and students.

This book was conceptualized with the vision of imparting up-to-date information and advanced data in this field. To ensure the same, a matchless editorial board was set up. Every individual on the board went through rigorous rounds of assessment to prove their worth. After which they invested a large part of their time researching and compiling the most relevant data for our readers.

The editorial board has been involved in producing this book since its inception. They have spent rigorous hours researching and exploring the diverse topics which have resulted in the successful publishing of this book. They have passed on their knowledge of decades through this book. To expedite this challenging task, the publisher supported the team at every step. A small team of assistant editors was also appointed to further simplify the editing procedure and attain best results for the readers.

Apart from the editorial board, the designing team has also invested a significant amount of their time in understanding the subject and creating the most relevant covers. They scrutinized every image to scout for the most suitable representation of the subject and create an appropriate cover for the book.

The publishing team has been an ardent support to the editorial, designing and production team. Their endless efforts to recruit the best for this project, has resulted in the accomplishment of this book. They are a veteran in the field of academics and their pool of knowledge is as vast as their experience in printing. Their expertise and guidance has proved useful at every step. Their uncompromising quality standards have made this book an exceptional effort. Their encouragement from time to time has been an inspiration for everyone.

The publisher and the editorial board hope that this book will prove to be a valuable piece of knowledge for researchers, students, practitioners and scholars across the globe.

List of Contributors

Jiahui Chen, Qinghe Jing, Yating Tang, Dongjin Qian, Yi Lu and Yongxiang Jiang
Department of Ophthalmology and Vision Science, Eye and ENT Hospital of Fudan University, Shanghai, China
Key Laboratory of Myopia of State Health Ministry and Key Laboratory of Visual Impairment and Restoration of Shanghai, Shanghai, China

Hong Chen, Hang Lu, Dongmei Wei and Lin Wang
Center of Integrative Research, The First Hospital of Qiqihar City, Qiqihar, Heilongjiang 161005, China

Jinglin Cui
Center of Integrative Research, The First Hospital of Qiqihar City, Qiqihar, Heilongjiang 161005, China
Department of Orthopedic Surgery and BME-Campbell Clinic, University of Tennessee Health Science Center, Memphis, TN 38163, USA

Yan Jiao
Department of Orthopedic Surgery and BME-Campbell Clinic, University of Tennessee Health Science Center, Memphis, TN 38163, USA

Weikuan Gu
Department of Orthopedic Surgery and BME-Campbell Clinic, University of Tennessee Health Science Center, Memphis, TN 38163, USA
Research Service, Veterans Affairs Medical Center, 1030 Jefferson Avenue, Memphis, TN 38104, USA

Fangtian Dong
Department of Ophthalmology, Peking Union Medical College Hospital, Beijing 100730, China

Steve Charles
Department of Ophthalmology, University of Tennessee Health Science Center, Memphis, TN 38163, USA
Charles Retina Institute, Germantown, TN 38138, USA

San-Ni Chen
Department of Ophthalmology, Changhua Christian Hospital, Changhua, Taiwan
Department of Optometry, Da-Yeh University, Changhua, Taiwan
College of Medicine, Chung-Shan Medical University, Taichung, Taiwan

Chung-May Yang
Department of Ophthalmology, National Taiwan University Hospital, Taipei, Taiwan
College of Medicine, National Taiwan University, Taipei, Taiwan

Andreas F. Borkenstein and Eva-Maria Borkenstein
Private Practice, Privatklinik der Kreuzschwestern Graz, Kreuzgasse 35, 8010-Graz, Austria

Hiroaki Kanno, Wataru Yamada, Ikumi Shiraki and Kiyofumi Mochizuki
Department of Ophthalmology, Gifu University Graduate School of Medicine, 1-1 Yanagido, Gifu-shi, Gifu 500-1194, Japan

Kyoko Ishida
Department of Ophthalmology, Toho University Ohashi Medical Center, 2-17-6, Ohashi, Meguro-ku, Tokyo 153-8515, Japan

Hiroki Murase
Murase Eye Clinic, 17-1 Hanaike, Hagiwaracho, Gero-shi, Gifu 509-2515, Japan

Yuka Yamagishi
Department of Infection Control and Prevention, Aichi Medical University, 1-1 Karimata, Iwasaku, Nagakute-shi, Aichi 480-1195, Japan

Chun-Hsiu Liu, Chung-YingHuang, Wei-Chi Wu, Ling-Yuh Kao and Meng-Ling Yang
Department of Ophthalmology, Chang Gung Memorial Hospital, Chang Gung University College of Medicine, No. 5, Fuhsing Street, Kweishan, Taoyuan 333, Taiwan

Sherine Jue Ong
Ching Ming Eye Clinic, No. 32, Zhongshan 2nd Rd., Luzhou, New Taipei 247, Taiwan

Yi Liu
Department of Ophthalmology, Nanjing Hospital of Chinese Medicine, The Third Affiliated Hospital of Nanjing University of Chinese Medicine, Nanjing, Jiangsu 210001, China

Guo-Bin Zhuang
Department of Ophthalmology, Quanzhou First Hospital, Quanzhou, Fujian 362000, China

Xue-Zhi Zhou
Department of Ophthalmology, Xiangya Hospital, Central South University, Changsha, Hunan 410078, China

Jin Young Kim
Department of Ophthalmology, Jeju National University Hospital, Jeju National University School of Medicine, Jeju, Republic of Korea

Ju Byung Chae, Jisoo Kim and Dong Yoon Kim
Department of Ophthalmology, Chungbuk National University Hospital, College of Medicine, Chungbuk National University, Cheongju, Republic of Korea

Alfredo Niro, Giancarlo Sborgia, Alessandra Sborgia, Luigi Sborgia, Claudio Furino, Nicola Recchimurzo and Giovanni Alessio
Department of Medical Science, Neuroscience and Sense Organs, Eye Clinic, University of Bari "A. Moro", Bari, Italy

Dominika Wróbel-Dudzińska, Ewa Kosior-Jarecka, Beata Rymgayłło-Jankowska, Agnieszká Cwiklińska-Haszcz and Tomasz Zarnowski
Department of Diagnostics and Microsurgery of Glaucoma, Medical University of Lublin, Lublin, Poland

Jorge Alio
Department of Cornea and Refractive Surgery, Vissum Corporation, Alicante, Spain
Research and Development Department, Vissum Corporation, Alicante, Spain

Alejandra Rodriguez
Research and Development Department, Vissum Corporation, Alicante, Spain

Ewa Suchodoła-Ratajewicz
Department of General Ophthalmology, Medical University of Lublin, Lublin, Poland

Liangcheng Wu, Chenghai Weng and Fei Xia
Department of Ophthalmology, Jing'an District Centre Hospital of Shanghai, Fudan University, Shanghai, China

Xiaoying Wang
Department of Ophthalmology, Jing'an District Centre Hospital of Shanghai, Fudan University, Shanghai, China
Department of Ophthalmology and Vision Science, Eye and ENT Hospital, Shanghai Medical College, Fudan University, Shanghai, China

Xingtao Zhou
Department of Ophthalmology and Vision Science, Eye and ENT Hospital, Shanghai Medical College, Fudan University, Shanghai, China

Kamakari Smaragda, Kokkinou Vassiliki, Koutsodontis George and Stamatiou Polixeni
Ophthalmic Genetics Unit, OMMA Ophthalmological Institute of Athens, Athens, Greece

Giatzakis Christoforos
DNAbiolab, Cretan Center for Research and Development of Applications on Genetics and Molecular Biology, Heraklion, Crete, Greece

Anastasakis Anastasios
Department of Clinical Electrophysiology of Vision, Athens Eye Hospital, Glyfada, Athens, Greece

Aslanides Ioannis Minas
Department of Ophthalmology, Emmetropia Mediterranean Eye Institute, Heraklion, Crete, Greece

Koukoula Stavrenia
Ophthalmica Institute of Ophthalmology and Microsurgery, Thessaloniki, Greece

Panagiotoglou Theoni and Tsilimbaris K. Miltiadis
Department of Ophthalmology, University of Crete School of Medicine, Heraklion, Greece

Datseris Ioannis
Department of Retinal Disorders, OMMA Ophthalmological Institute of Athens, Athens, Greece

Tânia Gisela Biberg-Salum
Ribeirao Preto Medical School, University of São Paulo, University for Development of Pantanal Region (UNIDERP), São Paulo, SP, Brazil

Maria de Lourdes Veronese Rodrigues and Jayter Silva de Paula
Department of Ophthalmology, Otorhinolaryngology and Head and Neck Surgery, Ribeirao Preto Medical School, University of São Paulo, São Paulo, SP, Brazil

Ana Paula Morais Fernandes
Department of General and Specialized Nursing, Nursing School of Ribeirao Preto, University of São Paulo, São Paulo, SP, Brazil

Neifi Hassan Salum Deghaide
Molecular Immunology Laboratory and HLA Hemocentro, Ribeirão Preto Medical School University Hospital, Ribeirão Preto, Brazil

Eduardo Antonio Donadi
Molecular Immunology Laboratory and HLA Hemocentro, Ribeirão Preto Medical School University Hospital, Ribeirão Preto, Brazil
Division of Immunology, Department of Internal Medicine, Ribeirao Preto Medical School, University of São Paulo, São Paulo, SP, Brazil

Erick C. Castelli
School of Medicine, Department of Pathology and Molecular Genetics and Bioinformatics Laboratory, São Paulo State University, Botucatu, SP, Brazil

Celso Teixeira Mendes-Junior
Departamento de Química, Laboratório de Pesquisas Forenses e Genômicas, Faculdade de Filosofia, Ciências e Letras de Ribeirão Preto, Universidade de São Paulo, 14040-901 Ribeirão Preto, SP, Brazil

Eoi Jong Seo and Joo Yong Lee
Department of Ophthalmology, Asan Medical Center, University of Ulsan College of Medicine, Seoul, Republic of Korea

Klemens Fondi, Doreen Schmidl, Ahmed M. Bata, Katarzyna J. Witkowska and Gerhard Garhöfer
Department of Clinical Pharmacology, Medical University of Vienna, Vienna, Austria

Piotr A. Wozniak
Department of Clinical Pharmacology, Medical University of Vienna, Vienna, Austria
Department of Ophthalmology, Medical University of Warsaw, Warsaw, Poland

Leopold Schmetterer
Department of Clinical Pharmacology, Medical University of Vienna, Vienna, Austria
Center for Medical Physics and Biomedical Engineering, Medical University of Vienna, Vienna, Austria
Singapore Eye Research Institute, Singapore National Eye Centre, Singapore
Lee Kong Chian School of Medicine, Nanyang Technological University, 59 Nanyang Drive, Singapore 637459
Visual Science Academic Clinical Programme, Duke-NUS, Singapore

Alina Popa-Cherecheanu
Carol Davila University of Medicine and Pharmacy, Bucharest, Romania
Department of Ophthalmology, Emergency University Hospital, Bucharest, Romania

Yvan Jamilloux, Audrey De Parisot, Christiane Broussolle and Pascal Sève
Department of Internal Medicine, Hôpital de la Croix Rousse, Hospices Civils de Lyon, Universit´e Claude Bernard Lyon 1, Lyon, France

Aude Taleb
Department of Internal Medicine, Hôpital de la Croix Rousse, Hospices Civils de Lyon, Universit´e Claude Bernard Lyon 1, Lyon, France
Department of Ophthalmology, Hôpital de la Croix Rousse, Hospices Civils de Lyon, Universit´e Claude Bernard Lyon 1, Lyon, France

Laurent Kodjikian
Department of Ophthalmology, Hôpital de la Croix Rousse, Hospices Civils de Lyon, Universit´e Claude Bernard Lyon 1, Lyon, France

Laurent Pérard
Department of Internal Medicine, Hôpital Edouard Herriot, Hospices Civils de Lyon, Universit´e Claude Bernard Lyon 1, Lyon, France

Carole Burillon
Department of Ophthalmology, Hôpital Edouard Herriot, Hospices Civils de Lyon, Universit´e Claude Bernard Lyon 1, Lyon, France

Grace M. Wang, Lev Prasov, Colin E. R. Marrs, Sahil Tolia, Laurel Wiinikka-Buesser and Brenda L. Bohnsack
Department of Ophthalmology and Visual Sciences, W.K. Kellogg Eye Center, The University of Michigan, Ann Arbor, MI 48105, USA

Hayder Al-Hasani and Julia E. Richards
Department of Ophthalmology and Visual Sciences, W.K. Kellogg Eye Center, The University of Michigan, Ann Arbor, MI 48105, USA
Department of Epidemiology, The University of Michigan, Ann Arbor, MI 48109, USA

Yuying Ji, Miaoling Li, Xiongze Zhang, Yuting Peng and Feng Wen
State Key Laboratory of Ophthalmology, Zhongshan Ophthalmic Center, Sun Yat-sen University, 54 South Xianlie Road, Guangzhou 510060, China

Yuan Qiu, Jing Hong and Rongmei Peng
Department of Ophthalmology, Peking University ird Hospital, Beijing, China

Mohammad A. Rashad, Samah Mahmoud Fawzy, Ahmed Abdel Meguid Abdel latif and Mahmoud Abdel Meguid Abdel latif
Ophthalmology Department, Faculty of Medicine, Ain Shams University, Cairo, Egypt

Khaled M. Abd Elaziz
Community Department, Environmental and Occupational Medicine, Faculty of Medicine, Ain Shams University, Cairo, Egypt

Xhevat Lumi and Marko Hawlina
Eye Hospital, University Medical Centre Ljubljana, Ljubljana, Slovenia

Mateja M. Jelen, Daša Jevšinek Skok, Emanuela Boštjančič, Metka Ravnik-Glavač and Damjan Glavač
Department of Molecular Genetics, Institute of Pathology, Faculty of Medicine, University of Ljubljana, Ljubljana, Slovenia

Yavuz Oruc, Sinem Keser, Elif Yusufoglu and Fatih Celik
Department of Ophthalmology, Elazig Research and Education Hospital, Health Science University, 23119 Elazig, Turkey

Meltem Yardim and Suleyman Aydin
Department of Medical Biochemistry and Clinical Biochemistry, Firat Hormones Research Group, Medical School, Firat University, 23119 Elazig, Turkey

Ibrahim Sahin
Department of Medical Biochemistry and Clinical Biochemistry, Firat Hormones Research Group, Medical School, Firat University, 23119 Elazig, Turkey
Department of Medical Biology, Medical School, Erzincan Binali Yildirim University, 24100 Erzincan, Turkey

Mohammed A. Hussein
Internal Medicine Department, Rheumatology and Clinical Immunology Division, Cairo University, Cairo, Egypt

Iman M. Eissa and Ahmed A. Dahab
Ophthalmology Department, Cairo University, Cairo, Egypt

Pade Colligris
Universidad Alfonso X, Madrid, Spain
Ocupharm Diagnostics SL, Madrid, Spain

Maria Jesus Perez de Lara, Basilio Colligris and Jesus Pintor
Ocupharm Diagnostics SL, Madrid, Spain
Universidad Complutense de Madrid, Madrid, Spain

Ming-zhen Yuan, Ruo-an Han, Chen-xi Zhang and You-xin Chen
Department of Ophthalmology, Peking Union Medical College Hospital, Chinese Academy of Medical Sciences and Peking Union Medical College, Beijing, China

Heng Miao and Xianru Hou
Department of Ophthalmology, People's Hospital, Peking University, Beijing, China

De-Kuang Hwang
Department of Ophthalmology, Taipei Veterans General Hospital, Taipei, Taiwan
Department of Ophthalmology, School of Medicine, National Yang-Ming University, Taipei, Taiwan

Yong Tao
Department of Ophthalmology, Beijing Chaoyang Hospital, Capital Medical University, Beijing, China

Zsuzsanna Szepessy, Kinga Kránitz and Zoltán Zsolt Nagy
Department of Ophthalmology, Semmelweis University, Budapest, Hungary

Arpád Barsi
Department of Photogrammetry and Geoinformatics, Budapest University of Technology and Economics, Budapest, Hungary

Katarzyna Krysik and Anita Lyssek-Boron
Department of Ophthalmology with Pediatric Unit, St. Barbara Hospital, Trauma Center, Medykow Square 1, 41-200 Sosnowiec, Poland

Dariusz Dobrowolski
Department of Ophthalmology with Pediatric Unit, St. Barbara Hospital, Trauma Center, Medykow Square 1, 41-200 Sosnowiec, Poland
Department of Ophthalmology, District Railway Hospital, Panewnicka 65 St., 40-760 Katowice, Poland
Chair and Clinical Department of Ophthalmology, School of Medicine with the Division of Dentistry in Zabrze, Medical University of Silesia in Katowice, Panewnicka 65 St., 40-760 Katowice, Poland

Ewa Wroblewska-Czajka
Department of Ophthalmology, District Railway Hospital, Panewnicka 65 St., 40-760 Katowice, Poland

Edward A. Wylegala
Department of Ophthalmology, District Railway Hospital, Panewnicka 65 St., 40-760 Katowice, Poland
Chair and Clinical Department of Ophthalmology, School of Medicine with the Division of Dentistry in Zabrze, Medical University of Silesia in Katowice, Panewnicka 65 St., 40-760 Katowice, Poland
Hebei Provincial Eye Hospital, Xingtai, China

Index

Lightning Source UK Ltd.
Milton Keynes UK
UKHW050236070322
399559UK00002BA/37

9 781632 418968